MUSCLEMAG *International*.

TEEN FIT FOR GUYS

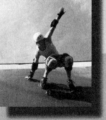

Your Complete Guide to Fun, Fitness and Self-Esteem

By Gerard Thorne & Phil Embleton

Published by MuscleMag International
5775 McLaughlin Road
Mississauga, ON
Canada L5R 3P7

Designed by Jackie Thibeault
Edited by Sandy Wheeler

National Library of Canada Cataloguing in Publication

Thorne, Gerard, 1963-
        Teen fit for guys : your complete guide to fun, fitness and
self-esteem / by Gerard Thorne and Phil Embleton.

Includes index.
ISBN 1-55210-030-8

        1. Teenage boys--Health and hygiene. 2. Physical fitness for men.
3. Physical fitness for youth. I. Embleton, Phil, 1963- II. Title.

RA777.2.T48 2004   613'.04233   C2004-901577-X

Distributed in Canada by
Canbook Distribution Services
1220 Nicholson Road
Newmarket, ON
Canada L3Y 7V1

Distributed in the United States by
BookWorld Services
1941 Whitfield Park Loop
Sarasota, FL 34243

Printed in Canada

This book is not intended as medical advice, nor is it offered for use in the diagnosis of any health condition or as a substitute for medical treatment and/or counsel. Its purpose is to explore advanced topics on sports nutrition and exercise. All data is for information only. Use of any of the programs within this book is at the sole risk and choice of the reader.

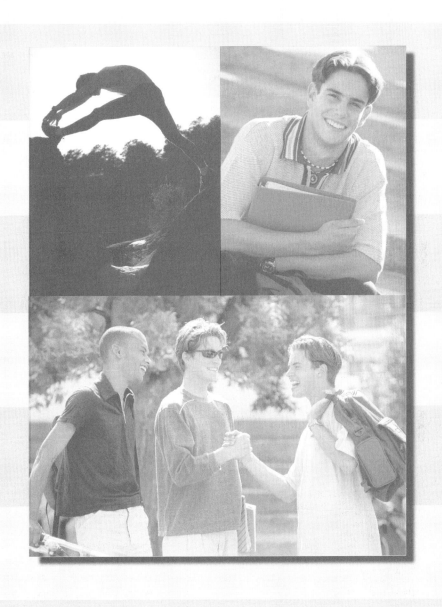

WHAT'S INSIDE

WHAT'S INSIDE

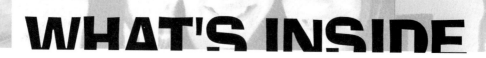

WHAT'S INSIDE

WHAT'S INSIDE

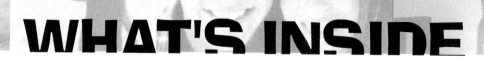

WHAT'S INSIDE

WHAT'S INSIDE

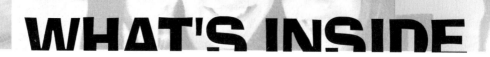

WHAT'S INSIDE

WHAT'S INSIDE

WHAT'S INSIDE

BOOK II

WHAT'S INSIDE

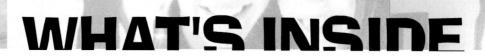

WHAT'S INSIDE

WHAT'S INSIDE

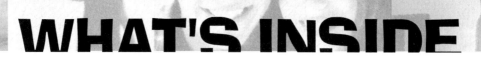

WHAT'S INSIDE

WHAT'S INSIDE

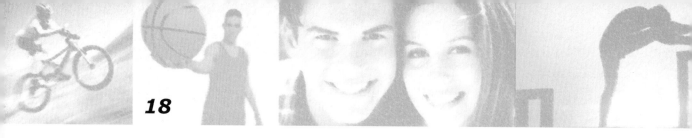

ACKNOWLEDGEMENTS

Seems like only yesterday we were putting the finishing touches on our first book, *MuscleMag International's Encyclopedia of Bodybuilding,* yet here we are, nearly six years later, proudly presenting our eighth publication. As with our previous works, we extend our sincere thanks to a number of individuals whose help has been invaluable.

To Jackie Thibeault and staff – thanks for another editing job well done. From photos and graphics to editing and layout, Jackie and gang bring our words to life.

Thanks to Katie Power for giving two "thirty-somethings" an insight into the almost forgotten teenage years. All the best in future endeavors, Katie.

Special appreciation goes to Daniel Campbell, owner of World Gym in Lake Forest, CA for allowing photographer Ralph DeHaan to invade his gym for two days for our exercise photo shoot. A big thanks to our physique and exercise model Joe Pride. Well done.

Finally, to Robert Kennedy... Just when we think maybe our careers with *MuscleMag* are over, there you are, waving another contract in our faces and throwing new ideas at us. Our sincere thanks for everything over the years. As long as you want us we are standing by with pen in hand. Our thanks to you all.

– Gerard Thorne and Phil Embleton

FOREWORD
By Robert Kennedy

To yearn for something is nothing more than wishful thinking. It means no more than having a desire for change. But change doesn't come without action and execution. It's never the idea, it's the *execution* of the idea that counts. Ideas come by the dozen. They're only worth a dime. However, if you morph your wishing into action – if you train regularly and correctly, if you eat the right foods, if you allow for proper recuperation – then your specific execution will give you the body of an Adonis, the fitness of a pro athlete, and the strength of Hercules.

Teen Fit For Guys provides everything you need to achieve ultimate fitness; and it's fun. No, you don't need 22-inch arms, and no, you don't need steroids. Anyone in normal good health can build a very impressive body. The type of body that guys respect and gals admire.

Picture yourself at the beach or relaxing by the pool. You are pale and skinny, or worse, you're flabby ... At the other end of the area a couple of guys and gals are throwing a Frisbee around. There's a lot of laughing, merriment, and all-round fun times. It's like they're in one of those beer commercials you see on TV.

You feel out of place because of your sad physical shape. You lay low and read your magazine, but you're not really reading that magazine, are you? You're checking out the action from behind your sunglasses. You secretly envy those guys and the fun they're having. Out of the blue the Frisbee lands near you. You ignore it because you don't want to stand up and expose your pitiful physique to the glances of the fun-loving group, especially the girls. It would be soooo embarassing.

Rewind ... Play it again, Sam. Okay, you're relaxing at the pool and you can't help but be aware of a group of fun-loving guys and gals playing Frisbee. Out of the blue the Frisbee lands near you. You jump up, grab it, and toss it back. The guys and gals are in awe of your tanned muscles; your broad shoulders, full pecs and six-pack abs stand out in the sun like diamonds in the sand. All of a sudden that Frisbee comes your way again, and yes, you're in the game. Life is good. You're in the beer commercial.

Robert Kennedy, Publisher
Oxygen, MuscleMag International
and *American Health and Fitness*

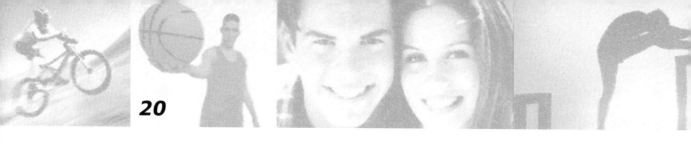

INTRODUCTION

"I Am Me!"

"I'm fat."
"I'm too skinny."
*"I'd be happy if I were taller,
shorter, had curly hair, straight hair,
smaller nose, bigger muscles, longer legs..."*
"Is there something wrong with me?"

Do any of these statements sound familiar? Are you in the habit of putting yourself down? If so, don't worry – you're not alone. As a teen you're going through a ton of physical changes, and as your body changes, so does your image of yourself. Read on to learn more about how body image affects your self-esteem and how you can develop a healthy body image.

Why Are Self-Esteem and Body Image Important?

You may have heard the term *self-esteem* on talk shows or seen it in your favorite magazine. But what does it mean? Self-esteem involves how much a person values himself and appreciates his own worth. Self-esteem is important because when you feel good about yourself you enjoy life more.

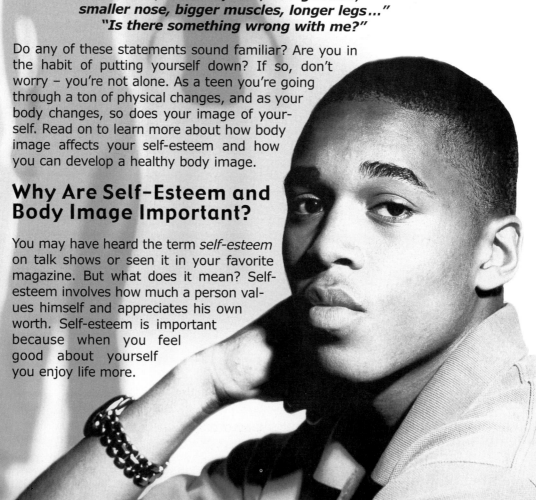

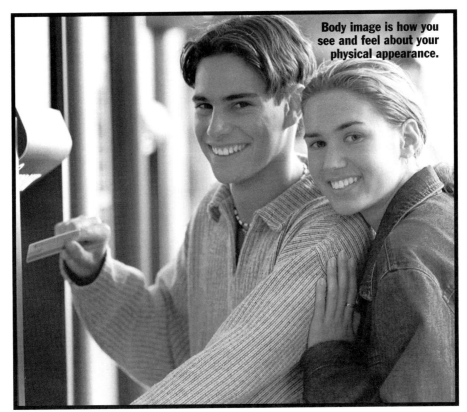

Body image is how you see and feel about your physical appearance.

Although *self-esteem* applies to every aspect of how you see yourself, the word is often mentioned in terms of appearance. Body image is how you see and feel about your physical appearance. We tend to relate self-esteem to body image for several reasons. First of all, most people care about what others think of them. Unfortunately, many people are judged by things like the clothes they wear, the shape of their body, or the way they wear their hair. If a person feels like he or she looks different than others, then body image and self-esteem may be affected negatively.

Teens with a poor body image may think negative thoughts like, 'I'm fat, I'm not good-looking, I'm not strong enough.'

What Shapes Self-Esteem?

The Effects of Puberty

Some teens struggle with self-esteem when they begin puberty. That's because the body undergoes many changes when puberty starts. These rapid changes and the desire for acceptance make it difficult for teens to judge whether or not they are "normal" when they look at other teens around them. And many people worry about what's normal during puberty. Compounding the problem, puberty begins at different ages. Some guys enter puberty at 10 or 12, while others may be in their early teens before changes start taking place.

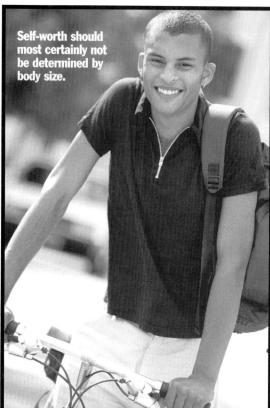

Self-worth should most certainly not be determined by body size.

The Effects of Culture

Media images from TV, movies, and advertising may affect self-esteem. Guys may struggle with images of teen actors and men who are unrealistically ripped and muscular. Sports individuals and other guys may put pressure on guys to gain muscle mass quickly, which can lead them to feel unhappy or dissatisfied with their bodies. Worse still, many teenage guys may turn to anabolic steroids and other dangerous performance-enhancing drugs to try to "bulk up."

Self-worth should most certainly not be determined by body size. It's more important to lead a healthy lifestyle by exercising regularly and eating nutritiously than to try to change your body to fit an unrealistic ideal. Later in the book we'll be looking at eating disorders, one of the hazards of striving for such unrealistic goals.

Sometimes low self-esteem is too much to bear. Instead of getting real help, some teens may drink or turn to drugs to help themselves feel better, especially in social situations. That is not the answer.

The Effects of Home and School

A young man's home or school life can also affect his self-esteem. Some parents spend more time criticizing than praising their children. Sometimes this criticism reduces a teen's ability to develop a positive body image – the teen may model his own "inner voice" after that of a parent, and learn to believe negative thoughts about himself.

It's hard to succeed at school when the situation at home is tense, so sometimes teens who suffer from abuse at home may also have problems in school, both of which contribute to poor self-esteem.

Maybe he also experiences negative comments and hurtful teasing or bullying from classmates and peers. This can definitely affect a person's self-esteem, but it's important to remember that the people who are being hurtful probably have low self-esteem as well, and putting others down may make them feel better about themselves.

Racial and ethnic prejudice is another source of hurtful comments. These comments come from ignorance on the part of the person who makes them, but sometimes the body image and self-esteem of the guy on the receiving end can be negatively affected.

Checking Your Own Self-Esteem and Body Image

If you have a positive body image, you probably like the way you look and accept yourself as you are – *I am me!* This is a healthy attitude that will allow you to explore other aspects of growing up, such as increasing independence from your parents, enhanced intellectual and physical abilities, and an interest in dating.

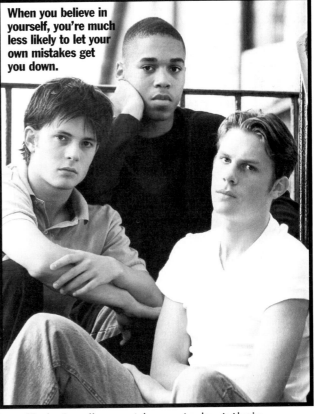

When you believe in yourself, you're much less likely to let your own mistakes get you down.

When you believe in yourself, you're much less likely to let your own mistakes get you down. You are better able to recognize your errors, learn your lessons, and move on. The same goes for the way you treat others. Teenagers who feel good about themselves are less likely to allow putdowns to hurt their self-esteem or to use harmful comments on anyone else.

A positive, optimistic attitude can help you develop better self-esteem – for example, say "Hey, I'm human" instead of "Wow, I'm such a loser" when you make a mistake; and avoid blaming others when things don't go as expected. Know what makes you happy and how to meet your goals. You will feel capable, strong, and in control of your life. A positive attitude and a healthy lifestyle – that's an excellent combination for developing good self-esteem.

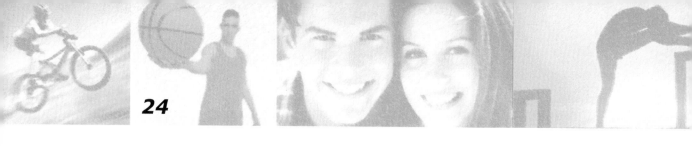

Tips for Boosting Your Self-Esteem

Some teens think they need to change their looks or the way they act to feel good about themselves. But here's the right answer. If you can train yourself to reprogram the way you look at your body, you'll be able to defend yourself from negative comments – both those that come from others and those that come from you. Remember: when others criticize your body, it's usually because they are insecure about the changes happening to themselves.

The first thing to do is recognize that your body is your own, no matter what shape, size or color it came in. If you are very worried about your weight or size, check with your doctor to verify that things are okay. But remember this: It is no one's business but your own what you look like – *ultimately you must be happy with yourself.*

Remember, too, that there are certain aspects you *cannot* change – such as your height and shoe size – and you should accept

> *Note: Your body is your own, no matter what shape, size or color it came in.*

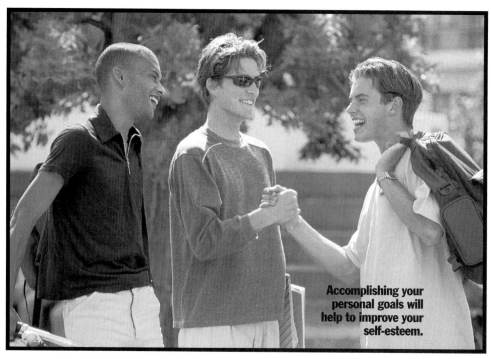

Accomplishing your personal goals will help to improve your self-esteem.

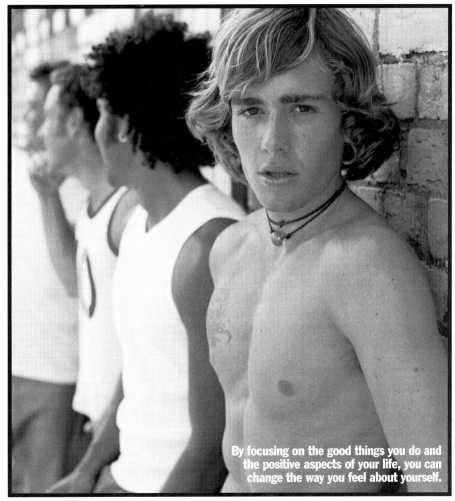

By focusing on the good things you do and the positive aspects of your life, you can change the way you feel about yourself.

and love these personal attributes. If you do want to make changes, be sure to set goals for yourself. For example, if you want to lose weight, commit yourself to exercising three or four times a week and eating healthy. Accomplishing your personal goals will help to improve your self-esteem.

When you hear negative comments from within, tell yourself to *stop.* Your "inner critic" can and must be retrained. Try these exercises: Give yourself three compliments every day. While you're at it, every evening list three things in your day that really gave you pleasure – anything from the way the sun felt on your face, to the sound of your favorite band, or the way someone laughed at your jokes. By focusing on the good things you do and the positive aspects of your life, you can change the way you feel about yourself.

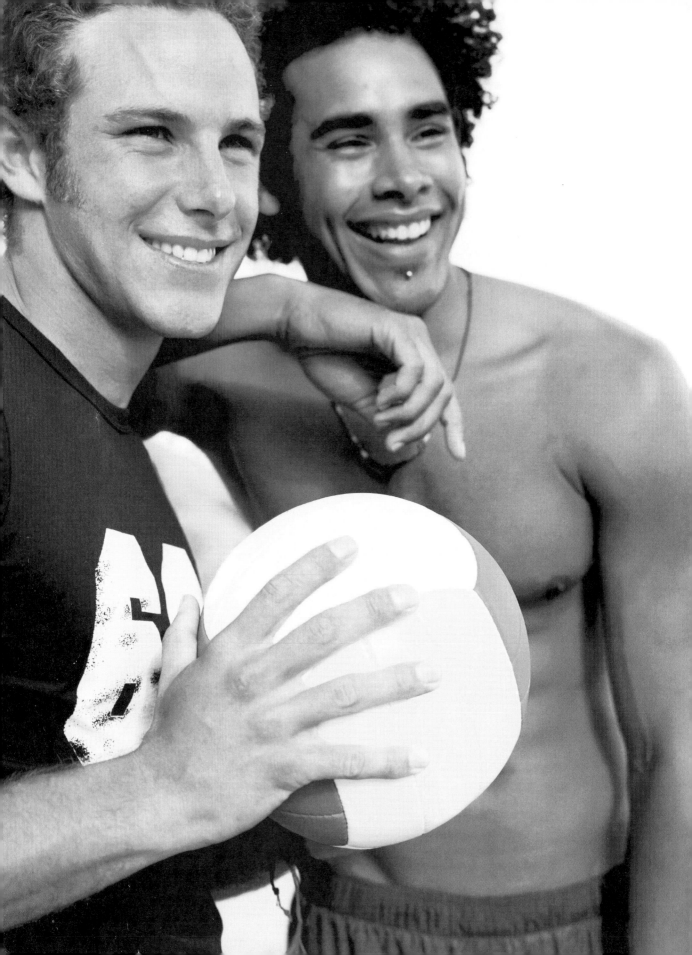

BOOK ONE

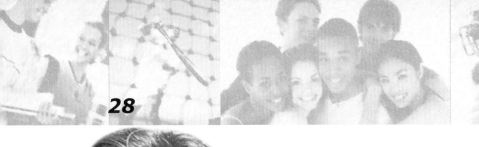

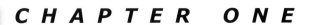

CHAPTER ONE

Prom night is one of the most important evenings in a man's life. A happy event by all accounts, it's not without its own stresses and strains. There's all the preparation – making sure the corsage arrives, confirming the dinner reservations, and of course, *the tuxedo.* These details can push the mind and body to the limit.

the Art of Looking Good

A guy also wants to look good on his prom night. Not only does he want to hide the telltale signs that pressure brings, but he wants to look his best for his date in the same way that his date wants to look her best for him. So how can a guy try to ensure that he succeeds in his quest? Read on.

Perfect Skin

Late nights, stress, an unhealthy diet, and too much sun all take their toll on the skin. It dries out, becomes flaky and cracked, and loses its vitality. What's missing from most people's diet? What does the skin need in abundance? Water! you need at least two litres a day, more in hot and humid weather.

To remain healthy the skin also needs *vitamin C* and this is readily available from citrus fruits, fortified breakfast cereals, and fortified bread. Potatoes are also a good source of vitamin C, too, and since this vitamin is found just below the skin, having a baked potato means the vitamin C doesn't end up in the trash lost in the peelings.

Moisturize your skin regularly, too, using a cream that contains vitamin E and UV protection. Many guys have facials nowadays to help revitalize their skin. There's no better excuse to start than for an upcoming big date.

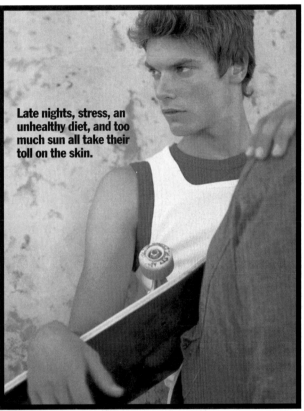

Late nights, stress, an unhealthy diet, and too much sun all take their toll on the skin.

Stealing the Limelight

Something else that the skin needs to keep it healthy is *zinc.* This vitamin also helps to boost the immune system (as does vitamin C) and keep it strong so that it can protect the body from infection. During the buildup to the big day it's easy to become run down and often the first sign that this is happening is the last thing you want, *a cold sore.*

Grabbing the limelight and occupying prize position in the prom photographs a cold sore is an uninvited guest. Stress, infection, being overtired, cold winds, and hot weather (since the UV radiation in sunlight is a common trigger for cold sores to appear) can all be responsible for waking up a cold sore when you would rather it remained asleep.

It's possible to avoid cold sores by getting enough rest, eating plenty of fresh fruit and vegetables, not smoking, and keeping alcohol to a minimum – with the stag night being an allowable exception of course! Of vital importance is to make sure that you take time to relax and unwind. Be sure to also apply a UV protection lip balm a few times each day to protect against the effects of cold winds and bright sunlight.

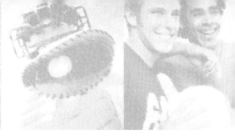

Tea-tree oil cream or aciclovir cream both have antiviral properties, and can shorten the duration and the severity of cold sores. Keep a tube of one or the other with all your prom night essentials, ready to use should the telltale tingle come your way.

Spot That

If it's not cold sores then it's *spots* that appear at the wrong time and in the wrong place. Once again these are more likely to occur if you have become run down. To try to avoid them, the same rules apply.

Don't pick them. That will not make them disappear and will only serve to make them look worse, and more obvious. Topical treatments from the pharmacist or tea-tree oil gel or cream will help to dry spots up.

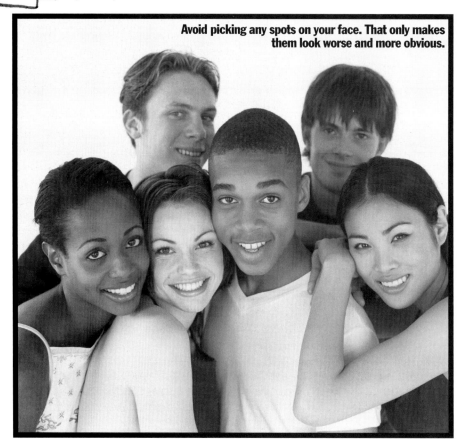

Avoid picking any spots on your face. That only makes them look worse and more obvious.

Now you may wish to sit down for this next bit of advice. To hide the spot that appears on the big day, use a blemish concealer or cover-up stick – it looks like a pencil. These are available from the make-up counter in large department stores, for example. Makeup specifically designed for men is now available, but if you're feeling more confident about making a speech than asking for makeup, then you can always say it's for your sister or girlfriend.

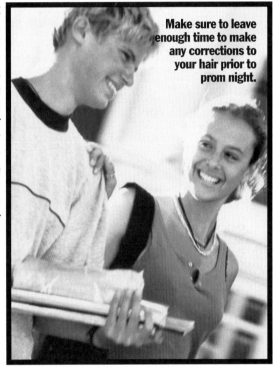

Make sure to leave enough time to make any corrections to your hair prior to prom night.

A well-balanced diet with lots of water helps keep the skin healthy looking.

Good Hair Day

The last thing you want is a bad hair day for prom night. If you are thinking about changing your hairstyle, then this is probably best done a few weeks before when there's a chance to correct it if it doesn't turn out to be what you had in mind. This suggestion is particularly important if color changes are involved.

If you simply want your usual style and just need things to be tidied up, then a week before the prom will probably be fine. Don't be frightened to ask the advice of a hair stylist either.

Looking Fine

So the big day arrives. You're relaxed, and enjoying the fact that everything is going to plan. You're looking and feeling good, so all that remains is for you to celebrate the big night you've been waiting for.

[Ref: www.bbc.co.uk/health/features/male_grooming.shtml]

CHAPTER TWO

Nutrition For Teenagers

The Importance of Nutrients

The science of nutrition is the study of "that which nourishes" the body. It can be studied from a molecular perspective (usually by adults in white lab coats) or from a more simplistic viewpoint. Let's look at it from the simplistic viewpoint.

Our bodies are made up of various systems, including the skeletal, digestive, circulatory and immune systems, which communicate with one another through the nervous and endocrine systems to maintain a state of *homeostasis* – healthy equilibrium.

Each of the organs that help the various systems perform must function properly. Organs are made up of tissues, which are groups of similar cells that perform similar functions. The cells are differentiated from one another in appearance and the way they work. All of your cells are made up of proteins, fats, carbohydrates, minerals, trace elements, hormones, enzymes, coenzymes and numerous other chemical compounds. (If you have taken an interest in nutrition, these terms are familiar.) Your cellular components are simply nutritional factors supplied by your diet.

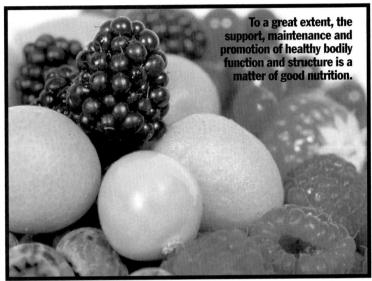

To a great extent, the support, maintenance and promotion of healthy bodily function and structure is a matter of good nutrition.

Good nutrition is crucial to cellular health ... Can you see why it is so critical that you supply your body with adequate levels of nutritional substances? Do you see why it is so important to eat right – to consume those fruits and vegetables that moms keep telling us to eat? To a great extent, the support, maintenance and promotion of healthy bodily function and structure is a matter of good nutrition. While it is true that stress, genetic and environmental factors, and lifestyle all influence your state of health, your cells *must have nutrients* to stay healthy. How could they possibly function without them?

The Digestive System

All right, it's now time to take a closer look at nutrition. Before we jump right into what you should and shouldn't eat, we need to explore that *wonder of human engineering* called the digestive system. Every time food passes your lips, it marks the beginning of an incredible journey...

Your Tastebuds

The moment food hits your tongue, your tastebuds come alive. You have roughly 10,000 tastebuds on your tongue. As nerve endings, they're responsible for sussing out the chemicals in the food you're eating and transmitting messages to your brain. Without them, you wouldn't be able to experience those salty, bitter, sweet or sour sensations.

While your tastebuds are busy at work, your teeth grind the food down into easily digestible pieces and your saliva moistens everything up, so that it doesn't scrape your digestive (gastrointestinal) tract on the way down.

34

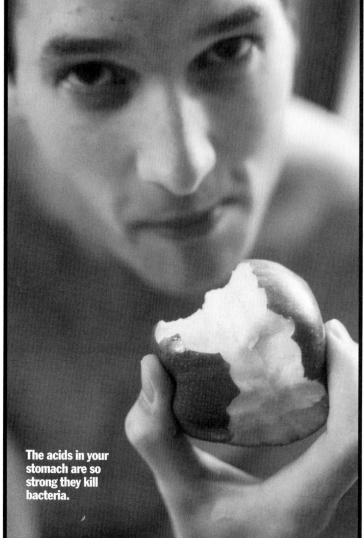

The acids in your stomach are so strong they kill bacteria.

Stomach

Once you've swallowed your food, it's carried down the esophagus to your stomach. Your stomach walls begin to churn the food up to make sure it mixes with your acidic digestive juices. The acids in your stomach are so strong, they kill bacteria – and are used in industry as metal cleaner! By the time your tummy has finished, the food is a creamy mixture called chyme (pronounced kime). Once it's liquefied, it can be squirted through a tiny hole into your small intestine.

Small Intestine

This is where most of the nutrient-digesting action happens. To help the small intestine cope with the acidity of the chyme, your pancreas releases an alkaline and lots of enzymes, which break down the food's carbohydrates, fat and protein. Meanwhile, your gallbladder donates some bile, to ensure that any fat is melted down thoroughly.

Once the food is reduced to tiny particles, it's absorbed through the walls of your small intestine and the nutrients are carried into your bloodstream.

Large Intestine

Any nutrients that *cannot* be digested end up here. Fiber is a nutrient with certain components that cannot be absorbed by the human body. Your large intestine begins at the cecum and progresses to the colon, where some of the remaining nutrients can be mopped up. After this point, anything that's left over is waste matter and is stored in the rectum, waiting for the journey's end. An average stool is 75 percent water. The remainder is made up of fiber, dead cells and bacteria.

[Ref: www.bbc.co.uk/health/nutrition/basics_digestive.shtml]

Nutritional Considerations

The teenage diet should sustain growth, promote health – and be enjoyable. In addition, during adolescence a number of physiological changes occur. These include a marked acceleration in growth (the pubertal growth spurt) and considerable gains in bone and muscle. These changes influence nutritional requirements.

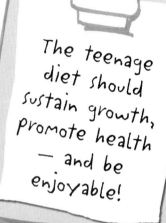

The teenage diet should sustain growth, promote health – and be enjoyable!

In July 2000 the British government's report into the eating and physical activity habits of children was published. *The National Diet and Nutritional Survey: Young People Aged 4 to 18 Years* provided detailed information on the nutritional intakes and physical activity levels of young people in the UK.

Alarmingly, during the seven-day recording period, more than half the young people in the survey had not eaten any citrus fruits (not eaten by 76 percent of boys and 72 percent of girls), any leafy green vegetables, such as cabbage, greens or broccoli (61 percent and 56 percent), any eggs (55 percent and 56 percent) or any raw tomatoes (68 percent and 58 percent).

What Are Minerals?
• Minerals are *inorganic substances* – they're found in the rocks and soil beneath your feet.
• Vegetables absorb mineral goodness as they grow and animals digest it through their diet.
• Minerals work together with vitamins to do good in your body.
• Just like vitamins, minerals can be divided into two groups – those that are needed in *minute quantities* and those that are needed in *larger quantities*.

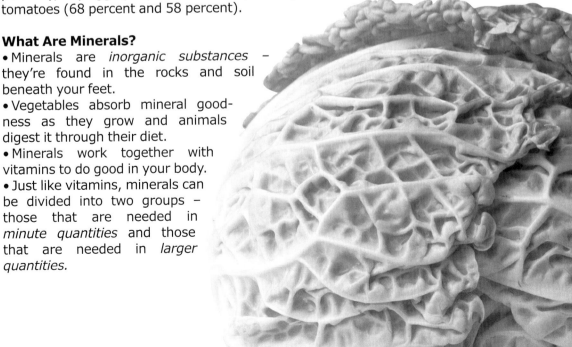

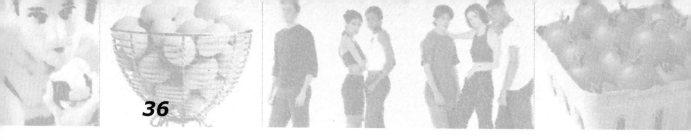

• Minerals needed in larger amounts – the *major* minerals – include calcium, magnesium, sodium, potassium and phosphorus.
• Minerals needed in tiny amounts are called trace minerals. This group includes iron, zinc, iodine, selenium and copper.

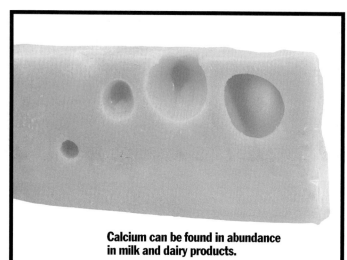

Calcium can be found in abundance in milk and dairy products.

Major Minerals

Why are minerals important? Where are major minerals found? What is the daily recommended intake? Read on.

Calcium – essential for healthy bones and teeth. It's in abundance in milk and dairy products. Very small quantities can be found in dark green leafy vegetables such as spinach and watercress. (daily recommendation is 700 mg for males and females)

Phosphorous – contributes to healthy cells, bones and teeth. You'll find it in milk, cheese, fish, meat and eggs. (550 mg for males and females)

Magnesium – helps your body to use energy and your muscles to function effectively. Get it from dark green leafy vegetables such as cabbage and broccoli. (300 mg for males and females)

Sodium – helps your body to regulate its water content and your nerves to function effectively. Available as table salt, added to food for flavor. (1600 mg for males and females)

Potassium – helps your cells and body fluids to function properly. It is in most foods, apart from fats, oils and sugar. (3500 mg for males and females)

Trace Minerals

Why are trace minerals important? Where are they found? What is the recommended intake? Here you go.

Iron – helps in the formation of red blood cells. Deficiency can lead to anemia. Available in red meat, fortified cereals and bread, some fruit and vegetables. (8.7 mg for males. 14.8 for females, but more if they experience a heavy menstrual flow)

Zinc – helps the body to reach sexual maturity and aids the repair of damaged tissue. Meat, fish, milk, cheese and eggs contain zinc. (9.5 mg for males. 7 mg for females)

Copper – helps your body to use iron properly. Green vegetables and fish give you copper. (1.2 mg for both males and females)

Selenium – ensures healthy cells. Selenium is in meat, fish, cereals, eggs and cheese. (75 mcg for males. 60 mcg for females)

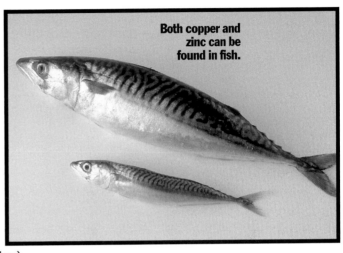

Both copper and zinc can be found in fish.

Iodine – helps to make thyroid hormones, which control metabolic activity. Seafood and dairy products are a source of iodine. (140 mcg for both males and females)

[Ref: www.bbc.co.uk/health/nutrition/basics_fruitveg3.shtml]

What Are Vitamins?

• Vitamins are *organic substances* – this means they're found in plants and animals.
• Most vitamins can't be made by your body, so they must be obtained from your diet. Vitamin D and the B vitamin niacin are exceptions.
• Nutritionists have divided vitamins into two groups – fat-soluble and water-soluble vitamins.
• The fat-soluble vitamins – A, D, E and K – are transported through your body by fat. They can also be stored in your fat cells and liver cells for a limited period of time.
• The water-soluble vitamins, B and C, are absorbed by and transported through your body *in water.* You need to eat them every day, as you can't store them for any length of time.

Fat-Soluble Vitamins

Why are they important? Where are they found? What's the daily recommendation?

Vitamin A – looks after your eyes, the lining of your nose, throat and lungs, and your skin cells. You get vitamin A from carrots, sweet potatoes, pumpkins, red chilies, tomatoes, "orange" fruits, such as apricots and mango, and dark green leafy vegetables. (600 mcg for females. 700 mcg for males)

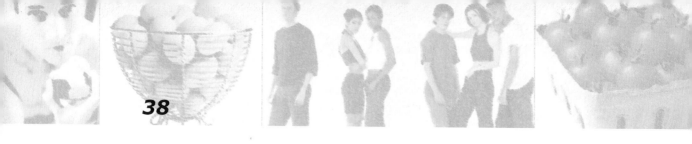

Vitamin D – helps your body to absorb calcium, needed to ensure strong bones and teeth. The most important source is the sun, but it's also found in tiny amounts in dairy products, cod liver oil and oily fish. No recommendations as sunlight is the main source.

Vitamin E – fights free radicals, unbalanced molecules that can cause damage to your cells. It also contributes to the healthy condition of your skin. Vegetables, poultry, fish, fortified breakfast cereals, vegetable oils, nuts and seeds. (up to 4 mg for adult males and up to 3 mg for adult females is considered a safe intake)

Vitamin K – helps your body to make a number of proteins, one of which helps your blood to clot. Dark green leafy vegetables such as Brussels sprouts, broccoli, cabbage, spinach and asparagus. It's also found in soya oil and margarine. (1 mcg for every kg of bodyweight is considered a safe intake for both men and women)

Water-Soluble Vitamins

Why are they important? Where do you get them? What is the recommended daily intake? Read on.

B-complex vitamins – help you to metabolize your food and help your blood cells to form and flow. Green vegetables, whole grains, meat, such as liver, kidneys, pork, beef and lamb, vegetable extracts, nuts and fortified breakfast cereals supply B-complex vitamins.

Eight vitamins make up the B-complex family: *B1 (thiamin)* – adult male 0.9 mg, adult female 0.8 mg; *B2 (riboflavin)* – adult male

Broccoli is a good source of vitamin K.

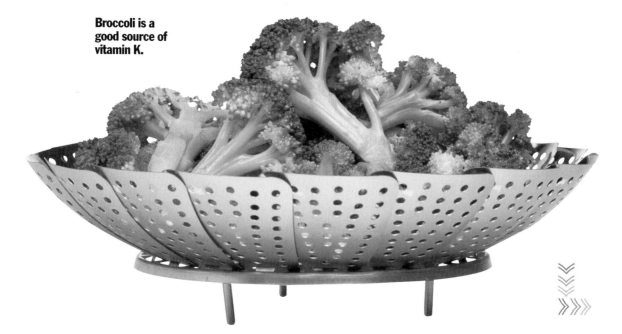

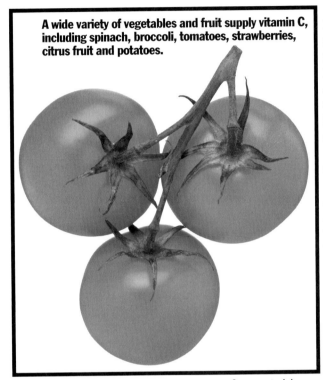

A wide variety of vegetables and fruit supply vitamin C, including spinach, broccoli, tomatoes, strawberries, citrus fruit and potatoes.

1.3 mg, adult female 1.1 mg; *B3 (niacin)* – adult male 17 mg, adult female 13 mg; *B5 (pantothenic acid)* – 3 to 7 mg is considered a safe intake for both sexes; *B6 (pyridoxine)* – adult male 1.4 mg, adult female 1.2 mg; *B9 (folate)* – 200 mcg for both adult males and females; *B12 (cobalamin)* – 1.5 mcg for both adult males and females; *Biotin* – 10 to 20 mcg is considered a safe intake for both sexes.

Vitamin C – helps your body to produce collagen (important for skin and bone structure) and to absorb iron. A wide variety of vegetables and fruit supply vitamin C, including spinach, broccoli, tomatoes, strawberries, citrus fruit and potatoes. (40 mg for both adult male and female)

[Ref: www.bbc.co.uk/health/nutrition/basics_fruitveg2.shtml#fat]

Iron

Iron deficiency is one of the most common nutritional deficiencies and adolescents are at special risk, since up to 13 percent of teenage boys and girls were found to have low iron stores in some studies. Rapid growth, coupled with a fast lifestyle and poor dietary choices, can result in *iron deficiency,* or anemia. Teenage girls need to pay special attention to nutrition as their iron stores are depleted each month following menstruation.

Iron is found in both red meat and non-meat sources, such as fortified breakfast cereal, dried fruit, bread and green leafy vegetables. The body does not quite as easily absorb iron from non-meat foods. However, vitamin C (found in citrus fruits, blackcurrants, green leafy vegetables) *enhances* the absorption of iron. In contrast, tannins found in tea *reduce* the absorption of iron. Eat iron rich and vitamin C-rich foods together. For example, choose a glass of *fruit juice* with a bowl of breakfast cereal rather than a cup of tea.

Calcium

The report also highlighted the fact that 25 percent of teens had a calcium intake below recommendations. This news has serious implications for the future, with respect to bone health. Osteoporosis is a disease that causes bones to become brittle and break very easily. Bones continue to grow and get stronger until the age of 30 – but the teenage years are the most important for development. Vitamin D, calcium and phosphorous are vital for this process. Calcium requirements for the teenage years range from 800 to 1000 mg per day.

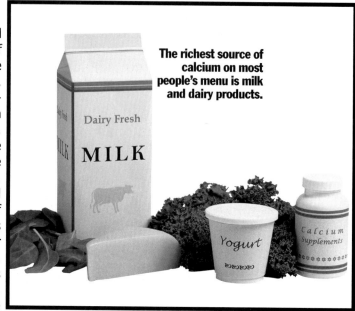

The richest source of calcium on most people's menu is milk and dairy products.

Calcium-rich foods should be consumed on a daily basis. The richest source of calcium on most people's menu is milk and dairy products (foods made from milk: cheese, yogurt etc., but not butter). Consuming a pint of milk per day, or eating other dairy products, will ensure a sufficient intake of calcium. Alternatively, try fortified soya milk. Here is the approximate calcium content of some common foods.

Food Calcium Content

Food	Calcium
1/3 pint (0.2 litre) whole milk	220 mg
1/3 pint (0.2 litre) semi-skimmed milk	230 mg
1/3 pint (0.2 litre) fortified soya milk	246 mg
2 oz. (60 g) tofu	304 mg
1 oz. (28 g) hard cheese	190 mg
1 carton low-fat yogurt	285 mg
2 oz. (60 g) sardines (including bones)	310 mg
3 large slices brown or white bread	100 mg
3 large slices whole-meal bread	55 mg
4 oz. (115 g) cottage cheese	80 mg
4 oz. (115 g) baked beans	60 mg
4 oz. (115 g) boiled cabbage	40 mg

Adolescence is a time for rapid growth, and the primary dietary need is for energy – *often reflected in a voracious appetite!* Ideally, foods contributing to dietary energy should comply with healthy eating principles. However, in practice this isn't usually the case. Average consumption of fat and sugars is high, while that of starchy carbohydrates and fiber is low. While undesirable, these poor eating habits won't do much harm – in the short term – but becomes a potential problem when this type of diet persists into adulthood.

Foods to Choose

Most teenagers are probably aware of what they should be eating. Putting this knowledge into practice is another issue! Regular meals are often replaced by "grazing" – eating snacks and fast foods throughout the day, depending on hunger and availability. As with other age groups, teenagers should be encouraged to choose a variety of items from all the basic food groups:

- *Plenty of carbohydrates* – bread, rice, pasta, breakfast cereals and potatoes.
- *Plenty of fruit and vegetables* – at least 5 portions every day.
- *Lots of dairy products* – like milk, yogurt and cheese.
- *Enough of all proteins* – like meat, fish, eggs (well-cooked), beans and pulses.
- *Not too much of* – fatty and sugar rich foods.

Other important factors during adolescence include:
- Aim to drink at least 8 glasses of fluids per day.

Foods contributing to dietary energy should comply with healthy eating principles.

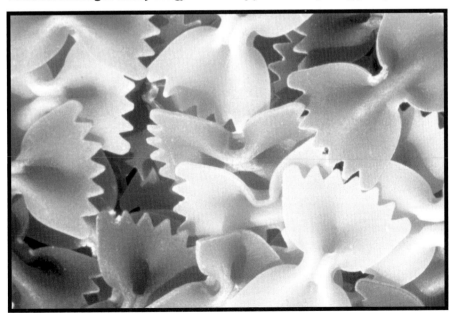

• Eat breakfast – breakfast can provide essential nutrients and improve concentration in the morning. Choose a fortified breakfast cereal with semi-skimmed milk, and a glass of fruit juice.

• Exercise – regular physical exercise is important for overall fitness and cardiovascular health, and it also helps in bone development.

Alcohol

Experimenting with alcohol is often part of growing up and asserting independence. Now we are not going to preach to you about the evils of alcohol, but if you do drink, be sensible. Don't binge drink, and don't overdo it. Keep your intake within a sensible limit. And *under no circumstances* get into a car with someone who has been drinking.

[Ref: www.bbc.co.uk/health/nutrition/life_adolescence.shtml]

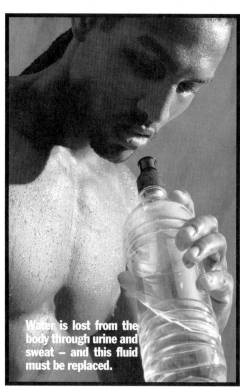

Water is lost from the body through urine and sweat – and this fluid must be replaced.

Why Do We Need Water?

Water is essential for the growth and maintenance of our bodies, as it's involved in a number of biological processes. Although water is not a nutrient, it is an important component of your daily diet. In adults water comprises 50 to 70 percent of total bodyweight. Without fluid, our survival time would be limited to a matter of hours or days.

Water is lost from the body through urine and sweat – and this fluid must be replaced. Many people do not consume enough fluids, and as a result may become dehydrated, with symptoms like headaches, tiredness and loss of concentration. Chronic dehydration can contribute to a number of health problems, such as constipation and kidney stones.

How Much Water Do We Need?

The body gets its water from three sources:

1. water as a beverage in itself, or water present in other beverages
2. water present in solid foods
3. water produced as a byproduct of chemical reactions within the body

The British Dietetic Association guidelines state that the average adult should consume 2.5 litres of water per day. Of this, 1.8 litres must be obtained directly from beverages, the equivalent of 6 to 7 glasses of water per day. Intake needs to be increased during periods of hot weather, as well as during and after periods of physical activity, in order to avoid dehydration.

Water is the major ingredient of all drinks – for example, carbonated and still drinks are 65 percent water, diluted squashes are 86 percent water (after dilution) and fruit juices are 90 percent water. All in all, drinking plain water is still the most effective way of replacing fluids lost from the body. Increase your daily water intake with the following steps.

1. Start as you mean to go on, with a glass of water when you wake.
2. Keep a supply of fresh water close by, at work or on your desk at school, if possible, so that it's within easy reach throughout the day.
3. If you're out and about during the day, carry a bottle of water with you and take a drink whenever you want.
4. Increase your intake of fresh fruit and vegetables. They have a high water content, along with many other health benefits.

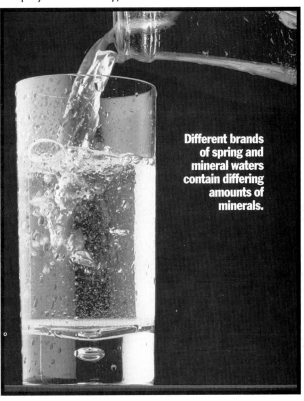

Different brands of spring and mineral waters contain differing amounts of minerals.

What About Bottled Waters?

There are two types of bottled water – spring water and mineral water. *Spring water* is collected directly from the spring where it arises from the ground, and must be bottled at the source. *Mineral water* is water that emerges from under the ground, and then flows over rocks before it's collected. As a result, mineral water has a higher content of various minerals picked up as it flows over rock. Unlike spring water, natural mineral water cannot be treated, except to remove grit and dirt. Different brands of spring and mineral waters will contain differing amounts of minerals, depending on where they have been sourced.

On June 30, 1999 new government regulations came into force covering the labeling requirements of bottled waters, in order to enable consumers to make informed decisions when choosing which products to buy. As a result of these regulations, the levels of all minerals in "natural mineral water" must be printed on the label.

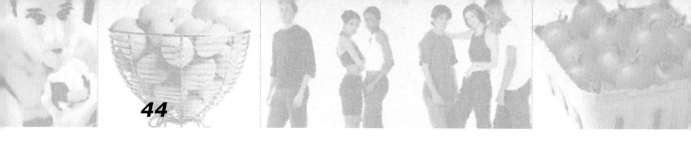

But wait. Why should we *pay for bottled water?* The drinking water available from our taps is perfectly adequate to replenish our fluid loss. After all, it undergoes many processes to bring it up to the standards set out in the Water Supply Regulations. There are certainly no proven health benefits of bottled water over tap water – so it's up to you. Basically it all comes down to personal taste and cost.

[Ref: www.bbc.co.uk/health/nutrition/drinks_water.shtml]

Fruit Juices

Pure unsweetened fruit juice is a particularly good source of vitamins and minerals, and a great way to replenish lost fluids in the body. The World Health Organization recommends that five portions of fruit and vegetables should be included in the daily diet to protect against a variety of diseases.

Pure fruit juices contain the same vitamins, minerals and special phytochemicals as fresh fruit (but not fiber or pectins), and are included in the "five-a-day" message. One glass of pure unsweetened fruit juice can count as one of your important five portions per day. So why not start the day off right and include a glass of pure fruit juice with your

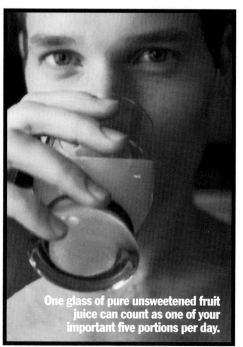

One glass of pure unsweetened fruit juice can count as one of your important five portions per day.

breakfast? If you're feeling particularly adventurous you could start the day off with a nutritious *fruit smoothie* – you can pack in at least three portions of fruit too! They're easy to make, full of important vitamins, and because they contain real fruit, they're filling too – making them the perfect breakfast drink.

Pure fruit juice should not be confused with fruit juice drinks – fruit-flavored drinks usually containing only 5 to 25 percent pure fruit juice. These types of drinks *do not* give you the same health benefits as pure fruit juice. Juice drinks are particularly popular among children but unlike pure fruit juice these drinks tend to have sugar added to them during processing, and are often blamed for the excessive sugar consumption in adults and children alike.

Tooth decay has also been linked to excessive consumption of sugary drinks. The sugar *added to* juice drinks is more harmful to teeth than the naturally occurring sugars found in fruits and pure fruit juice.

Dairy Drinks

Milk, milk-flavored drinks and yogurt drinks are great sources of calcium in the diet, and are needed for strong, healthy teeth and bones and the prevention of osteoporosis. The recent publication of *The National Diet and Nutrition Survey* has shown that calcium intakes of teenagers and children are at an all-time low, with a high percentage of teenagers taking in less than what is recommended.

Dairy products and milk are the best sources of easily absorbable calcium, and provide about half of our daily requirement. For most people, one glass of milk at every meal will be sufficient to ensure calcium needs are met. Some dairy products, including milk, can also contain quite a high proportion of fat, which has led to people cutting down on the consumption of these products in order to reduce fat intake. Although current advice is to reduce fat intake, with the increased availability of reduced-fat products, we can now enjoy the nutritional benefits of dairy foods without worrying about the fat.

Semi-skimmed and skimmed milk are much lower in fat than whole milk – and yet still contain the same amount of calcium. These types of milk are advised for the general population over 5 years. For children under the age of 5 years, whole milk should be encouraged. Semi-skimmed milk may be used at the age of 2 and above, if the diet supplies an adequate amount of energy.

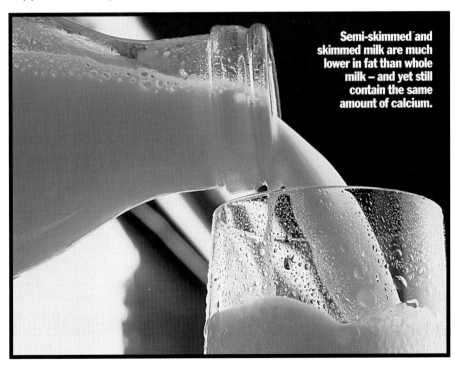

Semi-skimmed and skimmed milk are much lower in fat than whole milk – and yet still contain the same amount of calcium.

Carbonated Soft Drinks

We love them! Yet they're crammed full of sugars and acids that attack our teeth and may result in decay. Dental decay occurs when teeth are attacked by acid, and this can happen in two ways. Acid attacks can be a result of plaque bacteria acting on the sugars in your diet, or as a direct result of the acids in foods dissolving away the enamel on the surface of the tooth. As carbonated soft drinks tend to contain high amounts of both sugars and acids, they're the worst possible combination for dental health. Not only are sugary drinks detrimental to oral health, they are also calorific. These drinks provide little in the way of nutrients, so stay clear. At least use diet alternatives if you are watching your weight.

What about reduced-sugar alternatives?

Even those drinks that are labeled "sugar-free," "reduced sugar" and "low sugar" can still contain enough sugar to cause damage to your teeth. They also contain the same acids as the standard carbonated drinks. It's recommended, therefore, to replace carbonated drinks in the diet with other options where possible.

Energy Drinks

So-called "energy drinks" are becoming more and more popular throughout the world. Here are three basic types of energy drinks:

1. Refreshment energy – formulated to replenish energy levels for someone who is perhaps run down or recovering from illness.

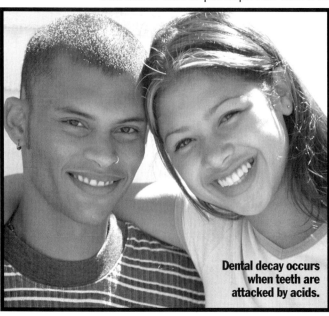

Dental decay occurs when teeth are attacked by acids.

2. Sports drinks – formulated to rapidly replace fluids during exercise and to maintain the body's blood glucose levels.

3. Functional energy – available for virtually anyone who wants to gain a quick burst of energy and alertness.

Energy drinks contain complex carbohydrates – a blend of slow, medium and fast acting sugars – to supply energy to the body over an extended period of time. Additionally energy drinks may also contain so-called "energy-enhancing" ingredients such as caffeine or taurine, to boost alertness.

The safety of energy drinks, in particular the additional energy-enhancing ingredients, has been investigated by a European committee. In relation to caffeine, while there is a wide range of caffeine levels, the majority of energy drinks have the same amount of caffeine as a cup of filtered coffee.

The committee felt that there was no concern about the contribution of energy drinks for nonpregnant adults. However, it is recommended that pregnant women should moderate their caffeine intake, from whatever source. Caffeine in energy drinks may also lead to overexposure in children, who do not normally consume much tea or coffee and are therefore more susceptible to the effects of caffeine on the body.

[Ref: www.bbc.co.uk/health/nutrition/drinks_soft.shtml]

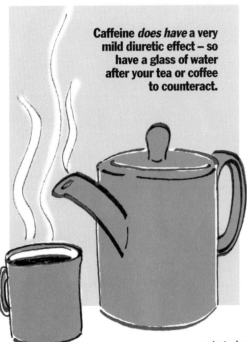

Caffeine *does have* a very mild diuretic effect – so have a glass of water after your tea or coffee to counteract.

Caffeinated Drinks

A number of our favorite thirst-quenchers now contain caffeine, a stimulant. Caffeine is added to many carbonated drinks for that familiar *kick* – but what about the health benefits in those most-loved hot drinks, tea and coffee?

Tea

It has been estimated that 196,000,000 cups of tea are drunk every day in the UK alone, and that the average person in the UK will consume no less than 80,000 cups of tea during his lifespan. These figures are quite spectacular – so what can tea do for us?

Tea does contribute slightly to our intake of some minerals, and it certainly will help to replace lost fluids, but the health interest in tea at the moment surrounds its proposed role in lowering coronary heart disease risk. Tea contains a group of antioxidant substances called flavonoids. These flavonoids have been shown to be able to slow down or inhibit the chemical reactions that are thought to take place during the development of coronary heart disease. *So sup up!* But remember that fresh water is still the best way of rehydrating your body. For every cup you have, try to drink a glass of water too.

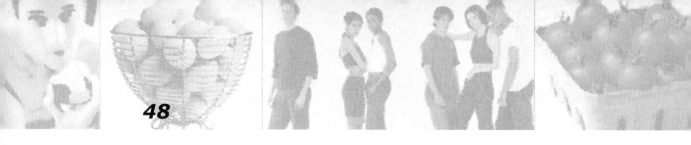

There has also been a lot of interest recently in the health advantages of green tea, with many claims that it can reduce blood cholesterol levels. However, scientific studies investigating the effect of green tea on blood cholesterol levels are divided. Some studies have found no effect at all; other studies have found low cholesterol levels in people who consume large quantities of green tea. However, we cannot rule out the possibility that the actual reason for the lower cholesterol levels is simply, people who drink green tea tend to have a healthier diet in general. There is certainly no definitive evidence that green tea reduces cholesterol levels.

Coffee

Coffee is a very popular drink with estimates suggesting 80 percent of adults drink coffee within the course of a week. But coffee has had some pretty bad press in the past, mainly due to its caffeine content. Coffee is not the only beverage to contain caffeine, but it does contain the most (although decaffeinated coffee is now widely available). Caffeine acts as a stimulant to the heart and central nervous system. Caffeine is also known to increase blood pressure in the short term, although there is no conclusive evidence of long-term effects on blood pressure.

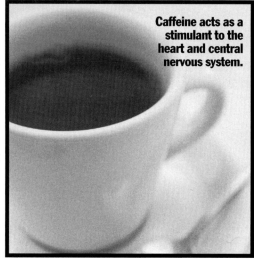

Caffeine acts as a stimulant to the heart and central nervous system.

The effects are most prominent when excessive quantities are taken and in highly sensitive people. In particular, those who are hypertensive. That is, people with habitual high blood pressure are advised to avoid caffeinated drinks, as are pregnant women.

Food Caffeine Content

Coffee (per cup)	instant	61 to 70 mg
	percolated, ground	97 to 125 mg
Tea (per cup)		15 to 75 mg
Hot chocolate (per cup)		10 to 17 mg
Chocolate bar		60 to 70 mg
Cola drinks (per 12 oz. can)		43 to 65 mg

Coffee has been linked to a number of the risk factors for coronary heart disease, including increased blood pressure and high blood cholesterol levels. However, no relationship has been found between drinking coffee and the likelihood of developing coronary heart disease. And there's good news for all you coffee drinkers out there. It has been found that coffee may be *beneficial* in some areas of health. Early research has found that coffee may reduce the risk of developing gallstones, kidney stones and colorectal cancer.

It's difficult to suggest a safe limit for coffee intake because there is huge variation in caffeine content of differing brands, and in the sensitivity to caffeine of each individual. However, considering the evidence we have to date, people with high blood pressure and pregnant women are advised to limit their caffeine consumption. For the rest of the population there is no evidence that coffee does any long-term harm. Caffeine *does have* a very mild diuretic effect – so have a glass of water after your coffee to counteract.

[Ref: www.bbc.co.uk/health/nutrition/drinks_caff.shtml']

Simple and Complex Carbohydrates

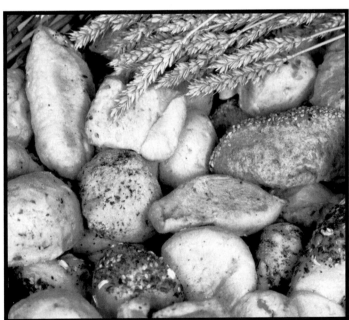

These are often confused with refined and unrefined carbohydrates, but the terms *simple* and *complex* refer to how complicated the chemical structure of a carbohydrate is, rather than whether or not it's whole grain. Complex carbs are the most common and there are three different kinds.

1. Glucose – Glucose is the blood sugar and is found in most carbohydrate foods. Glucose is a major fuel source that is stored as glycogen in the muscles and liver, and can be converted back to glucose when required for fuel.

The term *refined carbohydrates* refers to foods in which machinery has been used to remove the high-fiber bran and germ bits from the grain.

2. Starch – This is found only in plants. Contrary to popular belief, starch isn't fattening – it's the rich sauces, fats and oils often added to pasta, potatoes, rice, noodles and bread that are the culprits!

3. Fiber (non-starch polysaccharide) – Fiber is abundant in unrefined carbohydrates, fruit and vegetables, and important because it helps your body to process waste efficiently and helps you to feel

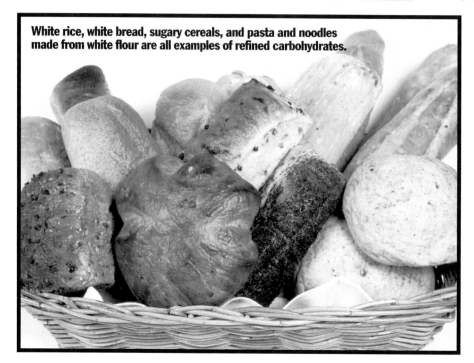

White rice, white bread, sugary cereals, and pasta and noodles made from white flour are all examples of refined carbohydrates.

fuller for longer. If you decide to increase the amount of fiber you eat, try to drink more water too. Your body doesn't digest fiber, so you need the extra water to help it flow through your digestive system with ease.

The term *refined carbohydrates* refers to foods in which machinery has been used to remove the high-fiber bran and germ bits from the grain. White rice, white bread, sugary cereals, and pasta and noodles made from white flour are all examples of refined carbohydrates.

Unrefined carbohydrates still contain the whole grain, including the bran and the germ, so they're higher in fiber. Examples include whole-grain rice, whole-meal bread, porridge oats, and whole-wheat pasta. You may try one of these "swaps" to increase your fiber intake, but this must be done slowly to avoid gastrointestinal discomfort – and always as part of an overall healthy balanced diet.

REFINED	"SWAP"	UNREFINED
Frosted flakes	⟷	Frosted bran flakes
White toast	⟷	Porridge oats
Rice cakes	⟷	Cereal bar
French bread	⟷	Whole-meal baguette
Normal pasta	⟷	Whole-meal pasta
Breadstick	⟷	Dark rye crispbread

How much is enough?

Nutritionists recommend that the bread, cereals and potatoes group makes up the bulk of your diet – roughly 50 percent. They also suggest that your dietary intake include 18 grams of fiber every day. An easy way to get that much fiber is to make sure that a food from this group forms the basis of every meal – and choose *fiber-rich, unrefined carbohydrates.* Here are three healthy choices to get you started.

1. Porridge oats with natural yogurt, raisins and sunflower seeds for breakfast.
2. Whole-meal bread banana sandwich or potato jacket and chili for lunch.
3. Seafood paella, made with brown rice, for dinner.

[Ref: www.bbc.co.uk/health/nutrition/basics_carbos.shtml]

Milk and Dairy Products

This food group includes milk, cheese, yogurt and fromage frais – but not butter, margarine or cream (which are in the fat and sugar group). The foods in this group contain many different kinds of nutrients, but they're particularly rich in calcium.

The Importance of Calcium

Calcium is a mineral that strengthens your bones and teeth and makes sure that everything runs smoothly with your muscles and nerves. It's especially important for growth, and calcium can continue to add to the strength of your bones until you reach about 30 to 35 years of age, when peak bone mass is reached. After that point, as a natural part of the aging process, your bones lose their density and grow weaker. If you haven't had enough calcium in your diet prior to this, there's an increased risk that your bones won't be strong enough to cope with any weakening – which can result in the brittle bone disease *osteoporosis.*

Health professionals estimate that one in three women and one in ten men suffer from osteoporosis, and there's concern that the diets of teenage girls and young women, in particular, aren't

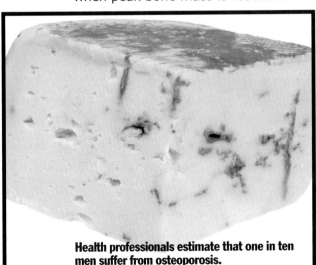

Health professionals estimate that one in ten men suffer from osteoporosis.

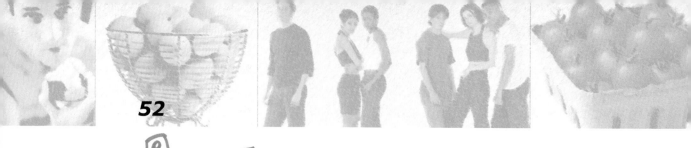

high enough in calcium. Some experts predict that the future could bring an osteoporosis epidemic in women.

Calcium for Vegans and the Lactose Intolerant

Of course, if your diet excludes milk and dairy products or if you can't tolerate the milk-sugar lactose, then you need to look for calcium alternatives. You can keep your bones healthy by:

- buying soya milks, yogurts and cheeses that are enriched with calcium
- eating lots of dark green leafy vegetables such as spinach, broccoli and watercress
- using almonds or sesame seeds as a topping on salads, cereals or desserts
- snacking on dried fruits – apricots, dates and figs all contain small amounts of calcium
- or ... if you're not vegan you can add sardines, prawns or anchovies to your main meal

Calcium is a mineral that strengthens your bones and teeth, and makes sure that everything runs smoothly with your muscles and nerves.

How much is enough?

The Department of Health recommends that both men and women get 700 mg of calcium every day to ensure good health. Realistically this means:

- a pint of milk
- 2 small tubs of plain or fruit yogurt
- roughly 80 grams of hard cheese

The good news is that, if you're concerned about your weight, getting the calcium you need doesn't have to mean eating or drinking full-fat dairy foods. There's exactly the same amount of calcium in skimmed milk as there is in

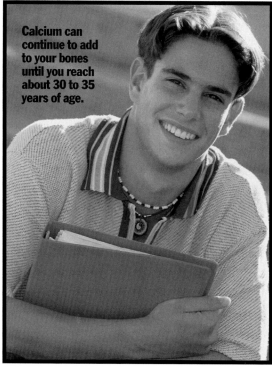

Calcium can continue to add to your bones until you reach about 30 to 35 years of age.

whole milk. The same goes for low-fat yogurt and reduced-fat cheese. So you don't have to buy their full-fat counterparts to look after your bones.

[Ref: www.bbc.co.uk/health/nutrition/basics_dairy.shtml]

Fatty and Sugary Foods

The foods in this group are best eaten sparingly because, although they're an energy source, they contain few nutrients. Don't be fooled into thinking that they're entirely "bad" for you, though. Fat is actually an important contributor to your good health.

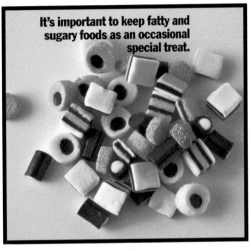

It's important to keep fatty and sugary foods as an occasional special treat.

Fat Facts
• Fat transports fat-soluble vitamins A, D, E and K through your body.
• Fat cushions your internal organs.
• Fat makes food taste better.
• Fat contains essential fatty acids (EFAs), which are thought to have a positive effect on the health of your heart and immune system.
• Fat is a concentrated source of energy.

And it's this last point that has gotten fat such a bad reputation. Just 1 gram of fat provides 9 calories – more than *double the calories* in 1 gram of protein or carbohydrate. This means that if you eat a lot of fatty foods, you're likely to put on weight. However, understanding the terms *unsaturated* and *saturated fats* can help.

Saturated and Unsaturated Fats
Fat can be divided into two groups – saturated and unsaturated.

Saturated fat is generally solid at room temperature and usually comes from animal sources. It's found in lard, butter, hard margarine, cheese, whole milk, and anything these ingredients are used in, such as cakes, chocolate, biscuits, pies and pastries. It's also the white fat you can see on red meat and underneath poultry skin. The less saturated fat you eat, the better – a high intake has been linked with an increased risk of coronary heart disease.

Unsaturated fat is usually liquid at room temperature and generally comes from vegetable sources. Monounsaturated and polyunsaturated fat are both included in this group. Unsaturated fat is a healthier alternative to saturated fat and can be found in vegetable oils

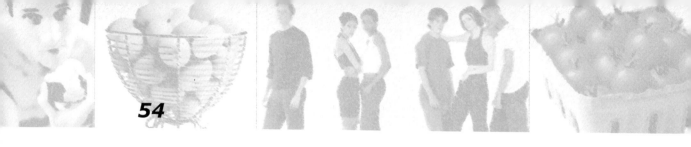

such as sesame, sunflower, soya and olive, oily fish such as mackerel, sardines, pilchards and salmon, and soft margarine.

In reality, many foods contain both saturated and unsaturated fats, but they're described as one or the other, depending on which they contain the most of. So, a healthier unsaturated fat like olive oil contains saturated fats, too.

Sugary Foods

Like fat, sugar is a concentrated source of energy and also has a bad reputation. The psychological benefits of eating foods like jam, sweets, cakes, chocolate, soft drinks, biscuits and ice cream are fairly obvious. They taste great and feel like a special treat. However, it's important to keep them as just that – an occasional special treat. *Why?* Because ...

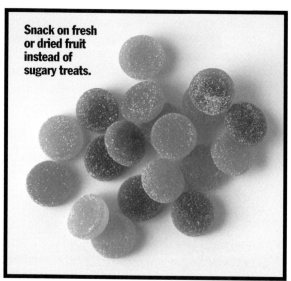

Snack on fresh or dried fruit instead of sugary treats.

a. Sugary foods often go hand in hand with fatty foods. (Think cakes, biscuits, chocolate and pies.)

b. Sugar interacts with the plaque on your teeth and has now been proven to cause tooth decay.

How much is enough?

Government guidelines recommend that fat should make up no more than 35 percent of your diet. For the average woman this means about 76 grams of fat per day, and for a male this means roughly 100 grams of fat per day. In reality, though, most of us have higher fat intake than that.

The recommendation for sugary foods is that we eat them sparingly. If you'd like to cut down on fatty and sugary foods, follow these suggestions:

• Snack on fresh or dried fruit rather than biscuits and chocolate.
• Trim any visible fat off meat and poultry, before cooking if possible.
• Buy lean cuts of meat and reduced-fat ground meats.
• Ditch the frying pan – try poaching, steaming, grilling and baking.
• Swap whole milk for semi-skimmed or skimmed.
• If you use lard, butter or hard margarine, switch to vegetable oil and low-fat spreads.

[Ref: www.bbc.co.uk/health/nutrition/basics_fatsugar.shtml]

Fruit and Vegetables

Fruit and vegetables are brimming with fiber, vitamins and minerals. And because they're low in calories, they provide a healthy addition to any diet.

Five a Day

Scientific studies have shown that people who eat a lot of fruit and vegetables may have a lower risk of getting illnesses such as heart disease and some cancers. For this reason, health authorities recommend that you eat at least five portions of fruit and vegetables every day – and it doesn't matter whether they're fresh, canned, frozen, cooked, juiced or dried.

But what does a portion look like?
- One medium-size piece of fruit – e.g., an apple, peach, banana or orange.
- One slice of large fruit, such as melon, mango or pineapple.
- A few handfuls of grapes, cherries or berries.
- A small handful of dried fruit.

Health authorities recommend that you eat at least five portions of fruit and vegetables every day.

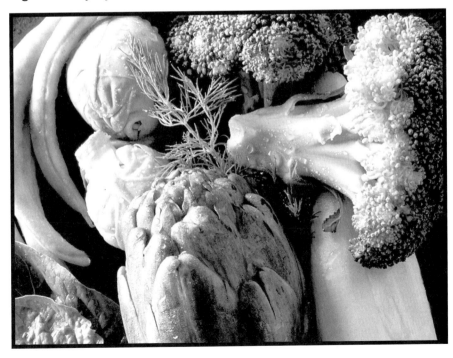

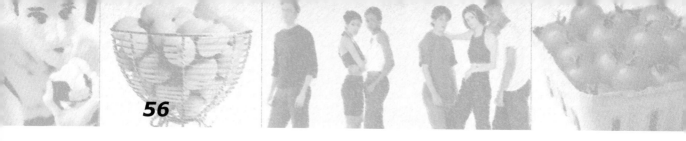

- A glass (roughly 100 ml) of fruit or vegetable juice.
- A small can (roughly 200 g) of fruit.
- A side salad.
- A serving (roughly 100 g) of vegetables – e.g. frozen or mushy peas, boiled carrots or stir-fried broccoli.
- The vegetables served in a portion of vegetable curry, stir-fry or casserole.

Right, but how does this translate to real life? How do you make sure you're getting your five a day? Here's a suggestion to get you started:

- Glass of pink grapefruit juice for breakfast = 1 portion
- Small pack of dried apricots for midmorning snack (instead of that chocolate bar or bag of chips) = 1 portion
- Side salad with lunch = 1 portion
- Sugar snap peas and asparagus, served with main meal = 1 portion
- Strawberries with dessert = 1 portion

If you're worried about getting the right amount of nutrients from fruits and vegetables, add a bit of color to your life. Many nutritionists recommend eating something *green,* something *red* and something *citrus* every day to guarantee a good mix of vitamins and minerals in your diet.

[Ref: www.bbc.co.uk/health/nutrition/basics_fruitveg.shtml]

Meat, Fish, Eggs and Other Alternatives

This food group includes poultry, pulses, beans, nuts, seeds, soya products and vegetable protein foods, such as quorn and seitan. They're all grouped together because they're rich in protein.

Protein – Highs and Lows

Protein plays an essential role in building and repairing your body. But whether it helps a fingernail to grow or heals a sore muscle, for example, depends very much on what the protein is made up of. You see, protein consists of smaller units called amino acids, which chain together in many different combinations to achieve different things. Some amino acid chains are created by your body, but some must come from your diet. These are called essential amino acids. Though all animal and plant cells contain some protein, the amount and the quality of the protein varies greatly.

High biological value foods contain enough indispensable amino acids for an adult diet and are considered to be good quality protein. Meat, fish and eggs are in this category. *Low biological value foods* don't contain enough indispensable amino acids. Plant foods such as pulses, nuts and seeds are in this group. So if you're vegetarian or vegan you need to do some clever protein-combining at meal times to ensure that the amino acid of one protein (e.g. soya milk) can compensate for the deficiencies of another (e.g. muesli with nuts and seeds).

Protein Combining for Vegetarians and Vegans

Because plant foods contain only some – *but not all* – of the protein elements needed by your body, they must be mixed together to ensure your good health.

Vegetarians

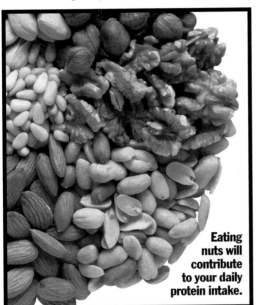

Eating nuts will contribute to your daily protein intake.

Foods such as eggs, nuts, seeds, beans, pulses, vegetable protein foods and soya products all contain protein. Plus, there are small amounts of protein in grains and dairy products. It's quite easy to combine two or three of these to make sure you're getting enough protein. Here are some ideas for tasty combinations:

• bran flakes with milk and sunflower seeds
(grain + dairy product + seed)
• grated cheese and baked beans on toast
(dairy product + bean + grain)
• egg-fried rice with chick peas (grain + egg + pulse)
• yogurt dip with aubergine curry and naan (dairy product + grain)

Vegans

If you're vegan and don't eat dairy products or eggs, there's no reason to feel limited. Here are some ideas for you:
• muesli with nuts, seeds and soya milk (nut + grain + seed + soya)
• tomato and lentil soup with bread (pulse + grain)
• stir-fried tofu, vegetables and rice (tofu + grain)

[Ref: www.bbc.co.uk/health/nutrition/basics_protein.shtml]

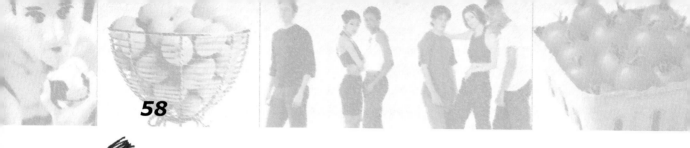

How much is enough?

Health professionals (those people in the white coats again) recommend that protein makes up 10 to 15 percent of your diet. They suggest that adult males eat 55.5 grams of protein every day and adult females eat 45 grams every day. In real terms, eating a moderate amount of protein – in one or two meals every day – should give you all the protein you need. Did you know that eggs contain all eight essential amino acids, making them a perfect source of protein? However, you'd have to eat at least eight eggs a day to get all the protein you need. Be sensible and include them as part of a well-balanced and varied diet.

The need to eat protein *every day* is worth emphasizing because your body cannot store it – you can't stock up by binging on protein once a week. Simply eat a variety of foods every day – that's all you need to do.

[Ref: www.bbc.co.uk/health/nutrition/basics_protein.shtml]

Weighty Issues: The Solution to Yo-Yo Dieting

Getting rid of the unhealthy pounds is only half the battle. The real challenge you face is learning how to lose the excess, then maintain your lower weight and avoid yo-yo dieting. The key to maintaining weight loss and breaking the up-and-down pattern is to get psychologically prepared for weight maintenance even before you begin a weight-loss program. To successfully make the transition from active dieting to active maintenance, you need to invest time anticipating, identifying and effectively planning realistic eating and exercise lifestyle changes.

The first question you must ask yourself before going on a diet is: Am I willing to change my unhealthy eating and exercise

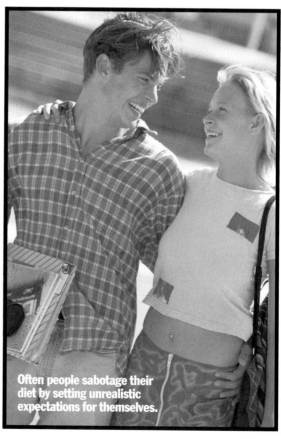

Often people sabotage their diet by setting unrealistic expectations for themselves.

habits for life? If the answer is *yes,* then you'll probably be able to prepare a realistic maintenance program that you'll be able to follow throughout your life. If on the other hand the answer is *no,* then you run the risk of continuing to be a career dieter, struggling to lose weight that you're essentially doomed to put back on.

Then again, if you feel unable to change your unhealthy eating and exercise habits, there is a third option: Refrain from rigorous dieting altogether until you are ready to make the necessary lifestyle changes. Instead of dieting, simply choose one unhealthy eating or exercise habit that you're willing to change right now, and slowly begin the process of preparing yourself for the time when you'll be psychologically ready to change the majority of your unhealthy eating and exercise habits for life.

Unrealistic expectations place too much pressure on both the dieter and the diet, which ultimately leads to self-sabotage.

Remember, old habits die hard! Be patient with yourself and learn to accept the fact that making *permanent* positive changes is a process. It's okay if you're not prepared to adopt a whole new lifestyle right away. By being honest with yourself about that fact and by accepting it, you'll be able to avoid the physical and emotional rollercoaster of yo-yo dieting, and start on the road to a healthier life – one step at a time.

[Ref: www.efit.com/servlet/article/weight/6014.html]

Diet Sabotage

Often people sabotage their diet by setting unrealistic expectations for themselves. Either they choose diets that involve too much personal sacrifice (forcing them to do without foods they believe they can't forgo) or they choose to diet because of something they hope to gain from weight loss, aside from the actual shedding of pounds. In either case, these unrealistic expectations place too much pressure on both the dieter and the diet, which ultimately leads to self-sabotage.

To break the unproductive cycle, you can benefit greatly by doing some self-investigation before beginning a weight-loss regimen. When you're clear about *why* you want to lose weight and *what* you need to do in order to be successful on a weight-loss plan, you're much more likely to see the diet through to your goal weight.

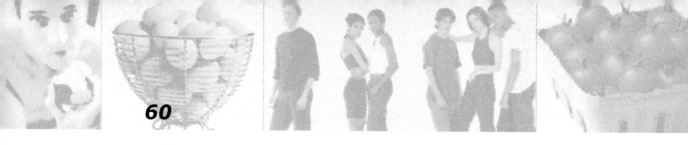

Ask Yourself what you really want out of each day.

For example, many people on high-protein diets report experiencing low levels of energy and carbohydrate cravings. They have a taste for a carbohydrate-rich food to satisfy their cravings and end up going off the diet entirely. Only these individuals can really know why they sabotage their diets, but had they been clear about their reasons for losing weight and the kind of structure and support they require to stick with the weight-loss program all the way to their goals, it's likely they would have chosen a different diet, one that wouldn't require them to give up so many of the foods they love.

People who lack *personal clarity* will be more vulnerable to diet sabotage. If you want to avoid the pitfalls of starting another diet you can't follow through on, ask yourself what you really want out of each day – and what you want out of your life in the bigger picture – before you begin. This information will help you set *realistic expectations,* which will lead you to diet success.

[Ref: www.efit.com/servlet/article/weight/800.html]

Flax in Your Diet

One of the wonders of flax stems from its fat content: 9 grams in a one-ounce serving. Sounds hefty, but don't worry. The majority of fat is in the form of alpha-linolenic acid, an omega-3 fatty acid, which is also found in fish such as herring, salmon and mackerel. Actually, flax is one of the richest sources of these "good fats" touted as having several heart-protecting effects, such as lowering blood pressure, making blood clots less likely to occur, and lowering the level of triglycerides in the blood.

In fact, studies seem to back flax as an important part of a heart-healthy diet. For example, a study of 11 healthy men who added about four tablespoons of flaxseed oil to their diets found that flaxseed decreased the blood's tendency to clot. Another study showed that 15 obese people who replaced regular margarine with one made from flaxseed oil had more flexible arteries after just one month.

Other research suggests omega-3 fatty acids found in flax and fish may be helpful in easing the symptoms of arthritis, multiple sclerosis, and skin conditions such as psoriasis and eczema. There is also some preliminary evidence that they may help inhibit the formation of cancerous cells.

Fiber – Although flax comes in both seed and oil form, *it's the seed* that seems to help lower cholesterol levels. One study showed that women who ate flaxseed muffins containing about two tablespoons of ground flaxseed daily for one month reduced their total cholesterol by an average of 9 percent and their bad LDL cholesterol by 18 percent. The seeds themselves contain a good amount of *soluble fiber,* a substance known for its cholesterol-lowering properties, but no study has proven whether it is flax's fiber content, its level of omega-3s, or the combination of the two that provides the benefit.

While we're on the subject of fiber, whole flaxseeds are also good for relieving constipation. In addition to soluble fiber, flaxseed also contains the *insoluble* variety, the kind that helps improve laxation and prevents constipation by increasing fecal bulk and reducing bowel transit time. However, keep in mind when it comes to flaxseed and laxation: Eat the whole flaxseed, not ground, since it's the outer covering of a seed that facilitates this whole process.

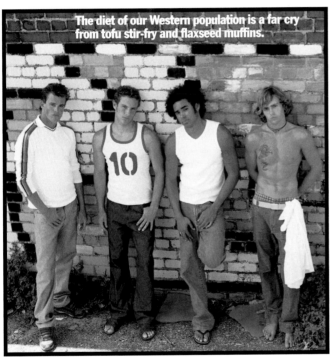
The diet of our Western population is a far cry from tofu stir-fry and flaxseed muffins.

Lignans – Flaxseed is also a rich source of lignans, a type of phytoestrogen found in plants. You may have heard of phytoestrogens before; they're also found in soybeans in the form of daidzein and genistein. Lignans, as well as other phytoestrogens, may protect against certain cancers, particularly hormone-sensitive cancers such as those of the breast, endometrium and prostate. Lignans seem to interfere with sex hormone metabolism, which often goes awry in hormone-sensitive cancers. Although research is ongoing in this area, keep in mind that populations with high intakes of phytoestrogens tend to have lower rates of cancer than our Western population, whose diet is a far cry from tofu stir-fry and flaxseed muffins.

You can find flax in most health food stores, where it is available in basically two forms – oil and whole. Keep in mind, however, that if you use whole flaxseeds you may want to grind them first because a whole

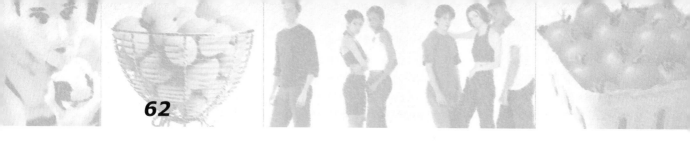

seed will pass right through you without leaving behind any of its health benefits. You can purchase ground flaxseeds, or you can grind them yourself in a coffee grinder. Sprinkle flaxseed in cereal, soups or salads. You can use flax oil any way you want – except in cooking, because at high temperatures the fatty acids break down and are not as beneficial. Store flax oil (as well as ground or whole flaxseed) in the refrigerator.

[Ref: www.efit.com/servlet/article/nutrition/18142.html]

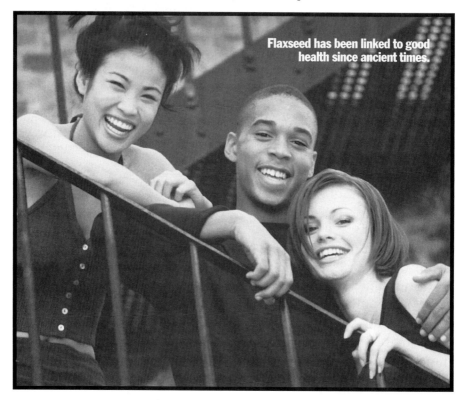

Flaxseed has been linked to good health since ancient times.

What is Flax?
Flax is a blue flowering crop grown on the prairies of Canada for its oil-rich seeds. The seeds of flax are tiny, smooth and flat, and range in color from light to reddish brown. They serve a variety of purposes, including baking and other food uses. People have eaten flaxseed since ancient times. Taste – a pleasant, nutty flavor – is one reason; good nutrition is another.

Flaxseed as a Food
Because of its link to good health, flaxseed is fast becoming a new food in many diets. Bakers and commercial food companies use flaxseed as a unique ingredient in everything from yeast breads to bagels and

cookie mixes. Not only do muffins and breads baked with flax taste great, but studies have shown that these foods provide health benefits.

Omega-3 enriched eggs from hens fed rations containing flaxseed are also very popular. These eggs contain eight to ten times more omega-3 fatty acids than regular eggs. Health Canada states that two of these enriched eggs supply more than half the recommended daily intake of omega-3 for adult men and women.

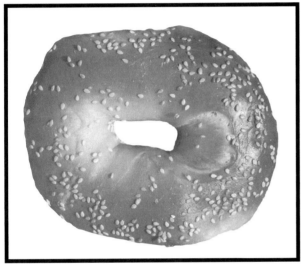

Bakers and commercial food companies use flaxseed as a unique ingredient in everything from yeast breads to bagels and cookie mixes.

Why Flaxseed is Good Medicine

Current nutrition research continues to identify various substances in foods that appear to act as protectors against chronic illnesses like cardiovascular disease and cancer. Flaxseed, a popular food ingredient in Europe and Canada, is no exception. The reasons are many.

• Several studies confirm that flaxseed can be a cholesterol-lowering agent like oat bran, fruit pectin and other food ingredients that contain soluble fiber. By packaging both omega-3 fatty acids and soluble fiber together, flaxseed presents two ingredients that favor healthy blood lipid patterns.

• Flaxseed contains healthy amounts of both soluble and insoluble fiber. Scientists at the American National Cancer Institute singled out flaxseed as one of six foods that deserved special study.

Nutrient Profile

While flaxseed is rich in protein, research suggests that the health benefits probably have more to do with its fatty acid and fiber profile. Here is the nutrient profile of flaxseed.

Proximate: 100 grams (3-1/2 ounces)
Food energy: 450 kilocalories (calories)
Fat: 41.0 grams
Total dietary fiber: 28.0 grams
Protein: 20.0 grams

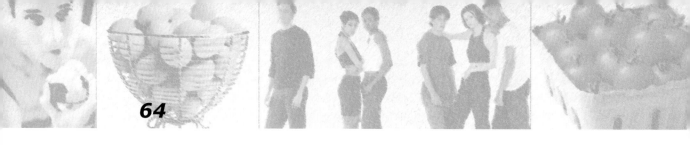

A Focus on Fatty Acids

Fats and oils have earned such a bad reputation in recent years – and that's partly because people eat too much fat, too much *saturated fat* in particular. (Saturated fats raise blood cholesterol levels and increase the risk of heart disease.)

Although about 41 percent of flaxseed is oil, very little of that is saturated. More than 70 percent of fat in flaxseed is of the healthful polyunsaturated type. In fact, a unique feature of flaxseed is the high ratio of alpha-linolenic acid (an omega-3 fatty acid) to linoleic (omega-6 fatty acids). Nutritionists consider these two polyunsaturated fatty acids as *essential* because the body cannot manufacture them from any other substances. (Normally the body converts carbohydrates, proteins and fats into fatty acids as needed.) That means they must be eaten as part of the diet.

While other plant seeds – corn, sunflower, peanuts – contain omega-6 polyunsaturated fatty acids, flaxseed is the only one that contains so much of the essential omega-3 fatty acids. Understanding how these two types of polyunsaturated fats differ can help underscore the reasons why flaxseed has so many unique health benefits.

Fatty Acid Composition of Flaxseed Oil

Saturated fatty acids	9%
Monounsaturated fatty acids	18%
Polyunsaturated fatty acids	
Omega-3	57%
Omega-6	16%

Omega-3 fatty acids — More than half the fat in flaxseed is of the omega-3 essential fatty acid type. Scientific studies reporting the health benefits of omega-3 show that these fatty acids are required for proper infant growth and development, and that cholesterol can be reduced by adding flaxseed to the diet. New research also suggests that alpha-linolenic acid, an omega-3 fatty acid which is abundant in flaxseed, offers protective effects against both coronary heart disease and stroke. Omega-3 has also been shown to protect against hypertension and inflammatory and autoimmune disorders. Long-term studies of flaxseed effects on breast cancer are now under way.

Omega-6 fatty acids — An essential fatty acid, linoleic is the chief polyunsaturated fat in the North American diet. Most omega-6 fatty acids in the diet come from vegetable oils.

Ratio of omega-3 to omega-6 — Studies of hunter-gatherer populations show their diets contained roughly equal amounts of omega-6 and omega-3 fatty acids. Currently, researchers and nutrition experts recommend people replace some omega-6 fatty acids in their diet with omega-3 fatty acids like those found in flaxseed.

An Overview of Health Benefits

Recent scientific reports point out that flaxseed can have a positive influence on everything from cholesterol levels to laxation to cancer and heart disease. Here are some highlights:

• *Relief from constipation* – Eating 50 grams of flaxseed per day (baked into muffins) helped increase the frequency of bowel movements and the number of consecutive days with bowel movements in a group of older Canadian adults.

• *A lower risk for heart disease* – Total cholesterol levels dropped 9 percent and LDL (the "bad" cholesterol) decreased 18 percent when a group of nine healthy women ate 50 grams of milled flaxseed a day for four weeks (as flour or cooked into bread) along with their regular diets, according to a report from the University of Toronto. In a similar study with men and women, 50 grams of flaxseed (eaten daily in muffins) lowered total cholesterol and showed a constant trend of about 11 to 16 percent toward lower serum lipids (fat in the blood).

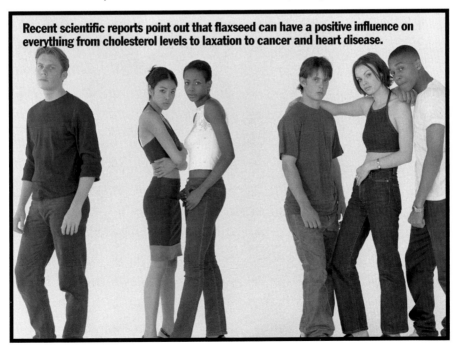

Recent scientific reports point out that flaxseed can have a positive influence on everything from cholesterol levels to laxation to cancer and heart disease.

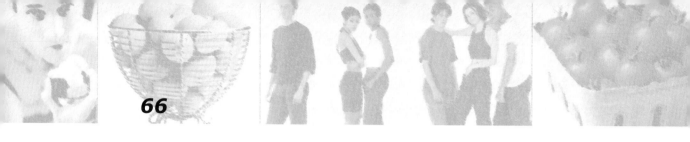

• *Cancer prevention* – Lignans and alpha-linolenic acid are found abundantly in flaxseed. Population studies of diet and disease risk suggest an anticancer role for flaxseed. Long-term studies of flaxseed effects in women with breast cancer are under way.

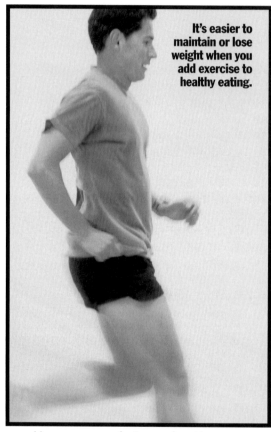

It's easier to maintain or lose weight when you add exercise to healthy eating.

What's the best advice on nutrition?

Follow North American dietary recommendations. These suggestions for a healthful diet offer guidelines for healthy people two years of age and over. By following the dietary recommendations, you can enjoy better health and reduce your chances of getting certain diseases – such as heart disease, high blood pressure, stroke, some cancers, and the most common type of diabetes. These guidelines form the best, most up-to-date advice from nutrition experts.

• Eat a variety of foods.
• Maintain healthy weight.
• Choose a diet low in fat, saturated fat and cholesterol.
• Choose a diet with plenty of vegetables, fruits and grain products.
• Use sugars only in moderation.
• Use salt and sodium only in moderation.
• If you drink alcoholic beverages, do so in moderation.

Eating: Rules of Thumb

• Don't eat when you're not hungry. (This problem is common. Some people eat when they are bored or depressed, when they're by themselves, and well, just 'cuz it tastes good.)
• Eat slowly. (It takes your body some time to digest and realize that you are full.)
• Drink lots of water. (This does all sorts of good things to wash your system clean – sometimes food cravings are really caused by your being thirsty, so have a drink of water before you start eating.)

• Keep the extra sugar and carbs to a minimum. (Avoid that Snickers bar, don't overdo it on the bread and pasta, and include salad and veggies in your diet regularly.)

• Try to stay as close to foods in their natural state as possible. (The fewer preservatives the easier for your body to break the food down.)

• There are tons of different diets out there, but staying in shape really comes down to the number of calories you consume.

• Your metabolism slows in the late evening, so don't have all your calories at the end of the day. (Especially avoid that 2 a.m. pizza run!)

• Ditch the mayo for mustard, and start trying salsa as a spread.

• Change the TV station when tempting food commercials come on – they're evil.

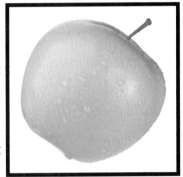

• Eating out all the time adds about 300 calories a day. (They always sneak in tons of butter and oil.)

• Don't deny yourself everything you love, but have it in moderation.

• It's easier to maintain or lose weight when you add exercise to healthy eating.

• If you are determined to lose weight, try to stay close to 1200 to 1400 calories a day and limit your fat intake to about 10 to 15 grams.

[Ref: www.beautyq.com/adeating2.html]

Eating: Sample Meal Choices
Here are some ideas for each meal.

Breakfast:
☐ English muffin w/low-sugar or "lite" jam
☐ One packet of instant oatmeal and fruit
☐ One bowl of cereal and toast
☐ Yogurt and fruit
☐ Poached egg (or hard boiled egg) w/Canadian bacon
☐ Spinach and tomato frittata

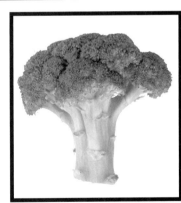

Lunch:
☐ Big salad with all sorts of stuff like lettuce, tomatoes, cucumber, potatoes w/a little oil and vinegar, salt and pepper, plus a banana
☐ Turkey burger and salad
☐ Ham and cheese or roast beef sandwich
☐ Turkey or tuna sandwich
☐ Tortilla w/black beans and rice
☐ Pita sandwich
☐ Soup and salad
☐ Baked potato w/fat-free chili and salad
☐ Chicken breast w/roll and fruit

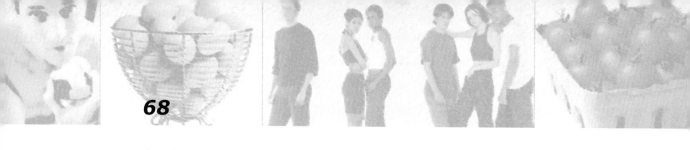

Snack:
☐ One packet of raisins
☐ One apple
☐ Ginger snaps
☐ Apple sauce
☐ Snackwell's

Dinner:
☐ Broiled chicken topped w/mustard and Good Seasons salad
    dressing mix w/a zucchini, squash, mushrooms, onions combo
☐ Grilled salmon, swordfish, tuna or sea bass w/steamed string beans
☐ Chicken and vegetable stir-fry over rice w/asparagus
☐ Pasta w/tomato sauce (or marinara) w/steamed green veggie
☐ Beans and rice, asparagus and salad
☐ Flank steak w/beans and rice

Note:
If you go "over the top" in the first half of the day,
end with a salad or something lighter and with less carbs.

[Ref: www.beautyq.com/adeating5.html]

Vegetarian Nutrition

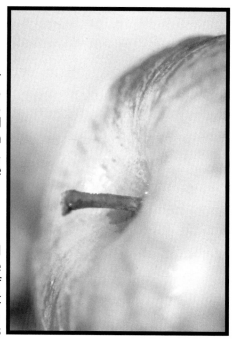

More and more teenagers are choosing not to eat meat, poultry or fish. They are becoming vegetarians. Teenage vegetarians are often faced with pressures – pressures from parents concerned about their health, and pressures from within to continue on the path they have chosen.

Variety is the Key to a Healthy Vegetarian Diet

Probably the most frequently asked questions for teenage vegetarians are about the nutritional adequacy of their food choices. A vegetarian diet can be enjoyed by people of all ages. The key to a healthy vegetarian diet is *variety.* Just as your parents should be concerned if you eat only hamburgers, they should also worry if you eat only potato chips and salad. A healthy, varied vegetarian diet includes fruits, vegetables, plenty of leafy greens, whole-grain products, nuts, seeds and legumes. Some vegetarians also choose to eat dairy products and/or eggs.

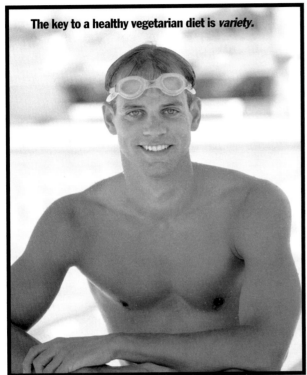

The key to a healthy vegetarian diet is *variety*.

Teenage vegetarians have nutritional needs that are the same as any other teenager. The years between 13 and 19 are times of especially rapid growth and change. Nutritional needs are high during these years. The nutrients that are of most concern are protein, calcium, iron and vitamin B12.

What about protein?

North American vegetarian teens eating varied diets rarely have any difficulty getting enough protein as long as their diet contains enough energy (calories) to support growth. Cow's milk and low-fat cheese are protein sources; however, beans, breads, cereals, nuts, peanut butter, tofu and soy milk are also some foods that are especially good sources of protein. Fruits, fats and alcohol do not provide much protein, and so a diet based only on these foods would have a good chance of being too low in protein.

The vegetarian must plan combinations of foods to obtain enough protein, or amino acids (components of protein). A mixture of plant proteins eaten throughout the day will provide enough of the essential amino acids.

Other Important Nutrients for Vegetarian Teenagers

Especially during adolescence, calcium is used to build bones. Bone density is determined in adolescence and young adulthood; so it is important to include three or more good sources of calcium in your diet every day. Cow's milk and dairy products do contain calcium. However, there are other good sources of calcium such as tofu processed with calcium sulfate, green leafy vegetables including collard greens, mustard greens and kale, and calcium-fortified soy milk and orange juice.

Iron requirements of teenagers are relatively high. By eating a varied diet, a vegetarian can meet his or her iron needs, while avoiding

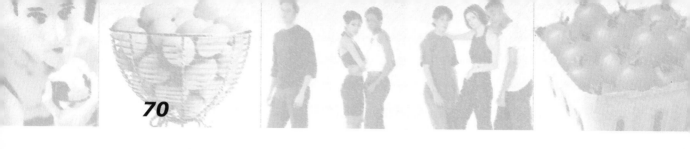

the excess fat and cholesterol found in red meats such as beef or pork. To increase the amount of iron absorbed from a meal, eat a food containing vitamin C as part of the meal. Citrus fruits and juices (for example, orange juice), tomatoes and broccoli are all good sources of vitamin C. Foods which are high in iron include broccoli, raisins, watermelon, spinach, black-eyed peas, blackstrap molasses, chickpeas and pinto beans.

Vitamin B12 is a vitamin which only vegans (vegetarians eating no dairy, eggs, meat, fish or birds) need to add to their diet. Some cereals and fortified soy milks have vitamin B12 (check the label). Red Star T-6635 nutritional yeast flakes (Vegetarian Support Formula) also supply vitamin B12.

What is a Vegan?
Vegetarians do not eat meat, fish or poultry. In addition to being vegetarian, vegans do not use other animal products and byproducts such as eggs, dairy products, honey, leather, fur, silk, wool, cosmetics, and soaps derived from animal products.

Why Choose Veganism?
People choose to be vegan for health, environmental, and/or ethical reasons. For example, some vegans feel that one promotes the meat industry by consuming eggs and dairy products. That is, once dairy cows or egg-laying chickens are too old to be productive, they are often sold as meat; and since male calves do not produce milk, they usually are raised for veal or other products. Some people avoid these items because of conditions associated with their production.

Many vegans choose this lifestyle to promote a more humane and caring world. They know they are not perfect, but believe they have a responsibility to try to do their best, while not being judgmental of others.

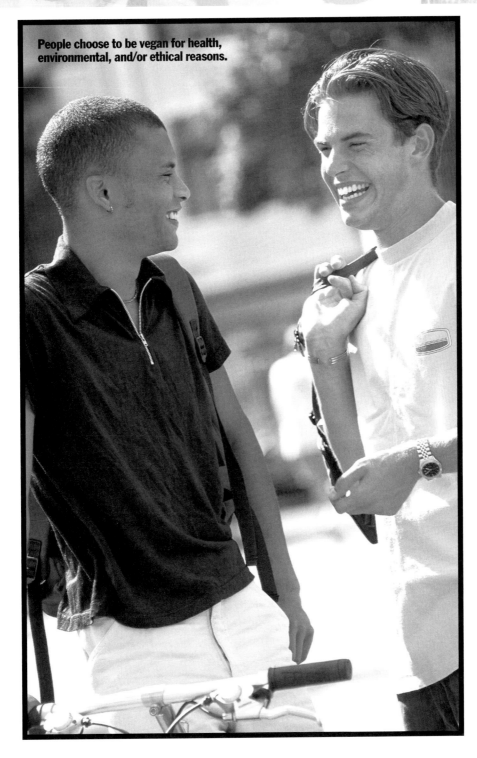

People choose to be vegan for health, environmental, and/or ethical reasons.

CHAPTER THREE

The key to a nutritionally sound vegan diet is *variety.* A healthy and varied vegan diet includes fruits, vegetables, plenty of leafy greens, whole-grain products, nuts, seeds and legumes.

Protein

It is very easy for a vegan diet to meet the recommendations for protein as long as calorie intake is adequate. Strict protein planning or combining is not necessary. The key is to eat *a varied diet.* Almost all foods except for alcohol, sugar and fats are good sources of protein. Vegan sources include: potatoes, whole-wheat bread, rice, broccoli, spinach, almonds, peas, chickpeas, peanut butter, tofu, soy milk, lentils, kale ...

Vegan Nutrition

For example, if part of a day's menu included the following foods, you would meet the Recommended Dietary Allowance (RDA) for protein for an adult male: 1 cup oatmeal, 1 cup soy milk, 2 slices whole-wheat bread, 1 bagel, 2 tablespoons peanut butter, 1 cup vegetarian baked beans, 5 ounces tofu, 2 tablespoons almonds, 1 cup broccoli, and 1 cup brown rice.

Fat

Vegan diets are free of cholesterol and are generally low in fat. Thus eating a vegan diet makes it easy to conform to recommendations given to reduce the risk of major chronic diseases such as heart disease and cancer. High-fat foods, which should be used sparingly, include oils, margarine, nuts, nut butters, seed butters, avocado and coconut.

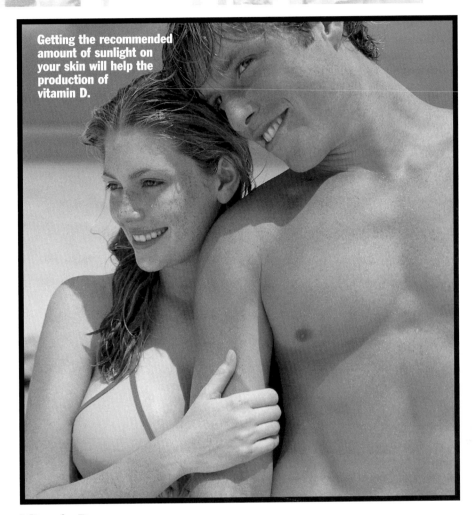

Getting the recommended amount of sunlight on your skin will help the production of vitamin D.

Vitamin D

Vitamin D is not found in the vegan diet but can be made by humans following exposure to sunlight. At least 10 to 15 minutes of summer sun on hands and face two or three times a week is recommended for adults so that vitamin D production can occur.

Calcium

Calcium is needed for strong bones and is found in dark green vegetables, tofu processed with calcium sulfate, and many other foods commonly eaten by vegans. Calcium requirements for those on lower-protein, plant-based protein diets may be somewhat lower than requirements for those eating a higher-protein, flesh-based diet. However, it is important for vegans to eat foods high in calcium and/or use a vegan calcium supplement every day.

Calcium Content of Selected Foods
Following are some good sources of calcium:

Soy or rice milk, commercial, calcium-fortified, plain	8 oz.	150-500 mg
Collard greens, cooked	1 cup	357 mg
Blackstrap molasses	2 tbsp.	342 mg
Tofu, processed with calcium sulfate	4 oz.	200-330 mg
Calcium-fortified orange juice	8 oz.	300 mg
Tofu, processed with nigari	4 oz.	80-230 mg
Kale, cooked	1 cup	176 mg
Tahini	2 tbsp.	128 mg
Almonds	1/4 cup	97 mg

Other sources of calcium include: okra, sesame seeds, turnip greens, soybeans, figs, tempeh, almond butter, broccoli, bok choy, commercial soy yogurt ... The recommended intake for calcium for adults 19 through 50 years is 1000 milligrams/day.

Note: It appears that oxalic acid, which is found in spinach, rhubarb, chard and beet greens, binds with calcium and reduces calcium absorption. Calcium is well absorbed from other dark green vegetables.

Zinc

Vegan diets can provide zinc at levels close to or even higher than the RDA. Zinc is found in grains, legumes and nuts.

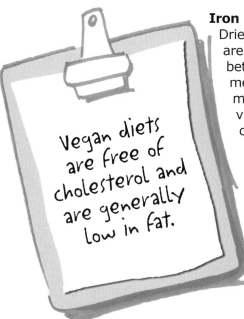

Vegan diets are free of cholesterol and are generally low in fat.

Iron

Dried beans and dark green vegetables are especially good sources of iron, better on a per-calorie basis than meat. Iron absorption is increased markedly by eating foods containing vitamin C along with foods containing iron.

Sources of Iron

Soybeans, lentils, blackstrap molasses, kidney beans, chickpeas, black-eyed peas, seitan, Swiss chard, tempeh, black beans, prune juice, beet greens, tahini, peas, figs, bulghur, bok choy, raisins, watermelon, millet, kale ...

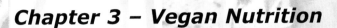

Comparison of Iron Sources

Here are the iron contents of selected foods:

1 cup cooked soybeans	8.8 mg
2 tbsp. blackstrap molasses	7.0 mg
1 cup cooked lentil	6.6 mg
1 cup cooked kidney beans	5.2 mg
1 cup cooked chickpeas	4.7 mg
1 cup cooked lima beans	4.5 mg
1 cup cooked Swiss chard	4.0 mg
1/8 medium watermelon	1.0 mg

Vitamin B12

The requirement for vitamin B12 is very low. Non-animal sources include Red Star nutritional yeast T6635, also known as Vegetarian Support Formula (about two teaspoons supplies the adult RDA). It is especially important for pregnant and lactating women, infants, and children to have reliable sources of vitamin B12 in their diets. Numerous foods are fortified with B12, but sometimes companies change what they do. Always read labels carefully or even write to the company for more information.

Tempeh, miso and seaweed are often labeled as having large amounts of vitamin B12. However, these products are not reliable sources of the vitamin because the amount of B12 present depends on the type of processing the food has undergone.

Other sources of vitamin B12 are fortified soy milk (check the label as this is rarely available in the US), vitamin B12-fortified meat analogues, and vitamin B12 supplements. There are supplements which do not contain animal products. Vegetarians who are not vegan can also obtain vitamin B12 from dairy products and eggs.

Common Vegan Foods

Oatmeal, stir-fried vegetables, cereal, toast, orange juice, peanut butter on whole-wheat bread, frozen fruit desserts, lentil soup, salad bar items like chickpeas and three-bean salad, dates, apples, macaroni, fruit smoothies, popcorn, spaghetti, vegetarian baked beans, guacamole, chili ...

Vegans Also Eat ...

Tofu lasagna, homemade pancakes without eggs, hummus, eggless cookies, soy ice cream, tempeh, corn chowder, soy yogurt, rice pudding, fava beans, banana muffins, spinach pies, oat-nut burgers, falafel, corn fritters, French toast made with soy milk, soy hot dogs, vegetable burgers, pumpkin casserole, scrambled tofu, seitan ...

When Eating Out Try These Foods

Pizza without cheese, Chinese moo shu vegetables, Indian curries and dahl, eggplant dishes without the cheese, bean tacos without the lard and cheese (available from Taco Bell and other Mexican restaurants), Middle Eastern hummus and tabouli, Ethiopian injera (flat bread) and lentil stew, Thai vegetable curries ...

Egg and Dairy Replacers

As a binding ingredient, substitute the following for each egg:
• 1/4 cup (2 oz.) soft tofu blended with the liquid ingredients of the recipe, or ...
• 1 small banana, mashed, or ...
• 1/4 cup applesauce, or ...
• 2 tablespoons cornstarch or arrowroot starch, or Ener-G Egg Replacer or another commercial mix found in health-food stores.

The following substitutions can be made for dairy products:
• Soy milk, rice milk, potato milk, nut milk, or water may be used (in some recipes).
• Buttermilk can be replaced with soured soy or rice milk. For each cup of buttermilk, use 1 cup soymilk plus 1 tablespoon of vinegar.
• Soy cheese is available in health-food stores. (Be aware that many soy cheeses contain casein, which is a dairy product.)
• Crumbled tofu can be substituted for cottage cheese or ricotta cheese in lasagna and similar dishes.
• Several brands of nondairy cream cheese are available in some supermarkets and kosher stores.

[Ref: www.vrg.org/nutshell/vegan.htm]

Recipes

Rigatoni Combination
(Meatless Meals for Working People –
Quick and Easy Vegetarian Recipes)
1/3 pound rigatoni or other pasta
1 onion, chopped
1 clove garlic, minced
1/2 green pepper, chopped
1 teaspoon olive or vegetable oil
1 small can tomato sauce
1 pound of canned kidney beans, drained
1 teaspoon soy sauce (optional)
1/4 teaspoon salt (optional)
1/2 teaspoon chili powder
Black pepper to taste

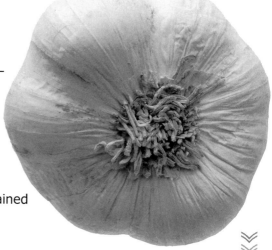

Cook pasta according to package instructions. Saute onions, garlic, and green pepper in oil 4 to 5 minutes or until soft. Stir in tomato sauce, kidney beans, soy sauce, salt, chili powder and black pepper. Simmer several minutes. Drain pasta when done and stir into sauce. Serve as is, or add 1/2 cup crumbled tofu or low-fat cottage cheese to each serving to make a lasagna-like dish. Add hot sauce if desired. (To decrease fat content – saute in water instead of oil or just brush the pan lightly with an oiled paper towel.) Serves 4.

Sweet Sauteed Red Cabbage
(Simply Vegan – Quick Vegetarian Meals)
1/2 red cabbage, shredded
1 apple, chopped
Small onion, chopped
1/2 cup water
1/2 cup raisins
1/2 teaspoon cinnamon

Use a nonstick pan, if possible. Heat ingredients, stirring occasionally, over medium-high heat for 10 minutes. Serves 4.

Spicy Potatoes, Cabbage and Peas Over Rice
(Simply Vegan – Quick Vegetarian Meals)
2 cups rice
4 cups water
5 medium potatoes, peeled and thinly sliced
2 cups water
1/2 green cabbage
10 ounce frozen peas (or equivalent fresh)
2 teaspoons curry powder
1 teaspoon turmeric
1/2 teaspoon ginger
1/2 teaspoon garlic powder
1/8 teaspoon cayenne pepper
Salt to taste (optional)

Cook rice in 4 cups water in a covered pot over medium-high heat until done. In a separate pan, add sliced potatoes to 2 cups of water and heat over medium-high heat. Shred cabbage and add to potatoes. Add peas and spices. Cover pan. Continue heating, stirring occasionally, until potatoes are tender. Serve over rice. Serves 6.

Garbanzo Bean Burgers
(Simply Vegan – Quick Vegetarian Meals)
2 cups cooked garbanzo beans (chickpeas), mashed
1 stalk celery, finely chopped
1 carrot, finely chopped
1/4 small onion, minced
1/4 cup whole-wheat flour
Salt and pepper to taste
2 teaspoons oil

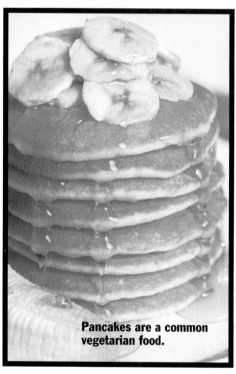

Pancakes are a common vegetarian food.

Mix the ingredients (except oil) in a bowl. Form 6 flat patties. Fry in oiled pan over medium-high heat until burgers are golden brown on each side. Serve alone with a mushroom or tomato sauce, or as a burger with lettuce and tomato. Makes 6 burgers.

Vegetarian Foods
Common vegetarian foods: macaroni and cheese, spaghetti, cheese pizza, eggplant parmesan, vegetable soup, pancakes, oatmeal, grilled cheese, bean tacos and burritos, vegetable lo mein, French toast, French fries, vegetable pot pie, fruit shakes, bread, yogurt, cheese lasagna, peanut butter and jam, fruit salad, corn flakes ...

Some vegetarians also eat: tofu, tempeh, bulgur, lentils, millet, tahini, falafel, nutritional yeast, whole-wheat flour, wheat germ, sprouts, chickpeas, tamari, kale, collards, carrot juice, barley, rice cakes, carob, split peas, kidney beans, soy burgers, kiwi fruit, papaya, blintzes, curry, nut loaf ...

Decreasing Fat Consumption
Vegetarian diets may be lower in fat than the typical American diet. However, for those people who need to be particularly cautious about the fat they eat, below are a few tips for reducing fat. Extremely low-fat diets are not appropriate for everybody, especially children and pregnant women.
• Saute *in water* instead of oil. Use soy lecithin sprays or rub a little oil on the pan using a paper towel. You can use half the amount of oil called for in most recipes – or even less. The oil can be just omitted, or replaced by juice or juice concentrate to make the item sweeter – or simply substitute water.

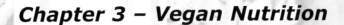

Remember: Only animal products (including dairy and eggs) contain cholesterol. Vegetable products contain no cholesterol. However, some vegetable products, such as coconut and palm oil, are high in saturated fat and may raise blood cholesterol levels.

Egg Replacers (Binders)

Any of the following can be used to replace eggs in a recipe:

• substitute 1 banana for 1 egg (great for cakes, pancakes, etc.)

• 2 tablespoons cornstarch or arrowroot starch for 1 egg

• Ener-G Egg Replacer (or similar product available in health-food stores or by mail order)

• 1/4 cup tofu for 1 egg (blend tofu smooth with the liquid ingredients before they are added to the dry ingredients)

Dairy Substitutes

The following can be used as dairy substitutes in cooking:

• soy milk (found in health-food and Oriental food stores)

• soy margarine

• soy yogurt (found in health-food stores)

• nut milks (blend nuts with water and strain)

• rice milks (blend cooked rice with water)

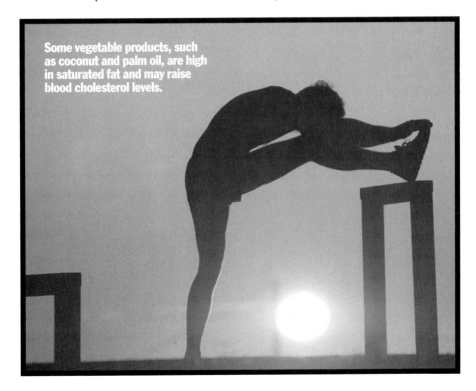

Some vegetable products, such as coconut and palm oil, are high in saturated fat and may raise blood cholesterol levels.

Meat Substitutes in Stews and Soups

The following can be used as a substitute for meat in soups and stews:
• tempeh (cultured soybeans with a chewy texture)
• tofu (freezing and then thawing gives tofu a meaty texture; the tofu will turn slightly off white in color)
• wheat gluten or seitan (made from wheat and has the texture of meat; available in health-food and Oriental stores)

[Ref: www.vrg.org/nutshell/nutshell.htm]

Healthy Steps to Your Ideal Weight

Many teenagers are concerned about losing or gaining weight. To lose weight, look at your diet. If it has lots of sweet or fatty foods, replace them with fruits, vege-tables, grains and legumes. If your diet already seems healthy, try to get more exercise – by walking, running or swimming daily, for example.

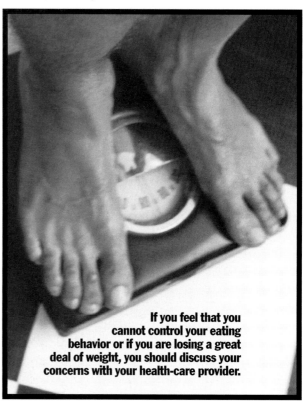

If you feel that you cannot control your eating behavior or if you are losing a great deal of weight, you should discuss your concerns with your health-care provider.

If you are trying to gain weight, you will need to eat more food. Perhaps eating more often or eating foods somewhat higher in calories and lower in bulk will help. Try to eat three or more times a day whether you are trying to gain weight or lose weight. It is hard to get all of the nutritious foods you need if you only eat one meal a day.

If you feel that you cannot control your eating behavior or if you are losing a great deal of weight, you should discuss your concerns with your health-care provider.

Quick Foods for Busy People

With the demands of school and outside activities, it may often seem there is just not enough time to eat. Here are some foods that require little or no preparation. Some of these foods can be found in fast-food restaurants – check the menu. Apples, oranges, bananas, grapes, peaches, plums, dried fruits, bagels and peanut butter, carrot or celery sticks, popcorn, pretzels, soy cheese pizza, bean tacos or burritos, salad, soy yogurt, soy milk, rice cakes, sandwiches, frozen juice bars.

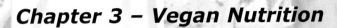

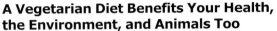

A Vegetarian Diet Benefits Your Health, the Environment, and Animals Too

Vegetarianism represents a positive move toward a cleaner and more compassionate world, a reduction in global hunger, and improved personal health. If you are concerned about the environment, consider the negative impact of meat production on tropical rain forests, soil stability, and air and water quality. If you are concerned about animal rights, think about the billions of chickens and other animals slaughtered for food each year in the United States and the conditions in which animals killed for food are raised. If you are concerned about your own health, consider this: Vegetarians are generally at lower risk than non-vegetarians for heart disease, high blood pressure, some forms of cancer, and obesity.

Some Famous Vegetarians ...

Clara Barton, Lisa Bonet, Albert Einstein (Nobel Prize winner), Daryl Hannah, Janet Jackson, Howard Jones, Tony LaRussa, Prince, Madonna, John Lennon, Paul McCartney, George Harrison, Ringo Starr, Natalie Merchant, Monie Love, Phylicia Rashad, Leonardo da Vinci, Leo Tolstoy, George Bernard Shaw, Mahatma Gandhi, Isaac Bashevis Singer (Nobel Prize winner), Mr. Rogers, k.d. lang, Alex Baldwin and Kim Basinger, Drew Barrymore (vegan), David Duchovny, Michael J. Fox, Woody Harrelson, Dustin Hoffman, Jennie Garth, Brad Pitt, Brooke Shields, Alicia Silverstone, Jonathan Taylor Thomas, Liv Tyler, Fiona Apple, Jeff Beck, All of the members of Blur, Bob Dylan, Lenny Kravitz, Sarah McLachlan, Moby (vegan) and Lisa Simpson.

Vitamin B12 in the Vegan Diet

Vitamin B12 is needed for cell division and blood formation. Plant foods do not contain vitamin B12 except when they are contaminated by microorganisms. Thus, vegans need to look to other sources to get vitamin B12 in their diet. Although the minimum requirement for vitamin B12 is quite small, one millionth of a gram (1 microgram) a day for adults, a vitamin B12 deficiency is a very serious problem leading ultimately to irreversible nerve damage. Prudent vegans will include sources of vitamin B12 in their diets. However, vitamin B12 deficiency is actually quite rare even among long-term vegans.

Normally, vitamin B12 is secreted into the small intestine along with bile and other secretions and is reabsorbed, but this does not add to the body's vitamin B12 stores. Since small amounts of vitamin B12 are not reabsorbed, it is possible that eventually vitamin B12 stores will be used up. However, we may be quite efficient at reusing vitamin B12 so that deficiency is rare.

Bacteria in the human intestinal tract do make vitamin B12. The majority of these bacteria are found in the large intestine. Vitamin B12 does not appear to be absorbed from the large intestine.

Possible Sources of Vitamin B12

A vitamin B12 deficiency is a very serious problem leading ultimately to irreversible nerve damage.

Some bacteria in the small intestine do produce vitamin B12. The amount of vitamin B12 which is produced does not appear adequate to prevent vitamin B12 deficiency, although some vegans may get vitamin B12 from inadequate hand washing, this is not a reliable vitamin B12 source. Vegans who previously ate animal-based foods may have vitamin B12 stores that will not be depleted for 20 to 30 years or more. However, long-term vegans, infants, children and pregnant and lactating women (due to increased needs) should be especially careful to get enough vitamin B12.

Reliable Vegan Sources of Vitamin B12

A number of reliable vegan food sources for vitamin B12 are known. One brand of nutritional yeast, Red Star T-6635+, has been tested and shown to contain active vitamin B12. This brand of yeast is often labeled as Vegetarian Support Formula with or without T-6635+ in parentheses following this new name. It is a reliable source of vitamin B12. Nutritional yeast, Saccharomyces cerevisiae, is a food yeast, grown on a molasses solution, which comes as yellow flakes or powder. It has a cheesy taste. Nutritional yeast is different from brewer's yeast or torula yeast. It can often be used by those sensitive to other yeasts.

Another source of vitamin B12 is fortified cereal. We recommend checking the label of your favorite cereal since manufacturers have been known to stop including vitamin B12.

Other sources of vitamin B12 are vitamin B12-fortified soy milk, vitamin B12-fortified meat analogues (food made from wheat gluten or soybeans to resemble meat, poultry or fish), and vitamin B12 supplements. There are vitamin supplements which do not contain animal products.

Vegans who choose to use a vitamin B12 supplement, either as a single supplement or in a multi-vitamin should use supplements at least several times a week. Even though a supplement may contain many times the recommended level of vitamin B12, when vitamin B12 intake is high, not as much appears to be absorbed – meaning, in order to meet your needs, you should take the vitamin several times a week.

If you are thinking about becoming a vegetarian, it's important to do a little research first and make sure you plan and maintain a healthy diet. We have met so many junk-food vegetarians (a self-proclaimed vegetarian who doesn't eat meat, but doesn't eat anything healthy or remotely close to a vegetable, unless potato chips and French fries count) – no wonder most people think eating vegetarian isn't healthy. It is extremely important to make sure your nutritional intake is balanced, especially since you have to find alternatives to getting your protein, iron and zinc from something other than meat.

As the previous reflection indicates, the key to successful vegetarianism is making sure that you take in healthy doses of beans/pulses and rice (or grains) together to get the full complement of essential amino acids. Without the beans, some essential protein

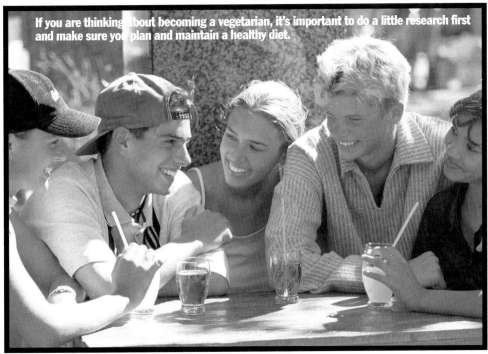

If you are thinking about becoming a vegetarian, it's important to do a little research first and make sure you plan and maintain a healthy diet.

building blocks are missing and the body will not be able to make proper muscle tissue, and other tissues in the body, and you could lose muscle and gain fat. *Soy protein* is a good way to get the protein needed. Veggie soy dogs and soy burgers are often the easiest way with a busy schedule! To meet these needs it is recommended that vegetarians:

• Eat at least 5 servings of a calcium-rich food every day.

• Get at lest 20 to 30 minutes of direct sunlight two or three times each week for vitamin D.

• Eat a food item that is *fortified* with vitamin B-12 and iron every day. This means that a vitamin or mineral has been added to a food item. A good source would be a fortified breakfast cereal.

• Eat a variety of whole-grain products every day to boost your intake of zinc.

• Enjoy a vitamin C fruit or juice with meals to help absorb iron.

Types of Vegetarians

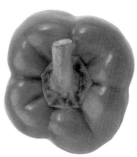

Veganism – Excludes the consumption of all food of animal origin except human breast milk.

Rastafarian veganism – In general the diet excludes all red meat, milk, fats and oils of animal origin, but it may include fish depending on the nationality of the Rastafarian.

Macrobiotic – A diet that does not totally exclude but strictly limits foods of animal origin.

Fructarianism – The diet is confined to foods such as fruit, nuts and certain vegetables, where harvesting allows the parent plant to flourish.

Polo-vegetarianism – Form of vegetarianism that includes the consumption of chicken.

Lacto-vegetarianism – Form of vegetarianism that includes the consumption of milk.

Lacto-ovo-vegetarianism – Form of vegetarianism that excludes red meat, poultry and fish but includes the consumption of dairy products and eggs.

Pesco-vegetarianism – Form of vegetarianism that includes the consumption of milk and eggs, and occasionally fish.

Semivegetarian (demi-vegetarian; quasi-vegetarian) – A self-classification among people who claim to have eating

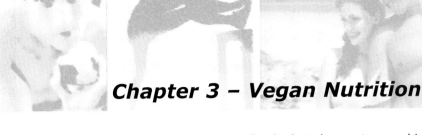
habits which focus on vegetarian foods, but they eat some kind of meat on an occasional basis. Red meats are usually excluded.

Reduced meat-eaters – People who classify themselves as reducing their overall meat consumption.

[Ref: www.fazeteen.com/summer2001/vegetarian.htm]

Lose Weight and Feel Great

1. Eat normal-sized meals. By eating meals that fill you up, you will be less likely to overeat later on during the day.
2. When you do snack, eat fruit, crackers, pretzels, vegetables, and other foods that are healthy and filling.
3. Keep healthy snacks handy. Pack a few extra good snacks with your lunch each day to eat when you get hungry – to help keep you away from those vending machines.
4. Drink a lot of water. A glass of water every few hours will help keep you full. If you don't like plain water, add lemon or a little bit of drink mix to it.
5. Brush your teeth after you eat. If your teeth feel clean, you are less likely to want to eat anything and get them dirty.
6. Keep a pack of gum handy at all times. A stick of gum will help satisfy your sweet tooth. If your school doesn't allow gum, chew it after school.
7. Use smaller portions of mayonnaise, cheese, and other fattening foods whenever possible.
8. Keep yourself busy all day. Don't give yourself time to sneak in a few extra snacks.
9. Find support. Hang around other people who are also trying to keep fit. If you hang with people who constantly snack, it will be very hard for you to resist eating.
10. Exercise. Walk up the stairs a few extra times a day, clean your house, or take the dog for a walk. The best thing you can do is find an exercise that you enjoy doing. Try jogging, and maybe once in a while do a little kickboxing.

[Ref: www.teenrefuge.com/fitness/health/loseweight.html]

CHAPTER FOUR

It's not easy being a teen these days. Between running to class, sports, homework, babysitting, after-school jobs, hanging out with friends and dating, who has time to think about whether or not the snacks you are eating are healthy and nutritious? But once you learn to tell the difference between a good snack and a bad snack, it will be easier to *take control* of your eating habits. After all, snacking can be a great way to get all of the vitamins and nutrients your body needs. Snacking helps to increase your rate of metabolism, as well as maintain a more balanced appetite.

Although you might think that gobbling down a large order of greasy fries at your local fast food joint is good for you, all it really does is give you a temporary boost. A high-fat

The Lowdown On Snacking

snack will actually *slow you down* in the long run. Teens should be taught how to read the labels on snack foods to determine if what they are about to eat really is good for them. And don't think that healthy snack foods are boring and tasteless, either. You'll be surprised at the types of healthy snack choices that are available.

Choosing Tasty Snacks

Snacking doesn't have to be boring as long as you have a variety of choices. Low-fat pretzels and spicy mustard, or flavored rice cakes topped with jam are tasty and easy. Instead of corn chips, try baked tortilla chips. Instead of ice cream, try nonfat frozen yogurt or fruit sherbet (sorbet). Salsa can take the place of cheese- or sour cream-based dips and low-fat angel food cake is a yummy substitute for pound cake. And if you're in a rush, a glass of 100 percent juice or skim milk is a good nutritious source of quick calories.

What does the word "healthy" really mean?

Choosing healthy snacks includes being cautious of food labels that make false or questionable claims. Many food manufacturers are now labeling their products as "all natural" and "pure." This *does not* mean the foods are nutritious. A food may contain all natural ingredients but may still be high in fat.

A good example is granola bars. If you're craving something sweet to munch on, you may think it's better to choose a granola bar over a chocolate bar. Although the granola bar may be a good source of certain vitamins and nutrients, it may also contain a surprisingly large amount of fat. On average, about 35 percent of the calories in a granola bar come from fat, unless the bars are of the low-fat variety. Check the package to be sure.

Smart Snacking Strategies

To become a healthy snacker you will need to make small adjustments to your eating habits. Try taking a snack break with a friend. By spending time with your bud, you can help to remind each other to catch up on skipped meals. Stash some fruit, pretzels or baby carrots in your backpack or workout bag so you always have something nearby.

Evenings can be a tempting time for indulging in fatty, sugary snacks. Don't ignore these cravings – if you're hungry, your body is probably telling you it needs nutrients. The trick is to *pick the right*

snacks to fill the hunger gap. Fig bars, rice cakes or air-popped popcorn are just a few good choices.

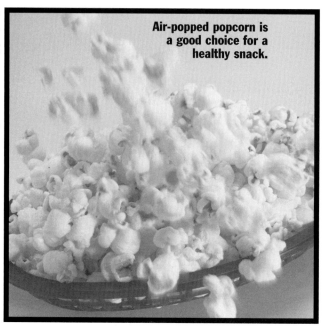
Air-popped popcorn is a good choice for a healthy snack.

• *Mini-pizzas* – Spread pizza sauce on top of half a bagel. Add low-fat mozzarella cheese and your favorite veggies and bake at a low temperature until the cheese has melted.

• *Low-fat pita and hummus* – Warm up a slice of pita bread or place in the toaster. Then cut into small pieces and dip into a tasty, low-fat hummus, which is available in delicious flavors like garlic and spicy red pepper.

• *Ants on a log* – Spread peanut butter on celery sticks and sprinkle a few raisins over the top. Or use cream cheese instead of peanut butter.

• *Trail mix* – Use your imagination to create a trail mix that is just right for your taste buds. In a large bowl, mix Rice Chex cereal, low-fat, unsalted peanuts and cashews, air-popped popcorn, pretzel sticks, raisins, and whatever else you want to throw in.

Don't forget to include fresh fruits and vegetables in your snack menu.

Don't forget to include fresh fruits and vegetables in your snack menu. Get into the habit of eating a handful of fresh seedless grapes when you come home from school or work, or slice up an apple and use some low-fat yogurt as a dipping sauce. And if you haven't tried carrot slices or baby carrots lately, you're in for a real treat.

It's easy to be tempted by fatty, sugary and salty snacks. Becoming a healthy snacker will take some small adjustments to your eating habits. Start by choosing a variety of foods when you need a snack. Avoid the rut of eating the same snack all the time, and *never* snack out of boredom, frustration or loneliness.

Smoothies

Strawberry Splash

5 large strawberries
6 oz. strawberry yogurt, frozen
1 teaspoon granola (optional)
Put all ingredients into blender, and blend until smooth.

Melon Madness

1 cup peach yogurt, frozen
1 cup milk
1/2 cup cantaloupe
1/2 cup honeydew melon
1/2 cup strawberries (or watermelon)
4 ice cubes
Put yogurt, milk, and strawberries into blender, and blend until smooth.
Then add in the cantaloupe, honeydew, and the ice. Blend again until
smooth.

Piña Colada

6 oz. coconut yogurt, frozen
1/2 frozen banana
10 oz. crushed pineapple (half a can)
1 cup milk
Put all ingredients into blender, and blend until smooth.

Apple Spice

2 cups apple sauce
1 cup apple cider
1 cup orange juice
2 tablespoons maple syrup
Sample ...
1/2 teaspoon cinnamon
Put all ingredients into blender, and blend until smooth.

Tropical Twist

1/2 cup frozen strawberries
1/2 cup frozen chopped peaches
1/2 cup frozen raspberries
1/2 cup crushed ice
3/4 cup pineapple or orange juice
2 scoops sherbet (sorbet), any flavor

[Ref: www.efit.com/servlet/article/weight/6014.html]

CHAPTER FIVE

This is an exciting time in your life because now is when you undergo various changes to become an adult ... The teen years may also be a tough period, but with the help and support of your family, friends and teachers, you should breeze through it!

Physical changes, mental changes, emotional changes – everything's changing! And if your friends seem to be maturing faster, don't worry! You will catch up with them in no time. In fact, think of it this way. They can give you tips on how to deal with the exciting changes!

Physical Changes

Before you plunge into puberty and all its changes, remember this: As you mature you should learn to think for yourself and make up your own mind about various matters. Don't be overly influenced by the opinions of your friends or the media – learn to think for yourself!

You begin to be conscious of your own identity and may try to express yourself through your clothes, hairstyle and choice of music. Making decisions about your future also becomes important, especially in relation to further studies and a career.

Anyway, just be careful to reflect *yourself* fully in all your decisions! As you cross the bridge to adulthood, your body and your feelings change. You may also begin to feel differently about your family, friends and classmates – and view the things that they do in whole new ways. You may consider changing what you do with them, the way you dress, and the things you talk about.

Puberty means *major changes,* but this stage is simply your body's transition from childhood to adulthood. You may even begin to wonder where you fit in. But these many physical and emotional changes are *normal!* This is also the time when you begin to be aware of your sexual feelings and responses. You start to become interested in the opposite sex!

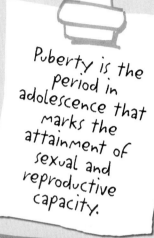

Puberty is the period in adolescence that marks the attainment of sexual and reproductive capacity.

Puberty is the period in adolescence that marks the attainment of sexual and reproductive capacity. The average female reaches puberty at the age of 12. In contrast, males usually attain puberty between 13 and 14. This is a very confusing and awkward time for all teenagers. Expect to feel weird. It's normal.

Male puberty: what happens?

The hormone that causes the changes in males is testosterone. Guys develop broader shoulders and a more muscular physique. Pubic, facial and body hair (face and chest hair) also develops. You find your voice "cracking" and getting deeper. You gain weight and grow taller – and you start sweating! The sweat glands

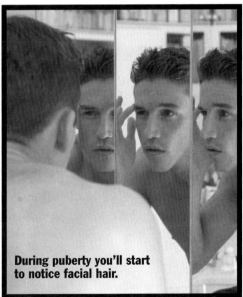

During puberty you'll start to notice facial hair.

around the genitals and armpits show the greatest development. Do be careful, that's when the danger of body odor lurks! You also may get acne. The oil-producing glands, especially around the face are activated ... and they pretty much go crazy during puberty.

A handful of other things happen. *Moodiness:* changes in estrogen (for females) or testosterone (for males) levels can cause mood swings. For females this is sometimes known as PMS (premenstrual syndrome). *Focus on appearances:* Adolescents are concerned about how their bodies look, how other people look and how they compare to themselves, and what other people think in general. Awkwardness or embarrassment often occurs, especially in times of change. Adolescents experience sexual attraction and arousal very easily.

Surviving Puberty

Puberty can be one of the toughest stages of life. With the help and support of relatives and friends, you can sail through it. Ask lots and lots of questions. If you're in doubt, simply ask trusted adults such as your family members, teachers, counselors or your family doctor. Get the answers. *Learn!* Look for more information about puberty from reliable resources at the library, bookstores, on the Web, or directly from a responsible older person you trust.

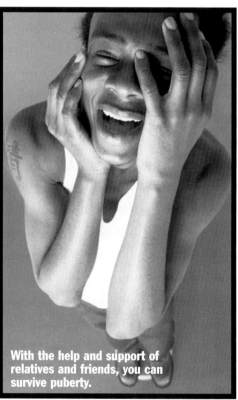

With the help and support of relatives and friends, you can survive puberty.

Respect your body. Don't smoke, use drugs or drink alcohol. Eat nutritious foods and get plenty of exercise. Love and accept your body. It is a work in progress. Remember that everyone goes through puberty, but don't compare yourself to anyone else – you're an individual.

If you feel sad, bad or totally weird, talk to somebody. Believe it or not, you already know someone you can talk to about your personal feelings and the changes you are going through. Don't suffer in silence. Give your parents and siblings a chance. They can really give you a lot of support and information if you let them in!

Anger, frustration, depression – they are all normal emotions during this period of time. Don't think you're abnormal or going mad or "losing it" ... It's just that you're dealing with a lot when you go through teenhood and puberty.

Believe us when we say that your family members, teachers or even professional counselors are more than happy to hear your concerns, or even just chat with you about life in general. Don't keep all your problems to yourself – things could get very bad ... and before you know it, you might develop serious problems. For example, some teenagers who experience depression may even attempt suicide. And if someone you know seems to be having difficulty, be supportive and understanding. Encourage him to get help from a counselor or doctor.

[Ref: www.teencentral.gov.sg/body_talk.htm]

How long does puberty last?
As with almost anything physical, it depends on the individual. Some boys and girls "finish" puberty in one year, while others may go through it for five or six years. It all depends on your body.

What happens to guys during puberty?
A boy undergoes a gradual physical transformation where his height increases, his sex organs develop and he starts to develop a deep voice. Body hair also starts to grow (on the chest and around the groin area).

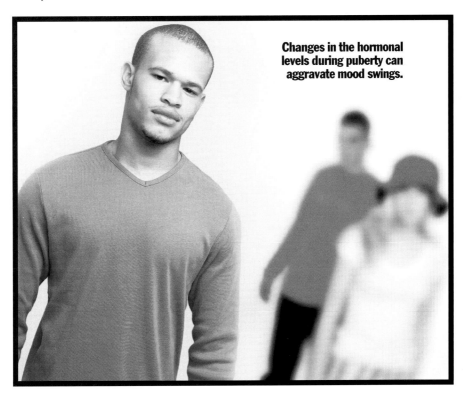

Changes in the hormonal levels during puberty can aggravate mood swings.

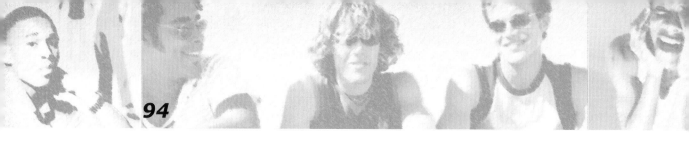

Is feeling moody part and parcel of puberty?

Yes, puberty involves both physical and emotional changes. Because puberty usually occurs during the teenage years when you are also experiencing many other changes in life, you may get stressed out and be upset. Changes in the hormonal levels during puberty (estrogen for females and testosterone for males) can also aggravate mood swings.

What is the function of the testicles?

A male's external sexual organs consist of a penis and a scrotum. The testicles are two small egg-shaped organs, one inside each compartment of the scrotum. The left scrotum usually hangs lower than the right. These organs contain cells that secrete the male sex hormone, testosterone. This is the hormone responsible for most of the sexual changes that occur in boys during puberty.

Is there an ideal or average length my penis should be?

The lengths of unerect penises vary from individual to individual and have no relation to body size.

[Ref: www.teencentral.gov.sg/faq03.htm, www.teencentral.gov.sg/sexual.htm]

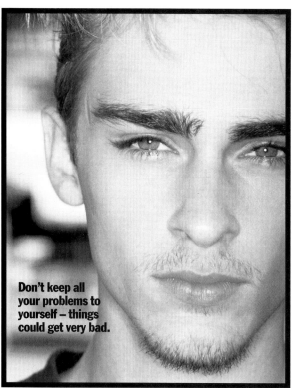

Don't keep all your problems to yourself – things could get very bad.

Feeling Blue

Just when you were happily fitting in with all your friends, your body starts to do funny things to you to make you feel different. If you dare not ask your dad, brother or a friend what's happening, or if you're worried that you've got some dreadful disease, read on about puberty and what it will do for you. You may be surprised but at least you'll know you are not alone.

Penis, Scrotum and Testicles

Early on in puberty you will find that your penis, scrotum and testicles begin to grow until they reach adult size. If the rest of you hasn't yet grown to match they may look out of proportion, but fairly soon you should start growing and it will

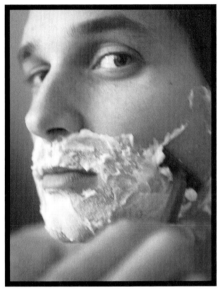

all seem normal. There is great variation in what is a "normal" size penis. *It just doesn't matter* – and is irrelevant to how successful you are in attracting and keeping a girlfriend!

With the development of your penis and testicles, you will find that they begin to start to work in a sexual way as well as being used to take a pee. The penis works sexually by going hard and getting longer – called an erection – when you think about girls. Then the sperm produced by the testicles will be pushed out in a spurt – called an ejaculation. If you are having sex with a girl and neither of you uses contraception, the sperm may fertilize her egg and she can become pregnant. Occasionally you may get an erection when you don't want to, though you won't ejaculate every time you have an erection. This is quite normal. Also normal is something called a wet dream (or nocturnal emission) where you ejaculate at night in your sleep. Though this may embarrass you, it is totally normal and does not mean anything.

Facial Hair

You have already developed many of the changes that come in puberty. This indicates that there is plenty of the male hormone, testosterone, in your blood stream, so it is unlikely that there is any real problem. The fact that you have yet to get any of the adult type facial hair shouldn't worry you as this, along with the chest, is often the last place to develop it. Acne can be just as much a problem for boys as for the girls, and like the girls it may affect the skin on the face, chest shoulders and back. The creams you use for your acne shouldn't be making a difference, although acne itself can make facial hair growth patchy. So don't worry, the hair will come, and in the meantime tell your dad its time he had a new look and lost the facial fuzz!

Mood Swings in Boys

Just like the girls, boys also experience extremes of emotional feeling as they go through puberty. Their hormones are just as powerful, and through cultural taboos it is harder for boys to admit they are having problems with their feelings. They are expected to either not feel the mood swings and lack of confidence or not want to talk about it. It may be hard to describe the way you feel, that you are lonely or don't fit in,

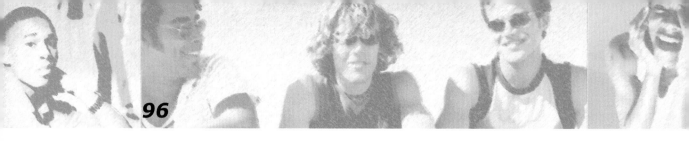

but if you ask an older friend or brother, or even your dad, he will most likely know what you mean. As you get more used to the "new you" life will become easier and your confidence will grow. Meanwhile just be yourself, don't feel you have to be the same as all the others, and be sure that no matter what happens, you are normal and everyone else out there will be going through the same problems.

[Ref: www.bbc.co.uk/health/body_chemistry/puberty_blues.shtml]

What is a hormone?

It is a chemical substance produced by a gland, secreted into the blood stream, and carried to a receptor, usually displaced far from the gland that secretes it.

Where do they come from?

The principal source is the pituitary gland at the base of the brain. This gland produces hormones that control:
• production of thyroxine by the thyroid gland (in the neck)
• production of cortisol from the adrenal glands (lying above the kidneys)
• production of testosterone and sperm from the testes, or of estradiol and eggs from the ovaries
• growth of children (growth hormone).
There are other important glands. One is the pancreas, which produces insulin.

How are hormones made?

There is a series of genes that control the processes leading to the synthesis of every hormone in the body. Hormones are usually released as granules into the circulation.

What do they do?

Hormones travel in the blood stream to cells that possess the relevant specific receptor for that hormone – and then bind to them.

How do they work?

The binding initiates a chain of events inside the cell, which causes the effect of the hormone to be expressed.

Why are they needed?

The maintenance of a constant internal environment is essential to the function of the body as a whole. Hormones regulate the processes designed to do this – because they are themselves closely monitored by the products of the cells they affect.

What happens if I have too much or too little of a hormone?

The effects depend on the hormone in question – but the result is usually to make one unwell in a rather nonspecific way. Sometimes the excess or lack can be life-threatening.

Making a diagnosis of a hormone (endocrine) disease is not difficult if the doctor thinks of a hormone imbalance as a possible diagnosis. Most problems arise when doctors forget the widespread nature of the complaints expressed by people with hormone imbalance.

[Ref: www.bbc.co.uk/health/body_chemistry/didyouknow.shtml]

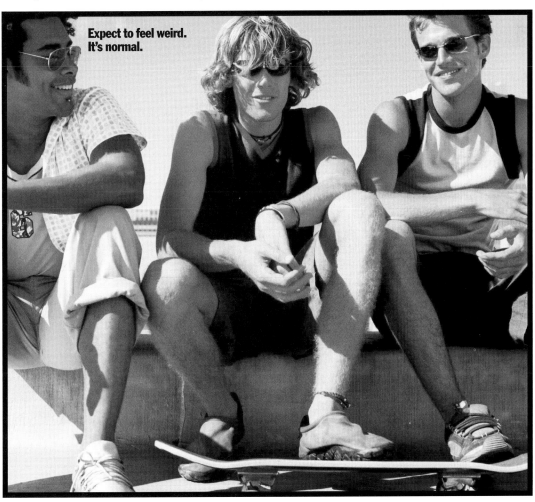

Expect to feel weird.
It's normal.

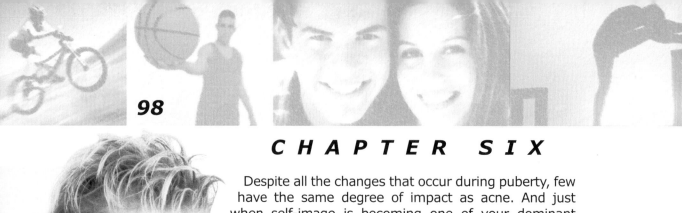

CHAPTER SIX

Despite all the changes that occur during puberty, few have the same degree of impact as acne. And just when self-image is becoming one of your dominant traits, those little black or white skin imperfections start rearing their ugly heads. Acne is a skin disorder. Acne occurs when excess oil (sebum) production combined with dead skin cells clogs the pores. Bacteria forms in the pores, resulting in red inflamed pimples, pus-filled whiteheads, or blackheads. There are many different forms of acne; however, acne vulgaris is the most common. An estimated 80 percent of teens have some form of acne at one point. Sometimes people will have perfect skin in their teens and will not develop acne until their adult years. Others may never develop it.

[Ref:www.absoluteacneinfo.com/acne.html]

What Is Acne?

What Causes Acne?

The causes of acne can be classified as bacteria, genetics, hormones and clogged pores. All four work together to cause acne. Bacteria is the single culprit required for acne. Genetics also play an important role. If one of your parents had acne sometime in their life, chances are you will too. Hormones (specifically testosterone) can cause increased oil (sebum) production, clogging the pores with dead skin cells.

[Ref: www.absoluteacneinfo.com/causes.html]

Four Myths About Acne

Myth #1 – Acne is curable. *No!* There is no cure for acne. However, through the consistent use of treatment and remedies, acne can be controlled or prevented.

Myth #2 – Sun is great for acne. *Wrong!* Sun may temporarily mask your acne, tighten up pores, or dry up the oil glands. However, the sun will also damage your follicular walls, clogging your pores. And that will only result in more acne that may not surface for 3 to 4 weeks after your sun exposure.

Myth #3 – Masturbation and sexual intercourse cause acne. *No!* It may reduce your stress levels and therefore eliminate the aggravating effect stress has on acne!

Myth #4 – Pizza, chocolate, and other junk food make you break out. A small population of individuals (perhaps less than 2 percent) may have food allergies that bring on acne. However, for the most part a balanced diet is important for a healthy body, and therefore will promote healthy skin. Iodine is one ingredient, though, with which some individuals may experience breakouts. So just to be safe, make sure the iodine in your diet isn't causing you problems.

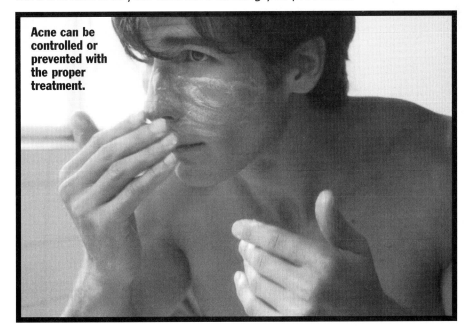

Acne can be controlled or prevented with the proper treatment.

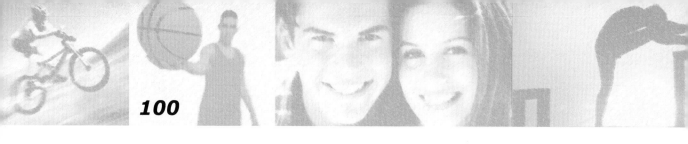

Basic Washing Routine

Before you attempt any other acne treatment techniques you must be sure that you are currently using the proper washing routine. Keeping your face clean requires that you wash it twice a day, three times at the most. You must be very careful not to overdo it. Skin must maintain the proper pH levels to remain healthy. Overwashing will make your face dry and irritated causing more breakouts. Many times individuals will vigorously scrub their skin when they wash it. We do not recommend you do this because such treatment will only serve to irritate the skin and cause more breakouts.

Note: acne is not caused by "dirty skin." It is the result of clogged pores infected with bacteria. Therefore, washing alone does not prevent acne. Washing is no mystery treatment. It simply serves to remove dirt and oil at the surface level. Nevertheless, the wrong type of washing can aggravate acne and make it worse.

Follow these tips: Wash your face by gently rotating your soap-lathered hands on your face. I do not recommend face cloths as they may irritate the skin. Use a mild nonabrasive soap. Rinse well with warm water. Using a clean soft towel, gently pat your face dry.

Methods of Treatment

You can treat and help prevent acne through one or more of the universal methods utilized to combat the problem. The methods are:
• Kill or avoid bacteria responsible for acne infection.
• Reduce the oil (sebum) production.
• Exfoliate dead skin cells to prevent clogged pores.

Experiment with the natural acne treatments and tips. Note that some of these treatments take time. Allow 2 to 4 weeks before discounting any acne treatment technique.

Touching – Perhaps one of the most often overlooked remedies. Stop putting your hands on your face! Also rubbing or bracing your chin when thinking is another common problem. Avoid rubbing, touching and scratching your skin. Your hands contain a lot of bacteria that can cause acne flare-ups. Also be careful of telephones. Clean them often with rubbing alcohol because they sometimes come in contact with the face, causing more acne.

Touching is probably one of the most difficult habits to break since much of the hand-to-face contact throughout the day we are unconscious of. Don't touch your face and be conscious to avoid bacteria at all times.

[Ref: www.absoluteacneinfo.com/treatments/index.html]

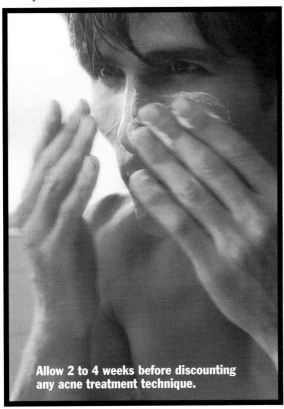

Allow 2 to 4 weeks before discounting any acne treatment technique.

Acne Therapy

The goal of acne therapy is to get rid of existing lesions and prevent the formation of new ones. Most treatments resolve existing acne lesions and, with continuous use, discourage new ones from forming. The following are some of the more popular treatments.

Benzoyl Peroxide – Benzoyl peroxide comes in cream, lotion or gel form and may be mixed with other useful ingredients such as antiseptics. It is not a new treatment and has been in use for over 20 years. It can reduce the number or troublesome skin bacteria by a factor of 100. After the first few days of use patients notice redness and scaling of the skin. This problem can be reduced by using a less-concentrated solution or not applying as often. This is normal and should settle down after a couple of weeks. Benzoyl peroxide will bleach clothes and hair. If you're applying it to the chest and back, wear old clothes.

Persevere – benzoyl peroxide is an underrated treatment. It actually releases oxygen into the hair follicle, killing bacteria. Start with 2.5 percent solution. If you find this is irritating the skin, apply for an hour or so and then wash off. Slowly increase the length of time you leave it on. You can progress to 5 percent if you do not have sensitive skin. Do not start treatment with 10 percent solution as this will result in excessive drying, redness and peeling.

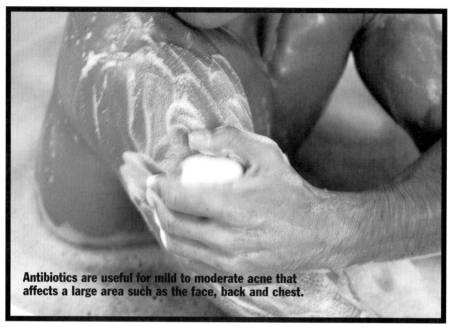

Antibiotics are useful for mild to moderate acne that affects a large area such as the face, back and chest.

Part of the therapeutic action of benzoyl peroxide is to dry the skin and also to shed the top layer of skin. It may take 2 weeks to see results, then you can reassess the strength you need. You can use an oil-free moisturizer. If you have tried benzoyl peroxide before, it is worth trying again under these guidelines. Benzamycin is one of the most popular treatments for acne in the States – it consists of benzoyl peroxide and the antibiotic erythromycin.

Azelaic Acid – Azelaic acid is a relatively new acne treatment applied as a cream once or twice a day for a maximum of six months. It is used to treat mild to moderate acne and is as effective as benzoyl peroxide, erythromycin cream or oral tetracycline against troublesome skin bacteria. A small percentage of users may notice redness, but that shouldn't last.

Topical Antibiotics – These are used for mild to moderate acne that mainly affects the face. They contain erythromycin (with or without zinc acetate), clindamycin or tetracycline. Some propionibacterium infections may become resistant to them. Topical antibiotics are less irritating than benzoyl peroxide. One or two solutions may fluoresce under ultraviolet light, and should not be worn to the disco!

Systemic Antibiotics – Four oral antibiotic treatments are available: tetracycline, doxycycline, minocycline and erythromycin. Very occasionally, trimethoprim may be used. Orally taken antibiotics are useful for mild to moderate acne that affects a large area such as the face, back and chest. They must be taken regularly for prolonged lengths of time, at least three to six months. Minocycline has several advantages over the other antibiotics used to treat acne. It can be given once a day, and can be taken with food (but not milk). It is less likely to induce bacterial resistance and has an anti-inflammatory action. The side effects of long-term administration of antibiotics affects bacterial balances in the intestinal tract and can lead to oral thrush, nausea, abdominal pain or diarrhea in around 5 percent of patients. Bacterial resistance may mean your antibiotics no longer work. If this happens consult your doctor for a different treatment. This also applies to topical antibiotics.

Acusal – Acusal is the brand name of a powerful pimple and blemish spot treatment specifically designed by Lex Advanced Skin Technologies to help treat and keep the skin clear by deeply penetrating pores. Acusal was designed specifically to help teens, fitness enthusiasts, and athletes combat those irritating and unsightly pimples and skin blemishes.

Alternative Acne Treatments
Acidophilus – You are probably wondering what this silly word acidophilus is, right? Well, let us tell you something about it. Acidophilus is a good bacteria that resides in the intestines. It's a good bacteria because it fights back against bad bacteria that can be harmful to your health. So you ask, what's the problem with acidophilus? The problem here is that certain actions will decrease the number of good bacteria within your intestines. The result is less good bacteria present will allow more bad bacteria to prosper in your intestines, increasing the possibility of diseases (acne included).

Chances are good that, if you are excessively using antibiotics and drugs, chlorinated water, junk and processed food in your daily life, then you need acidophilus supplementation to restore the levels of *good bacteria* in your system. Studies have illustrated that acidophilus supplementation assists in many illnesses. Acne is one disease that acidophilus is helpful in treating.

Acidophilus will fight against bacteria on the internal front. The best plan is to treat acne on multiple fronts: internal, external and fitness (physical and mental). Add acidophilus in conjunction with other internal and external treatments to receive the maximum results.

Avoid rubbing, touching and scratching your skin. Your hands contain a lot of bacteria that can cause acne flare-ups.

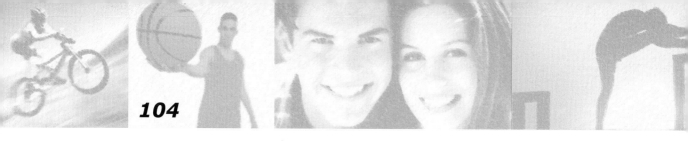

Herbs – Herbs can be one of your best natural acne treatments. Do not look for overnight results, though. Herbs work gently and build up in your system over time. Allow 3 to 4 weeks of consistent usage before examining effectiveness of treatment. Take prescribed doses as detailed on your bottle. Herbal supplements to include in the diet to balance the hormones are: saw palmetto berry extract for boys, and chaste tree berry extract for girls. Echinacea can be used to boost the immune system to fight against acne-causing bacteria.

Some other herbs that may help include: alfalfa, burdock root, cayenne, chaparral, dandelion root, the herbal combinations AKN and BFC, red clover, and yellow dock root. Green tea extract pills have also shown varied results in some individuals. The recommended dosage is generally 900 mg a day.

Vitamins – Some individuals have reported wonderful results from the following vitamin supplement stack: 1000 mg of vitamin C, 400 IU of vitamin E, and 100 mg of vitamin B complex.

Zinc – Zinc is one mineral that has shown to benefit acne in a scientific study. The results have been compared to tetracycline. *Warning:* high doses of zinc are toxic. Avoid going over 100 mg of zinc intake per day from food/supplement. Your daily intake should probably be at least 50 mg per day. You are also recommended to take a daily multivitamin because increased levels of zinc require more copper and manganese. Examine effectiveness after 14 weeks. Some individuals report results in as little as 3 weeks. Your acne may get worse before it gets better during your intake of zinc.

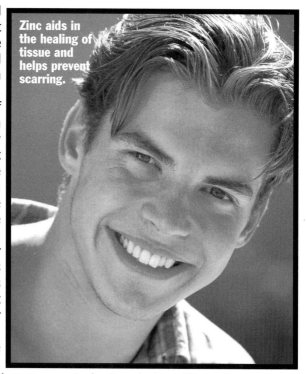

Zinc aids in the healing of tissue and helps prevent scarring.

Zinc is of course not the cure-all/end-all for your acne. However, some individuals have reported zinc being 75 percent effective for acne treatment. Zinc aids in the healing of tissue and helps prevent scarring. It is also important for the body in resisting infection and inflammation.

Distilled White Vinegar – You can use regular distilled white vinegar, but if you have sensitive skin you may find vinegar to be too strong. Dilute the vinegar with some water and then gradually strengthen the concentration until you find an appropriate level. Note, the solution should burn and sting a little. At night before going to bed, first gently wash your face with a mild soap and rinse well. Next, apply the vinegar to your face with cotton ball and let sit for 5 to 10 minutes, then rinse off with cool water. You may not notice results for the first 7 days. In fact your condition may even look worse. Give it time, allow 2 to 3 weeks to determine the effectiveness. A ton of individuals have reported amazing results from this treatment.

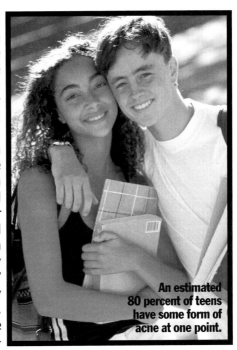

An estimated 80 percent of teens have some form of acne at one point.

Natural Exfoliates – Tomato, lemon, or actually any citric fruit makes an excellent natural exfoliate. They act as a natural sloughing treatment to remove dead skin cells from the clogged pores. Here's what you need to do. Wash your face and rinse thoroughly. Run to your fridge and get a fresh lemon. Squeeze it into a small bowl and dip a cotton ball into it. Apply wet cotton ball to your face. Repeat soaking of cotton ball in juice as needed. Let the lemon juice dry on face for about 10 minutes, then rinse with cool water. The lemon juice should make your face sting or mildly burn. If you have sensitive skin you may wish to dilute juice with water. Follow this procedure once or twice daily and you will notice amazing results within 14 days.

Facial Masks

Facial masks are good for guys as well as girls, and for a number of reasons. They can tighten your pores, remove excess oil from the skin, or moisturize and replenish dry skin. There are many types of masks. Here are a few you might want to try.

Pore-Cleaner Exfoliant Mask – Mix baking soda, hydrogen peroxide and water into a paste, and apply to your skin. Let dry on the skin, then wash off with cool water.

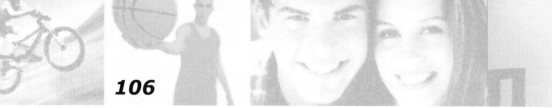
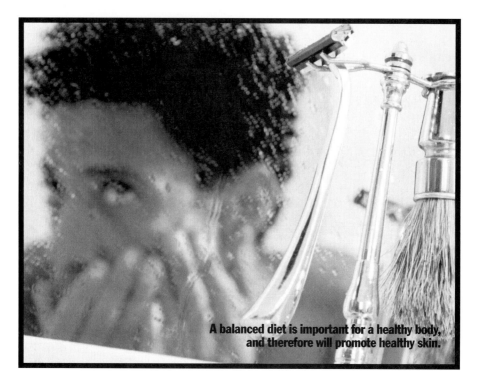

A balanced diet is important for a healthy body, and therefore will promote healthy skin.

Egg-Yolk Mask – This mask is great. It leaves your skin refreshed and feeling good. Take one beaten egg yolk and apply liberally to your face with a cotton ball. Let dry on the skin for 15 minutes, then rinse off with cool water. The egg yolk has a lot of protein and fatty acids in there that will help your skin. This mask will replenish your skin and tighten up your pores.

Honey Oatmeal Mask – Great for oily skin. Mix some honey and oatmeal into a paste, apply to skin, and leave on for 15 minutes. The oatmeal will absorb the excess oil of your skin.

Milk of Magnesia – Very nice mask for oily skin. You can apply a thin layer to your face and leave it on all day. Be sure to use flavorless milk of magnesia.

Emile's Natural Mask – Combine 1 teaspoon alcohol, 2 teaspoons of distilled water, 10 drops of natural lemon juice, 5 drops of honey, 1/4 teaspoon of baking soda, enough baby powder to mix it into a smooth paste. This mask is to be used only once a day, an hour before bedtime. Apply paste to your entire face area using cotton ball or your fingers. Leave it on your face for half an hour, then rinse very well with warm water. Dry well but without scrubbing. Results should show within one week.

John's German Mask – This is a German remedy used to tighten pores and clear blemishes. You take a little cube of yeast, and mix most of it in a bowl with water. Apply the mask to your face, wait until it is completely dry, then rinse.

Lynsi's Mask – This mask is excellent for oily skin. Mash 1/4 of a tomato (first remove skin and seeds) and add 2 teaspoons of plain

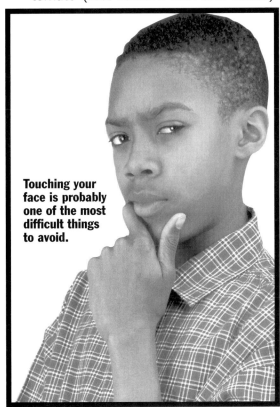

Touching your face is probably one of the most difficult things to avoid.

yogurt, 1 teaspoon of mashed cucumber, 2 teaspoons of aloe gel, 3 teaspoons oatmeal powder, and 2 mint leaves (crushed). Mix ingredients together in a bowl and apply to face. Leave on for about 10 minutes. Rinse with warm water. You may want to use a warm, damp face cloth to remove this one.

Rach's Mask – Take 1/2 a cup of natural yogurt, a couple of chopped strawberries, 1/2 a cup of oats ... and combine them in a blender until smooth. Then put the mask on your face with your fingers and lie back and relax for 15 minutes. For an extra boost, put cucumbers on your eyelids. You guys will be amazed at the difference you'll see in your complexion!

[Ref: www.absoluteacneinfo.com/masks.html]

Stress

Stress is something that needs to be reduced in your life since it tends to aggravate acne in many people. Teens experience very high levels of stress during final exams at school – and that results in increased levels of acne. So how do you lower your stress levels? Aside from eliminating things that cause you stress in your life, look into relaxation techniques. Relaxation techniques are great for stressful situations. You may even look into the practice of meditation or yoga to further reduce your stress levels.

[Ref: www.absoluteacneinfo.com/stress.html]

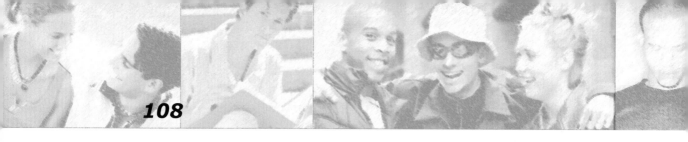

CHAPTER SEVEN

Mental Health
Issues

Today there is a huge focus on physical well-being. People are exercising more and trying to eat sensibly. These are positive pursuits and can contribute to a better quality of life. However, if we are to consider our *overall* well-being, we should not draw a line between our body and our head – it all works together! It's easy for many of us to overlook tending to our mental health. The topics covered in this area often still carry much taboo with them. Remember, the body does not stop at the neck, what is going on in your head is really important too!

The perception of mental illness has changed over time for many, but it can be difficult to recognize the signs that someone is struggling with their mental state of health. Everyone likes to think they are a strong person who doesn't need the help of others. Sometimes people, especially teenagers, feel that seeking help concerning a mental health issue makes them a weaker person. This is simply *not true!* Almost everyone needs help and guidance at some time in their life. There is no substitute for a skilled and compassionate therapist.

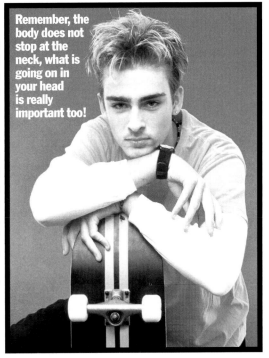

Remember, the body does not stop at the neck, what is going on in your head is really important too!

In dealing with our mental well-being, the key issues are what we do about it and the choices we make. The last thing a person in emotional pain wants to hear is that time will heal the hurt. In some cases this is true. If, however, the hurt is not going away and you feel a sense of hopelessness, then professional help is *essential.* There is help out there and you are by no means alone.

[Ref: www.coolnurse.com/mental_health.htm]

You Are in Control

Speaking from experience, it's hard enough that we acne victims must wear our disease on our faces and constantly protect ourselves from insensitive or irrational reactions and remarks from others. We shouldn't emotionally torment ourselves over our acne by thinking we are "damaged goods." We sometimes are our own worse enemies often convincing ourselves that "nobody will want to go out with me, marry me or love me." Powerless to change our appearance or cure acne, we may feel a sense of hopelessness and despair.

A lengthening history of unsuccessful treatments or permanent acne scarring may deepen our sense of hopelessness. We may even feel as if our chances at a normal life are gone. Only the most philosophical among us may have the strength to ride through an often long and painful journey without inflicting upon themselves lasting emotional scars. But, the more we learn to understand our self-defeating thought patterns, the better control we can achieve over them and over our inner happiness.

Even while we're still in pain, tormented by an unavoidable awareness of our less-than-perfect appearance, we must take control and arm ourselves against this self-destructive blame and hatred. Are you allowing the following self-defeating thoughts to eat away at your inner happiness and destroy you?

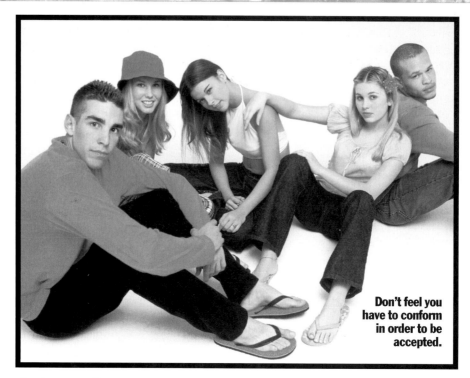

Don't feel you have to conform in order to be accepted.

Is this you? "Having acne is punishment for something else I did." Do you believe "everything happens for a reason," or do you falsely conclude that by having acne you're being punished for your sins or victimized by a malevolent fate?

Healthy inner view: Acne is a disease that can happen to anybody with an increased level of androgen in their body, resulting in overactivity of the sebaceous glands, plugging the oil glands. In other words, it's not your fault you have acne! Different treatments work better and faster on some than on others.

Is this you? "I allow criticisms and opinions from others to control my feelings about myself. Others make me feel ugly, so it must be true."

Healthy inner view: Remember, you create your own feelings and make your own decisions. People and events do not cause feelings, although they often *can* trigger your mental habits. Don't focus on the unrealistic expectations and standards of others, especially parents and society. Instead, focus on your abilities, talents and positive qualities. Be willing to risk the disapproval of others by trusting your own capabilities. Accept yourself. Don't feel you have to conform in order to be accepted.

Is this you? "I negatively label and blame myself for my condition." Don't be your own hardest critic, always finding fault with the way you look and feel. "I'm a loser and it's my fault."

Healthy inner view: Replace self-criticism with self-encouragement. Give yourself a compliment for your achievements. Visualize the positive. Say to yourself or even out loud, "So what if I have acne, I like who I am."

Is this you? "I become defensive and angry at the world and at myself." When your acne is pointed out to you, you feel as if you're under attack and become defensive. Having acne may provoke a deep anger against the disease and the world of "normal" people. The anger sometimes turns inward – a passion is allowed to disappear, a favorite hobby is abandoned, an opportunity for pleasure or success is ignored.

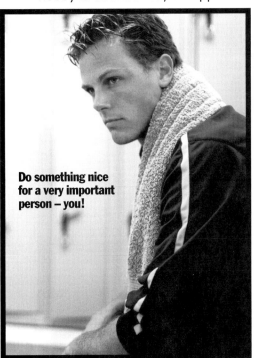

Do something nice for a very important person – you!

Healthy inner view: You're only human, so treat yourself with kindness, not abuse! Move ahead with a positive attitude. Take time to laugh at yourself. Explore the healing power of laughter. If you know you are doing everything in your power to take care of your acne, give yourself a break! You have very little control over what your body is going through.

Is this you? "I constantly seek approval from others." Always having love or approval from every significant person in your life is an unattainable goal.

Healthy inner view: It is more realistic and desirable to develop personal standards and values that are not completely dependent on the approval of others. Give yourself a pat on the back since you're doing the best you can to get through this. Don't wait to hear it from someone else. Tell *yourself* you're worthy. Do something extra nice for a very important person – you!

Is this you? "I am afraid to face the world." Acne sufferers frequently withdraw from social life, casting themselves as "damaged goods" who have no place among "good-looking" people, and the insensitive or irrational reactions of others compound the problem. Your circle of friends may diminish dramatically; you often don't try to make new friends after the acne appears. Even though you don't really want to, you may resign from clubs and organizations, exchanging social activities for solitary pursuits.

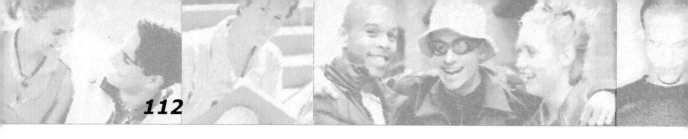
Healthy inner view: Don't drop out of life! Motivate yourself with choice, not fear. Visualize success and make decisions that fit with that image of success. For instance, picture yourself succeeding at a task and think of the satisfaction and good feelings you'll have when you meet your goals. Continue to do the things you know you are good at. You will most certainly receive praise and compliments for them.

Is this you? " I believe I can't do certain things because I have acne." You frequently say, "I can't go to the dance or go out in public like this." If you do this often enough, it will become a self-fulfilling prophecy and you will feel more powerless and out of control.

Healthy inner view: Believe in yourself and realize that you deserve the same opportunities as everyone else. Give yourself positive, encouraging statements. Work at feeling good about yourself and liking yourself.

Is this you? " I attribute everything to my acne, both the good and the bad." If someone pays a compliment, you may figure, "Yeah, but I still have acne, so I'll never be good enough" instead of simply accepting the compliment!

Healthy inner view: You have the choice, so why not accept the compliment for your achievement! Look at temporary setbacks as opportunities for growth. The positive appraisal helps you maintain your energy and gives you an improved outlook. Encourage positive self-talk from your inner voices.

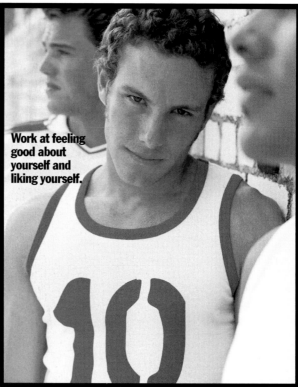

Work at feeling good about yourself and liking yourself.

Is this you? " I dwell on everything bad that was ever said or done to me. I can't forgive and forget, I just let all those negative thoughts convince me that everything anyone has ever said is true."

Healthy inner view: The only part of the past that affects you is your present interpretation of it. Only you are in charge of that. Try to reinterpret these past events in a positive way. Remember, everyone has their opinions, it doesn't make them truths. Forgiving is helpful and, at times, it's necessary to move forward. Don't forget to forgive yourself, too!

Building Self-Confidence

• *Emphasize your strengths.* Give yourself a pat on the back for every new thing you try. It's only possible to try to do things and to try to do them well. This attitude allows you to accept yourself while you keep striving to improve. By focusing on what you can do, praising yourself for efforts, you will gain self-confidence for those achievements.

• *Take risks.* Approach new experiences as opportunities to learn rather than occasions to win or lose. Doing so opens you up to new possibilities and can increase your sense of self-acceptance. If you never take risks, every possibility turns into an opportunity for failure, and inhibits personal growth.

• *Use positive self-talk.* Use positive self-talk as an opportunity to counter harmful assumptions. Substitute that inner negative voice with more reasonable assumptions. Remember, you do not have control over the attitudes and opinions of others, only over your own.

• *Evaluate yourself independently.* Doing so allows you to avoid the constant sense of turmoil that comes from relying exclusively on the opinions of others. Focus internally on how *you* feel about your own behavior, achievements, etc. – that will give you a stronger sense of self and will prevent you from giving your personal power away to others.

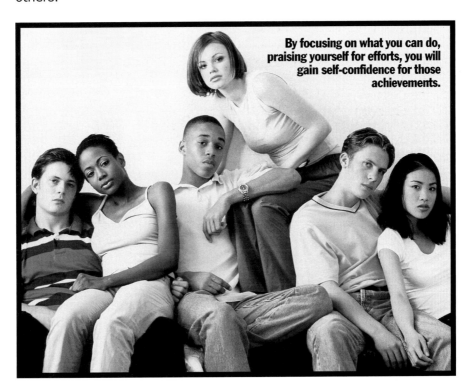

By focusing on what you can do, praising yourself for efforts, you will gain self-confidence for those achievements.

Remember, our happiness (or our misery) depends upon what we tell ourselves, how we treat ourselves, and how we interpret our world. It's an inside job that we must work through ourselves. When we are self-confident we trust our own abilities, have a general sense of control in our lives, and believe that, within reason, we will be able to do whatever we wish, plan and expect.

[Ref: www.absoluteacneinfo.com/skindeep.html]

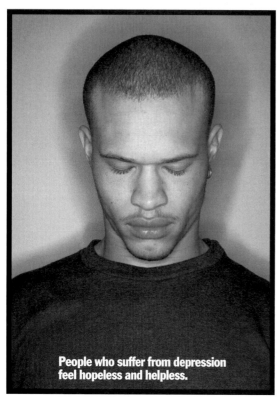

People who suffer from depression feel hopeless and helpless.

Depression

Did you know?
• Of the many millions of Americans who suffer from depression in any given year, 80 percent can be effectively treated, but only 30 percent seek help. And of that number, slightly more than half are accurately diagnosed and receive appropriate treatment.
• 30,000 suicide deaths occur every year nationally.
• The #1 cause of suicide is untreated depression.

[Ref: www.save.org]

Why do people kill themselves?
Most of the time people who kill themselves are very sick with depression or one of the other types of depressive illnesses, which occur when the chemicals in a person's brain get out of balance or become disrupted in some way. Healthy people do not kill themselves. A person who has depression does not think like a typical person who is feeling good. The illness prevents them from being able to look forward to anything. They can only think about *now* and they've lost the ability to imagine into the future. Many times they don't realize they are suffering from a treatable illness and feel they can't be helped. Seeking help may not even enter their mind. They do not think of the people around them, family or friends, because of their illness. They are consumed with emotional, and many times, physical pain that becomes unbearable. They don't see any way out. They feel hopeless and helpless. They don't want to die, but it's the only way they feel their pain will end. It is an irrational choice.

Getting depression is *involuntary* – no one asks for it, just like people don't ask to get cancer or diabetes. But, we do know that depression is a treatable illness, and that people can feel good again!

Please remember this: Depression plus alcohol or drug use can be lethal. Depressed people will sometimes try to alleviate the symptoms of their illness by drinking or using drugs. Alcohol and/or drugs will make the disease worse! There is an increased risk for suicide because alcohol and drugs decrease judgment and increase impulsivity.

Do people who attempt suicide do it to prove something?
Is it to show others how bad they feel and to get sympathy?

No, they don't do it necessarily to prove something, but it is certainly a cry for help which should not be ignored. This is a warning to others that something is terribly wrong. Many times people cannot express how horrible or desperate they're feeling – they simply cannot put their pain into words. There is no way to describe it. A suicide attempt must always be taken seriously. People who have attempted suicide in the past may be at risk for trying it again and possibly completing it, if they don't get help for their depression.

Can a suicidal person mask the depression with happiness?

We know that many people suffering from depression can hide their feelings, appearing to be happy. But can a person who is contemplating suicide feign happiness? Yes, he can. Most of the time a suicidal person will give clues as to how desperate he or she is feeling. The clues may be subtle, though, and that's why knowing what to watch for is critical. A guy may "hint" that he is thinking about suicide. For example, saying something like, "Everyone would be better off without me," or, "It doesn't matter. I won't be around much longer anyway." We need to "key in to" phrases like those and not dismiss them as just talk. An estimated 80 percent of people who died of suicide, mentioned it to a friend or relative before dying.

Depression is a treatable illness.

Other danger signs are a preoccupation with death, losing interest in what one cares about, giving away possessions, having a lot of "accidents" recently, or engaging in risk-taking behavior, like speeding or reckless driving, or general carelessness. Some people even joke about committing suicide – but it should always be taken seriously.

Is it more likely for a person to commit suicide if he or she has been exposed to it in their family or has had a close friend die of suicide?

We know that suicide tends to run in families, but it is believed that this is due to the fact that depression and other related depressive illnesses have a genetic component, and that if they are left untreated (or mistreated) can result in suicide. But talking about suicide or being aware of a suicide that happened in your family or to a close friend *does not* put you at risk for attempting it, if you are healthy. The only people who are at risk are those who are vulnerable in the first place – vulnerable because of an illness called depression or one of the other depressive illnesses. The risk increases if the illness is not treated. It's important to remember that not all people who have depression have suicidal thoughts, either – only some.

> Some people joke about committing suicide – but should always be taken seriously.

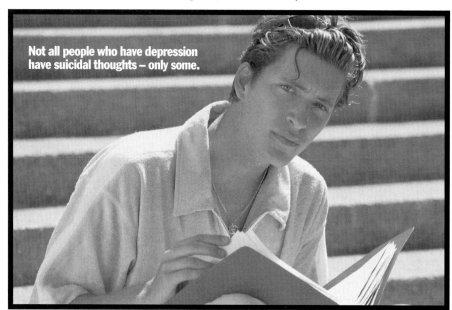

Not all people who have depression have suicidal thoughts – only some.

Why don't people talk about depression and suicide?

The main reason people don't talk about it is because of the stigma. Those who suffer from depression are afraid that others will think they are "crazy," which is so untrue. They simply may have depression. Society still hasn't accepted depressive illnesses the same way they've accepted other diseases. Alcoholism is a good example – no one ever wanted to talk openly about that, and now look at how society views it. It's a disease that most people feel pretty comfortable discussing with others if it's in their family. They talk of the effect it has had on their lives and different treatment plans. And everyone is educated on the dangers of alcohol and on substance abuse prevention.

As for suicide, it's a topic that has a long history of being taboo – something that should just be forgotten, kind of swept under the rug. And that's why people keep dying. Suicide is so misunderstood by most, and so the myths are perpetuated. Stigma prevents people from getting help, and prevents society from learning more about suicide and depression. If everyone were educated on these subjects, many lives could be saved.

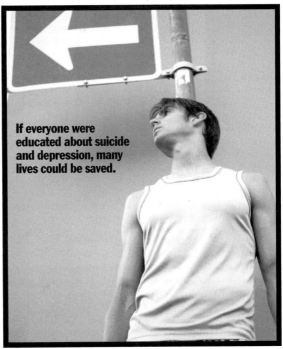

If everyone were educated about suicide and depression, many lives could be saved.

Will "talking things out" cure depression?

The studies that have been done on "talk therapy" vs. using antidepressant medication have shown that in some cases of depression, using well-supported psychotherapies (such as cognitive behavioral therapy or interpersonal therapy) may considerably alleviate the symptoms of depression. In other cases this simply wouldn't be enough. It would be like trying to talk a person out of having a heart attack. Studies continue to show that a combination of psychotherapy (talk therapies) and antidepressant medication is the most effective way of treating most patients who suffer from depression.

Why do people attempt suicide when they appear to have been feeling so much better?

Sometimes people who are severely depressed and contemplating suicide don't have enough energy to carry it out. But, as the disease

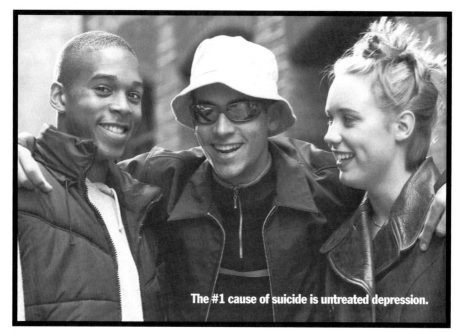

The #1 cause of suicide is untreated depression.

begins to "lift," they may regain some of their energy but will still have feelings of hopelessness. There's also another theory that these people just kind of "give in" to the anguished feelings (the disease), because they just can't fight it any longer. This in turn releases some of their anxiety, which makes them *appear* calmer. Even if they do die by suicide, it doesn't mean they chose that route. If they thought there was any way they could have the life back that they knew before the illness, they would choose life.

If a person's "mind is made up," can they still be stopped?

Yes! People who are contemplating suicide go back and forth, thinking about life and death ... the pain can come in "waves." They don't want to die, they just want the pain to stop. Once they know they can be helped, that there are treatments available for their illness, that *it isn't their fault,* and they are *not* alone, they become hopeful. We should never "give up" on someone just because we think they've made their mind up!

Is depression the same as the blues?

No. Depression is different from the blues. The blues are normal feelings that eventually pass, like when a good friend moves away or the disappointment that a person feels if something didn't turn out as expected. Eventually he will feel like his old self again. But the feelings and symptoms associated with depression *linger,* and no matter how hard a person tries to talk himself or herself into feeling better, that simply won't work. You can't just snap out of it. Depression is not a character flaw or a personal weakness. And it doesn't have a thing to do with willpower. It is an illness.

Why do depressive illnesses sometimes lead to suicidal thoughts?

There is a direct link between depressive illnesses and suicide. The #1 cause of suicide is untreated depression. Depressive illnesses can distort thinking, so a person can't think clearly or rationally. They may not know they have a treatable illness or they may think they can't be helped. Their illness can cause thoughts of hopelessness and helplessness, which could then lead to suicidal thoughts. They just can't see any other way out. That's why it is so important to educate people on the symptoms of depression and other depressive illnesses, and on the warning signs of suicide ... so that people suffering from these illnesses can get the help they need. They must understand that depression and other related depressive illnesses are *treatable* and that they can feel good again.

[Ref: www.save.org/Questions.shtml]

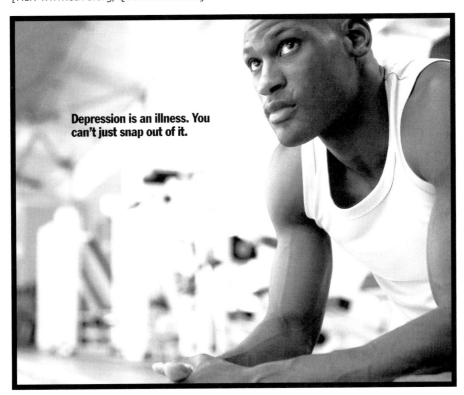

Depression is an illness. You can't just snap out of it.

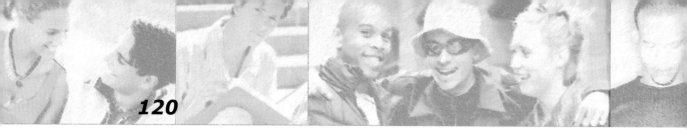

DEPRESSION CHECKLIST

- ☐ I feel sad.
- ☐ I often feel like crying.
- ☐ I'm bored.
- ☐ I feel so alone.
- ☐ I don't really feel sad, just "empty."
- ☐ I don't have any confidence in myself.
- ☐ I don't like myself.
- ☐ I feel scared a lot of the time, but I don't know why.
- ☐ I feel mad, like I could just explode!
- ☐ I feel guilty.
- ☐ I can't concentrate.
- ☐ I have a hard time remembering.
- ☐ I don't want to make decisions – it's too much work.
- ☐ I feel like I'm in a fog.
- ☐ I'm so tired, no matter how much sleep I get.
- ☐ I'm frustrated with everything and everybody.
- ☐ I don't have fun any more.
- ☐ I feel so helpless.
- ☐ I'm always getting into trouble.
- ☐ I'm so restless and jittery. I just can't sit still.
- ☐ I feel nervous.
- ☐ I feel disorganized, like my head is spinning.
- ☐ I feel so self-conscious.
- ☐ I can't think straight. My brain doesn't seem to work.
- ☐ I feel ugly.
- ☐ I don't feel like talking any more.
  I simply have nothing to say.
- ☐ I feel my life has no direction.
- ☐ I feel life isn't worth living.
- ☐ I consume alcohol or take drugs regularly.
- ☐ My whole body feels slowed down –
  my speech, my walk, my movements.
- ☐ I don't want to go out with friends any more.
- ☐ I don't feel like taking care of my appearance.
- ☐ Occasionally my heart will pound very hard, I can't
  catch my breath, and I feel tingly. My vision feels
  strange, and I think I might pass out. The feeling
  passes in seconds, but I'm afraid it will happen again
  (panic attack/anxiety attack).
- ☐ Sometimes I feel like I'm losing it.
- ☐ I feel "different" from everyone else.
- ☐ I smile, but inside I'm miserable.

- ☐ I have difficulty falling asleep or I awaken between 1 a.m. and 5 a.m. and then I can't get back to sleep.
- ☐ My appetite has diminished – food tastes so bland.
- ☐ My appetite has increased – I could eat all the time.
- ☐ My weight has increased or decreased.
- ☐ I have headaches.
- ☐ I have stomachaches.
- ☐ My arms and legs hurt.
- ☐ I feel nauseous.
- ☐ I'm dizzy.
- ☐ My vision seems blurred or "slow" at times.
- ☐ I'm clumsy.
- ☐ My neck hurts.

We're all going to feel these things from time to time – that's normal. But if you've checked several of the symptoms listed, and they have been present for 2 to 3 weeks or longer, you should see your doctor or psychiatrist for evaluation. Clinical depression is a chemical imbalance in the brain. It can be treated with antidepressant medication, psychotherapy or a combination of both. Remember, you don't have to feel this way. *You can feel good again.* Please note: There are other illnesses and certain medications that can mimic the symptoms of depression. Have a complete medical examination to rule them out.

[Ref: www.save.org/depcheck.shtml]

Common Misconceptions About Suicide

"People who talk about suicide won't really do it."
Not true. Almost everyone who commits or attempts suicide has given some clue or warning. Do not ignore suicide threats. Statements like "You'll be sorry when I'm dead," and "I can't see any way out," no matter how casually or jokingly said, may indicate serious suicidal feelings.

"Anyone who tries to kill himself must be crazy."
Not true. Most suicidal people are not psychotic or insane. They must be upset, grief-stricken, depressed or despairing, but extreme distress and emotional pain are not necessarily signs of mental illness.

"If someone is determined to kill himself nothing is going to stop him."
Not true. Even the most severely depressed person has mixed feelings about death, wavering until the very last moment between wanting to live and wanting to die. Most suicidal people do not want death; they want the pain to stop. The impulse to end it all, however overpowering, does not last forever.

"People who commit suicide are people who were unwilling to seek help."
Not true. Studies of suicide victims have shown that more than half had sought medical help within six month before their deaths.

"Talking about suicide may give someone the idea."
Not true. You don't give a suicidal person morbid ideas by talking about suicide. The opposite is true – bringing up the subject of suicide and discussing it openly is one of the most helpful things you can do.

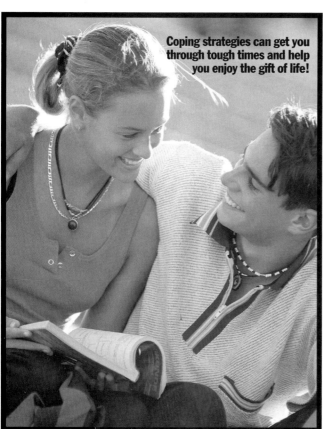

Coping strategies can get you through tough times and help you enjoy the gift of life!

Coping Skills

Developing coping skills before and during a crisis can make a big difference in your life. Of course this is easier said than done; some people never develop useful crisis coping skills. This is a good time in your life to begin to learn these skills, as crisis often comes when you least expect it.

Common Crises
Crises, although painful, are common. They include:
• Illness or accidents, especially if hospitalization is necessary.
• Divorce or separation in your family.
• Death of a parent, close relative or friend.
• Child abuse, including incest, violence, rape or emotional abuse.
• Abuse of a parent, either physical or emotional.

What You Can Do

A person in crisis needs extra attention, love and support. Spend special time with them; talking, listening, sharing physical affection, or just be there. If you are in crisis, let your friends and family know. Tell them, talk to them, share your thoughts and fears. They want to help, they have been through some crisis or another too.

A person's fears will decrease if they talk to others who have been through the same situation. Be honest, yet still sensitive to their way of thinking. Tell them their feelings are normal, and that a good cry is actually healthy.

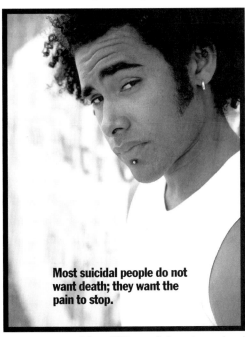

Most suicidal people do not want death; they want the pain to stop.

Get Help for Abuse

When there has been physical or emotional abuse, get help from social service agencies, guidance counselors, your clergy person or community groups. You and your family and friends will be able to get through these painful situations sooner if you use available resources.

Coping Strategies

Talk to yourself positively. Replace negative thoughts such as, "Nothing will be better from now on," or "Everything sucks!" with realistic ones: "How could I know that?" "Is there any real reason to say that?" "Something good is going to happen to me soon."

Challenge your unrealistic negative beliefs, such as "I'm not capable of anything," "I can't trust anybody," "Nobody likes me," and "This can't be happening to me." Analyze them as a scientist might. Try to find the evidence hidden in your life. You will find at least one thing that you are capable of doing. You will find at least one person you can trust. You will find at least one person who likes you.

Something bad can happen to you just as it can happen to other people. After saying to yourself, *This did happen to me, now what do I do?,* in time you will find a way to cope with it. Read these strategies, and then make them more suitable for your own situation and write them down. Read them now and read them again when you are feeling better. Coping strategies can get you through tough times and help you enjoy the gift of life!

[Ref: www.coolnurse.com/crisis.htm]

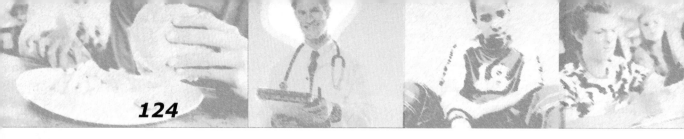

CHAPTER EIGHT

An eating disorder is a disturbance in eating behavior that compromises a person's physical and psychological health. Anorexia nervosa and bulimia are chronic problems in which there is a preoccupation with food, eating and weight loss. Eating disorders are a very dangerous type of illness no matter who you are. Men also get eating disorders. More and more young men are coming forward and admitting their obsessions with their weight and food.

Food Diary of a Bulimic Teenager – Age 16

7 a.m.	1 slice toast, plain
	1 cup of coffee, black
	1 cup bran cereal with 1/2 cup skim milk
Noon	One large salad with no dressing, but lemon juice
	1 diet cola
6 p.m.	Weight Watchers frozen dinner
	1 diet soda
10 p.m.	2 bags of cookies
	6 chocolate glazed donuts
	1 pint of ice cream
	1 loaf of garlic bread with butter
	1 large bag of corn chips
10:30 p.m.	*Self-induced vomiting!*

[Ref: www.something-fishy.org/whatarethey/be.php]

Eating Disorders

Anorexia Nervosa

Anorexia is characterized by a significant weight loss resulting from excessive dieting. Most women and an increasing number of men are motivated by the strong desire to be thin and a fear of becoming obese. Anorexics consider themselves to be fat, no matter what their actual weight is. Often anorexics do not recognize they are under-weight and may still "feel fat" at 80 pounds. Anorexics close to death will show you on their bodies where they feel they need to lose weight. In their attempts to become even thinner, the anorexic will avoid food and taking in calories at all costs, which can result in death.

An estimated 10 to 20 percent will eventually die from complications related to the illness. Anorexics usually strive for perfection. They set very high standards for themselves and feel they always have to prove their competence. They almost always put the needs of others ahead of their own needs.

Anorexics may also feel the only control they have in their lives is in the area of food and weight. If they can't control what is happening around them, they can control their weight. Each morning the number on the scale will determine whether or not they have succeeded or failed in their goal for thinness. They feel powerful and in control when they can make themselves lose weight. Sometimes focusing on calories and losing weight is their way of blocking out feelings and emotions. For them, it's easier to diet than it is to deal with their problems directly.

Anorexics usually have low self-esteem and some-times feel they don't deserve to eat. The anorexics usually deny that anything is wrong. Hunger is strongly denied. They usually resist any attempts to help them because the idea of therapy is seen only as a way to

More and more young men are coming forward and admitting their obsessions with their weight and food.

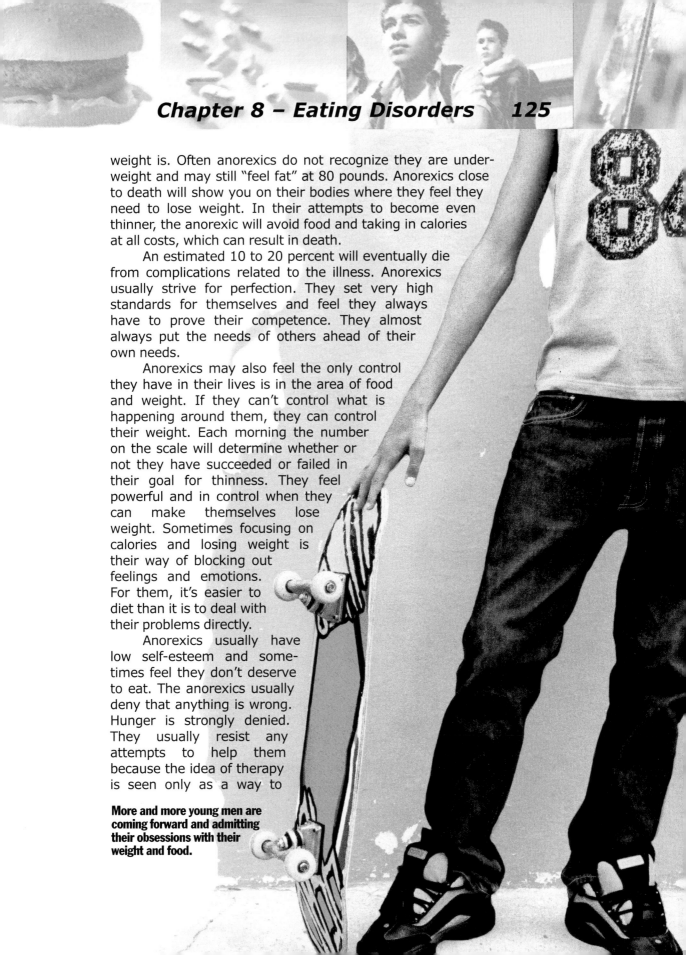

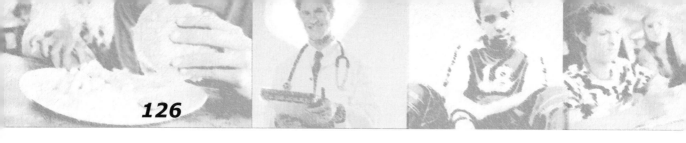

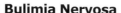

force them to eat. Once they admit they have a problem and are willing to seek help, they can be treated effectively through a combination of psychological, nutritional and medical care. Below are some signs to look for.

- Noticeable weight loss
- Becoming withdrawn
- Excessive exercise
- Fatigue
- Always being cold
- Muscle weakness
- Obsession with food, calories, recipes
- Excuses for not eating meals (ate earlier, not feeling well)
- Unusual eating habits (cutting food into tiny pieces, picking at food)
- Noticeable discomfort around food
- Complaining of being too fat, even when thin
- Cooking for others, but not eating themselves
- Restricting food choices to only diet foods
- Guilt or shame about eating
- Depression, irritability, mood swings
- Evidence of vomiting, laxative abuse, diet pills or diuretics to control weight

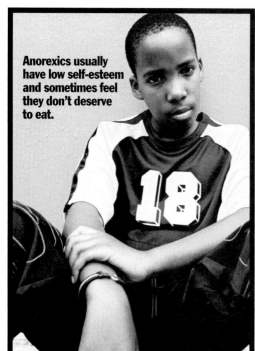

Anorexics usually have low self-esteem and sometimes feel they don't deserve to eat.

- Irregular menstruation
- Amenorrhea (loss of menstruation)
- Wearing baggy clothes to hide weight loss
- Frequently checking the scale
- Fainting spells and dizziness
- Difficulty eating in public
- Very secretive about eating patterns
- Pale complexion (almost a pasty look)
- Headaches
- Perfectionistic attitude
- Feelings of self-worth determined by what is or is not eaten
- No known physical illness that would explain weight loss

Bulimia Nervosa

Until the late Princess Diana revealed that she suffered from bulimia, this condition was relatively unknown by most of the population. Bulimia is characterized by a cycle of binge eating followed by purging to try to rid the body of unwanted calories. A binge is different for all

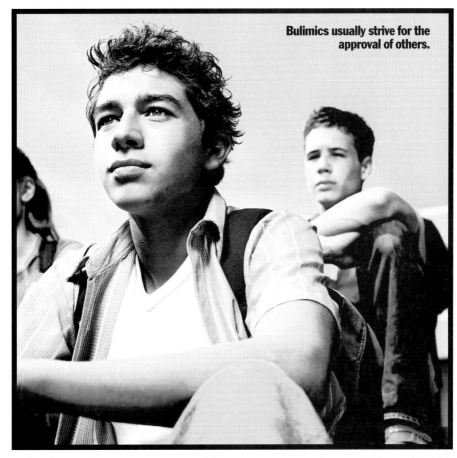

Bulimics usually strive for the approval of others.

individuals. For one person a binge may range from 1000 to 10,000 calories, for another, one cookie may be considered a binge. Purging methods usually involve vomiting and laxative abuse. Other forms of purging can involve excessive exercise, fasting, use of diuretics, diet pills and enemas.

Bulimics do not feel secure about their own self-worth. They usually strive for the approval of others. They tend to do whatever they can to please others, while hiding their own feelings. Food becomes their only source of comfort. Bulimia also serves as a function for blocking or letting out feelings. Unlike anorexics, bulimics do realize they have a problem and are more likely to seek help. Below are some signs to look for.

• Binge eating
• Secretive eating (food missing)
• Bathroom visits after eating
• Vomiting

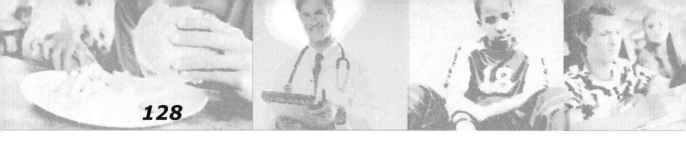

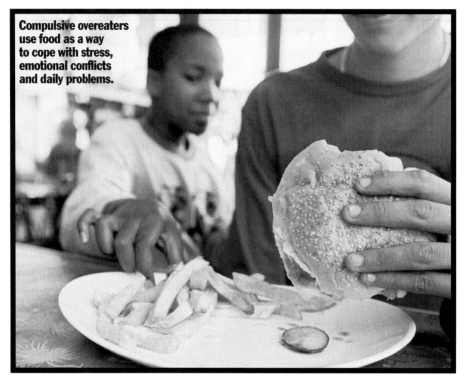

Compulsive overeaters use food as a way to cope with stress, emotional conflicts and daily problems.

- Laxative, diet pill or diuretic abuse
- Weight fluctuations (usually with 10 to 15 pounds)
- Swollen glands
- Broken blood vessels
- Harsh exercise regimens
- Fasting
- Mood swings
- Depression
- Severe self-criticism
- Self-worth determined by weight
- Fear of not being able to stop eating voluntarily
- Self-deprecating thoughts following eating
- Fatigue
- Muscle weakness
- Tooth decay
- Irregular heartbeats
- Avoidance of restaurants, planned meals or social events
- Complains of sore throat
- Need for approval from others
- Substance abuse
- Ipecac abuse

Compulsive Overeating

Compulsive overeating is characterized by uncontrollable eating and consequent weight gain. Compulsive overeaters use food as a way to cope with stress, emotional conflicts and daily problems. The food can block out feelings and emotions. They feel out of control and are aware their eating patterns are abnormal. Like bulimics, compulsive over-eaters do recognize they have a problem.

Compulsive overeating usually starts in early childhood when eating patterns are formed. Most people who become compulsive eaters are those who never learned the proper way to deal with stressful situations, and use food instead as a way of coping. Fat can also serve as a protective function for them, especially those who have been victims of sexual abuse. They sometimes feel that being overweight will keep others at a distance and make them less attractive.

Unlike anorexia and bulimia, there is a high proportion of male overeaters. The more weight that is gained, the harder they try to diet. And dieting is usually what leads to the next binge, which can be followed by feelings of powerlessness, guilt, shame and failure. Dieting and binge eating can go on forever if the emotional reasons are not dealt with. In today's society, compulsive overeating is not yet taken seriously enough. Instead of being treated for the serious problem they have, they are instead directed to diet centers and health spas.

Like anorexia and bulimia, compulsive overeating is a serious problem and can result in death. With the proper treatment, which should include therapy, medical and nutritional counseling, it can be overcome. Below are some signs to look for.

- Binge eating
- Fear of not being able to stop eating voluntarily
- Depression
- Self-deprecating thoughts following binges
- Withdrawing from activities because of embarrassment about weight
- Going on many different diets
- Eating little in public, while maintaining a high weight
- Believing they will be a better person when thin
- Feelings about self are based on weight
- Social and professional failures attributed to weight
- Feeling tormented by eating habits
- Weight is the focus of life

[Ref: www.fitteen.com/top]

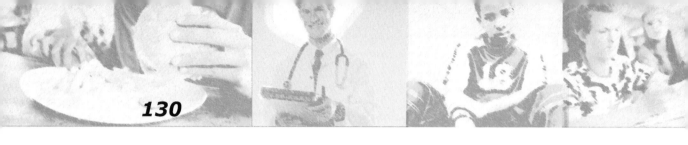

Associated Drug Abuse

Ipecac Syrup
Laxatives
Diuretics
Diet Pills
FDA Warning

Ipecac Syrup

Many people with eating disorders abuse a syrup called ipecac to help induce vomiting. Ipecac should only be used in cases of accidental poisoning. Repeated use can cause the heart muscle to weaken. It can cause irregular heartbeats, chest pains, breathing problems, rapid heart rate and cardiac arrest. Ipecac is very dangerous and it has been the cause of death in many people suffering with an eating disorder. If you are using this, we seriously urge you to speak to your doctor immediately.

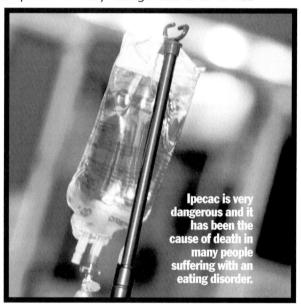

Ipecac is very dangerous and it has been the cause of death in many people suffering with an eating disorder.

Laxatives

Stimulant laxatives such as Ex-Lax and Correctol are the most common laxatives used by someone with an eating disorder. Laxatives have little or no effect on reducing weight because by the time they work, the calories have already been absorbed. The person usually feels like they have lost weight because of the amount of fluid that is lost. That feeling is only temporary because the body will start to retain water within a period of 48 to 72 hours. This usually leaves them feeling bloated and fearing they are gaining weight, and usually leads to repeated use of these products.

Laxative abuse can cause bloody diarrhea, electrolyte imbalances and dehydration. Many people find that after prolonged use they cannot have a bowel movement without them. A laxative abuser may also experience constipation, severe abdominal pain, nausea and vomiting.

Laxative abuse is very dangerous, can lead to permanent damage to the bowels, severe medical complications and even death. Laxatives are not always used for the sole purpose of trying to rid the body of calories that have been consumed. Just like vomiting is used as a way for someone to release built-up feelings and emotions, laxatives can also be used for the same reason. A person may also abuse laxatives as a way to harm themselves. The physical pain resulting from laxative abuse may actually be a reason a person continues to use them. They may believe they deserve the pain or they may find that dealing with physical pain is easier than dealing with emotional pain.

Diuretics, Water Pills

Diuretics are much like laxatives in the sense that they give the person a feeling of weight loss. When taken, a person will only lose vital fluids and electrolytes. Within a day or two the body will react and start to retain water, which is usually what causes someone to use them repeatedly. Abuse of diuretics usually leads to dehydration, which can cause kidney damage. Electrolyte imbalances can occur from repeated use – *and that is very serious.* Your body's electrolytes need to be in balance in order for your organs, such as the heart, kidney and liver, to function properly. Once the electrolytes go out of balance, the person is at a very high risk for heart failure and sudden death. Diuretics do not cause weight loss, but repeated use can cause serious medical complications.

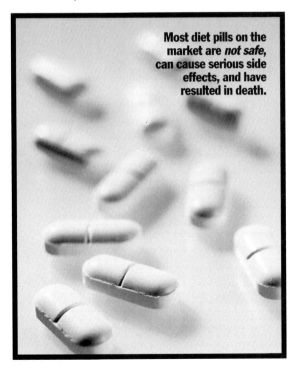

Most diet pills on the market are *not safe*, can cause serious side effects, and have resulted in death.

Diet Pills

The sale and use of diet pills continues to be on the rise in North America. Many people are led to believe this is a safe and effective way to lose weight. Most diet pills on the market *are not safe,* can cause serious side effects, and have resulted in death. Popular diet pills such as Acutrim and Dexatrim contain a combination of phenylpropanolamine and caffeine. Phenylpropanolamine is a stimulant and affects the central nervous system. It can produce symptoms such as increased heart rate, dizziness, high blood pressure, nausea, anxiety, irritability, insomnia, dry mouth and diarrhea.

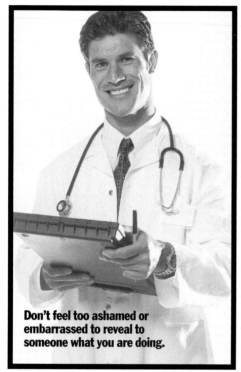

Don't feel too ashamed or embarrassed to reveal to someone what you are doing.

Fenfluramine, *Fen-Phen,* is also found in many diet pills and it is quite popular. Like all diet pills, it stimulates the central nervous system and can be addictive. Side effects can include diarrhea, high blood pressure, dry mouth, rash, palpitations and chest pains. Most doctors who prescribe Fen-Phen ignore the manufacturer's warnings about who should use these pills and how long they should be taken. People using them are usually not informed of the warnings either. The manufacturer of Fen-Phen states that it should only be used in treating obesity and when the person's weight is at a point where it is a serious threat to health. Many doctors claim that Fen-Phen is safe and can be taken for life. The manufacturer says these pills should not be taken for more than 3 months. Taking them for any longer can put you at risk for developing *primary pulmonary hypertension,* a rare but generally fatal lung disease. The life expectancy for someone who develops primary pulmonary hypertension is less than 3 years.

Getting Help for Your Diet Disorder

One of the hardest things to do is to admit and accept that you have an eating disorder. The next hardest thing is to reach out and ask for help. Many feel that, since this is their problem, they should deal with it on their own. People with eating disorders are very independent and are not used to sharing their feelings with anyone, especially not a therapist. They may feel too ashamed or embarrassed to reveal to someone what they are doing.

Please know that there is no shame in having an eating disorder. This problem is too big to correct on your own and you need the help of qualified individuals. There is help available. You don't have to be a prisoner to your eating disorder forever. Not only is it *okay* to ask for help, *it is necessary.* Having a good support system will make your fight toward freedom a little easier and you will know that you are not alone. Your treatment should probably include individual, family and group therapy, support groups, medical and nutritional counseling, in some cases medications, and sometimes there is a need for hospitalization.

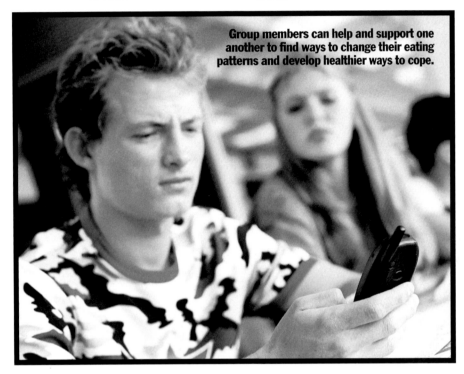

Group members can help and support one another to find ways to change their eating patterns and develop healthier ways to cope.

Individual Therapy

In individual therapy you will be able to develop a one-to-one relationship with your therapist. Once you begin to trust him or her, you will be free to start releasing all the feelings you have kept inside for so long. You will be able to start focusing on why you are doing this and what you need to do to stop. You will begin to understand why and how your eating disorder became your only means of coping, and learn new and healthier ways to cope. The frequency of visits will probably depend on the severity of the eating disorder. Some people are in daily therapy and others are in weekly therapy. The number of visits will probably depend on you and your therapist.

Group Therapy

Group therapy can be very beneficial to those who are trying to recover from an eating disorder. For the first time they are surrounded by others who know and understand exactly how they feel. For so long they probably felt like they were the only ones who had this problem – now they know they're not alone. Groups usually meet once a week and can discuss anything from the eating behavior itself and finding ways to change, to discussing the underlying issues that cause the disorder. Group members can help and support one another to find ways to change their eating patterns and develop healthier ways to cope.

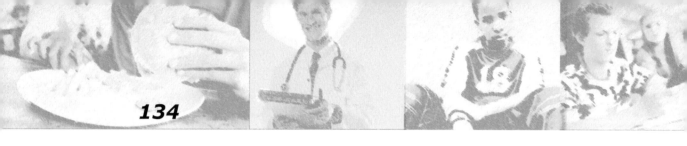

Family Therapy

Family therapy usually involves those who live with or are very close to the person with the eating disorder – possibly including parents, siblings, spouses and even grandparents. Usually an eating disorder indicates problems within the family. Some problems could include marital problems, substance abuse, physical or sexual abuse, lack of communication, or difficulty in expressing feelings. All these issues can be discussed and worked on in family therapy. In order to solve these problems, the families must be willing to participate in therapy and willing to make changes in their own behavior.

Support Groups

Support groups are usually not run by a professional. Usually the leaders are people who have experienced an eating disorder themselves. The groups meet anywhere from daily to once a month. Support groups can be very helpful because people with eating disorders realize they are not alone and that recovery is possible. The members also help and support each other during difficult periods. Each support group is different. Some groups are free to discuss what they feel and others may pick a topic to be discussed at each meeting.

Medical Treatment

It's important that your health be monitored by a physician who is aware of your eating disorder. There are many physical complications that can result from the eating disorder. If left untreated, they can lead to serious health problems or even death. We would also urge people suffering from eating disorders to be very open and honest about their behavior and symptoms with their doctor to ensure they receive the best medical treatment possible. It is also important to choose a doctor who is familiar with eating disorders and treats them properly. If you are bulimic, you may want to visit your dentist for a checkup. Frequent vomiting can lead to tooth decay as a result of enamel erosion from stomach acids.

Nutrition Counseling

A part of your recovery should include nutritional counseling. Many people with eating disorders have no idea what "normal eating" really is and a qualified nutritionist will be able to help you develop a healthy eating pattern.

Medications

In some cases medication has been useful in treating eating disorders. Antidepressants such as Prozac, Paxil and Zoloft have been prescribed to help with symptoms of severe depression. Antidepressants can sometimes help a person binge/purge less frequently. Medication should not be used as the sole source of treatment. It should be combined with all areas of treatment.

Hospitalization

If the person's weight is extremely low or if they are binging/purging several times a day, hospitalization may be necessary. Sometimes the individual needs more support than out-patient therapy has to offer. The hospital can provide them with a safe environment and will help control the eating behaviors. If hospitalization is necessary, they should be admitted to a ward that is familiar with treating eating disorders. Psychiatric wards are usually not equipped to handle eating disorder patients and the person can sometimes feel worse while in there. Some hospitals do have units that specialize in treating eating disorders, and should provide both psychological and physiological care.

If you should require more information, please check out the Internet for sites relating to eating disorders, such as www.eating-disorders.com. And remember – consult your doctor, parent or professional if you suspect you or someone you know has an eating disorder.

[Ref: www.fitteen.com, and www.something-fishy.org/isf/mentalhealth.php]

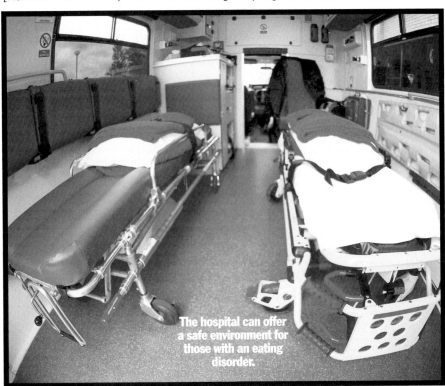

The hospital can offer a safe environment for those with an eating disorder.

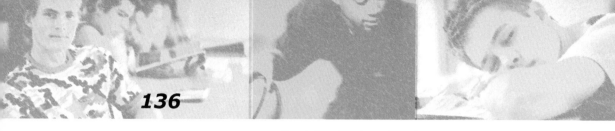

CHAPTER NINE
Sleep

You're busy with school, sports, after-school activities, homework, and possibly a job. So be honest – how high on your priority list is a good night's sleep? For many teens, *not very*. Perhaps you don't think you need much sleep ("I can get by on 6 hours"), or maybe you figure you can make up for it on the weekend ("I always sleep until noon on Saturday").

Although you may think getting the right amount of sleep isn't all that important, trust us – *it is.* In the same way that you make sure to get enough to eat, good sleep habits are a big part of staying healthy. And it's not just about making your parents and teachers happy. If you want to do well on tests, play sports without falling on your face, and hang out with your friends without turning into a zombie, you'll want to take a hard look at your sleep routine. Read on for some sleepy surprises – you'll be amazed what a few ZZZs can do for you!

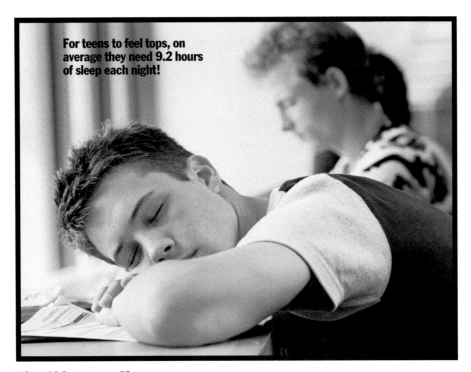

For teens to feel tops, on average they need 9.2 hours of sleep each night!

The Skinny on Sleep

Sleep isn't simply the opposite of being awake. In fact, while you're in sweet slumber, your brain is still active. As you sleep, your brain passes through stages that are necessary for you to stay healthy. Sleep is actually food for your brain! And like food, sleep is not an option – *it's a necessity.*

Many people – both teens and adults – believe that if they don't get enough sleep during the week, they can catch up on that lost sleep over the weekend and it will all even out. Although this seems like a simple trade-off, trying to pay back your sleep "debt" on weekends doesn't always work.

One of the most important stages of sleep is called REM (rapid eye movement) sleep, or the dream stage. REM is necessary because this is when your mind processes your experiences and helps you adjust to the world around you. REM sleep usually happens after you've already been asleep for about 4 hours. So if you only sleep for 6 hours a night and you use naps or weekends to make it up, you may not get the same *quality of sleep* that you would have if you had tacked on an extra 2 hours at the end of the 6 hours.

Some teens have sleep problems that go beyond the occasional late night out. If you experience any of the following symptoms that make you think you may have a problem, talk to your doctor.

Sleep Problems

Sleepwalking – This problem happens when you walk or move around during sleep. Because most sleepwalkers don't do it very often, sleepwalking doesn't usually become a serious problem. But some sleepwalkers move around almost every night, and they are at risk of getting hurt if they go into the kitchen where there are sharp items, for example, or if they go outside.

Sleep apnea – Sleep apnea is a disorder that causes a person to stop breathing temporarily during sleep. Causes of apnea include enlarged adenoids (tissues located in the passage that connects the nose and throat) and tonsils, and obesity. A person with sleep apnea may experience snoring, difficulty breathing, choking, and heavy sweating during sleep. Other symptoms include feeling extremely sleepy or irritable during the day.

Insomnia – Insomnia occurs when you have a lot of trouble falling asleep, especially when it happens often. The most common cause for insomnia is stress brought on by a big change in routine, such as starting at a new school or moving. Chronic insomnia lasts more than a month and may be caused by problems such as depression.

Narcolepsy – Narcolepsy *(pronounced: nar-kuh-lep-see)* is a sleep disorder in which the person has "sleep attacks" during the day during which he can't stay awake no matter how much sleep he has gotten the night before. This problem can be dangerous because someone with narcolepsy could fall asleep in a dangerous situation, such as while driving a car.

How many ZZZs do I need?

Do you think that as a teen you need less sleep than your younger sister or brother? Actually, research shows that for teens to feel tops, on average they need a whopping 9.2 hours of sleep each night! But this number can be hard to reach – you don't need to be a math wizard to figure out that, if you wake up for school at 6 a.m., you'd have to go to bed at 9 p.m. to reach the 9-hour mark. Recent studies have shown that many teens have trouble going to sleep that early – not because teens want to rebel against bedtime, but because their brains naturally work on a later schedule and they aren't ready for bed.

What happens if you don't get enough sleep? *Lots.* You would probably feel very sleepy during the day and you may have trouble staying awake in class. This can affect your ability to concentrate, make good judgments, and get good grades. Most importantly, you run the risk of falling asleep while driving your car, which could lead to a serious accident.

Some teens experience emotional problems such as depression if they don't get enough sleep. You might also feel irritable, cranky or more emotional than usual. Not getting enough sleep can also contribute to skin problems, such as acne.

Tips for Getting the Right Amount of Sleep

If you want to make good sleep a habit, take a look at your everyday schedule. Are you working so many hours at your after-school job that you end up staying up late to finish homework? Does football practice take up so much time that you never get to bed before 11? If so, think about ways to make your schedule more manageable. Can you work fewer hours if your job isn't essential? If football is especially important, can you drop another activity to make time for sleep?

If you are getting enough rest at night and you are still falling asleep during the day, it's a good idea to visit your doctor. He or she will look at your overall health and sleep

> Not getting enough sleep can also contribute to skin problems, such as acne.

habits and may do a test to find out whether anything is happening during the night to disturb your sleep, like sleep apnea. There are ways that may make it easier for you to fall asleep when you hit the sack. Here are some tips for good "sleep hygiene":

• Have a regular bedtime and try to arrange your schedule so that you can stick to the routine.
• Don't nap a lot during the day. If you absolutely must take a nap, limit it to 20 to 30 minutes.

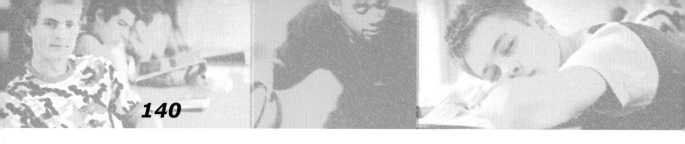

• Leave some time to unwind before bed. That may mean saving a little time for the stress-reducing techniques (such as meditation) that work best for you.

• Don't exercise right before bed. It's important to get enough regular exercise, but plan to do it early in the afternoon if possible.

• Avoid beverages that contain caffeine, such as coffee and soft drinks, after late afternoon.

• Try to stay on schedule even on weekends. Don't go to sleep more than an hour later or wake up more than 2 to 3 hours later than usual.

• Get into bright light as soon as possible in the morning, but avoid it in the evening. Bright light signals the brain that it's time to wake up.

• Say no to cramming for exams with all-nighters. The best way to prepare for a test is to spread your studying out over time and to get plenty of sleep.

The best way to prepare for a test is to spread your studying out over time and to get plenty of sleep.

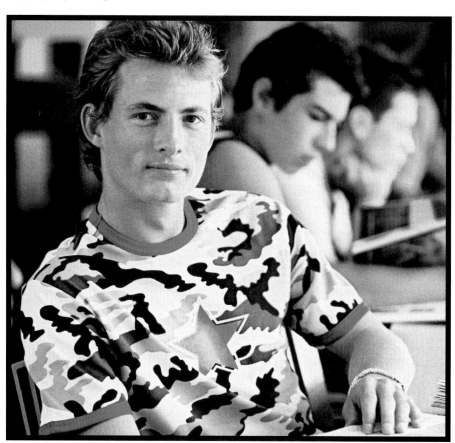

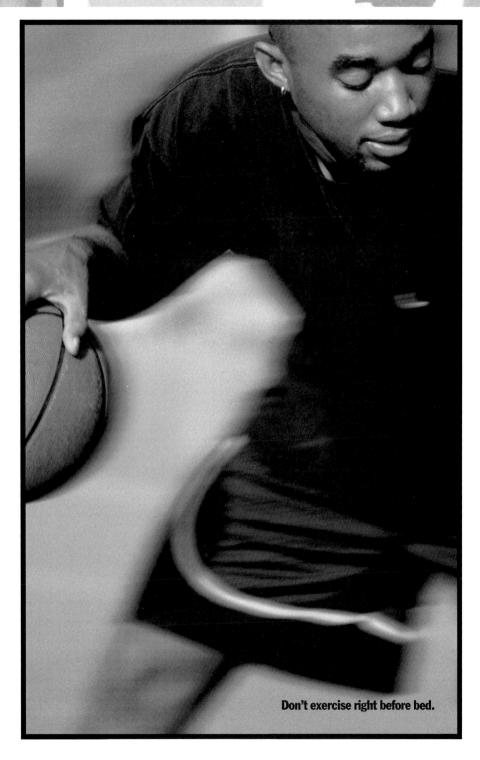

Don't exercise right before bed.

CHAPTER TEN

Great-Looking Teeth:
Something to
Smile
About

Are you getting braces and have no idea what to expect? Had braces for a while but wonder what's going on in there? Whatever your situation is, you're not alone. Millions of teens have braces. Braces are a totally normal and practically expected part of puberty (and many adults get braces, too).

Talking About Teeth

To better understand why braces and other orthodontic devices are needed, it will help to talk a bit about the teeth first. You probably don't remember your very first set of tiny teeth, but you had 20 of them when you were young. (The first ones probably came in when you were about 6 months old, and you most likely had all of them by the time you reached age 3.)

As you made your way through childhood, these teeth fell out one by one, to be replaced by permanent, adult teeth. If you're 14 or older, it's pretty likely that you have 28 of your permanent teeth in place; four more will grow in as you get a little older to create *a complete set of 32 teeth.* These last four teeth are commonly known as "wisdom teeth" (dastardly little devils that often cause trouble and must be removed).

The basic makeup of every tooth in your mouth is the same, and they all grow out of the same place: from within the jawbones, which are surrounded by the gums. And although some adult teeth grow out from the gums at the proper angle and with the right spacing, many don't. Some teeth may grow in crooked or overlapping. In others, teeth may grow in rotated or twisted. Some people's mouths are too small (as opposed to a few of your friends whose mouths are too big – *just kidding!),* and this crowds the teeth and causes them to shift into crooked positions. And in some cases, a person's upper jaw and lower jaw aren't the same size. When the lower half of the jaw is too small, the upper jaw hangs over when the jaw is shut, resulting in a condition called an overbite. When the opposite happens (the lower half of the jaw is larger than the upper half), it's called an underbite.

All of these different types of disorders go by one medical name: *malocclusion.* This word comes from Latin and means "bad bite." In most cases, a bad bite isn't anyone's fault; crooked teeth, overbites, and underbites are often inherited traits, just like brown eyes or big feet. In some cases, things like dental disease, early loss of baby or adult teeth, some types of medical problems, an accident, or a habit like prolonged thumb-sucking can cause the disorders.

Malocclusion can be a problem because it interferes with proper chewing – crooked teeth that aren't aligned properly don't work as well as straight ones. Because chewing is the first part of eating and digestion, it's important that teeth can do the job. Teeth that aren't aligned correctly can also be harder to brush and keep clean, which can lead to tooth decay and cavities. And finally, many people who have crooked teeth may feel self-conscious about the way they look. The

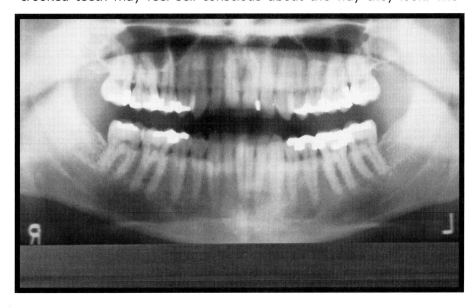

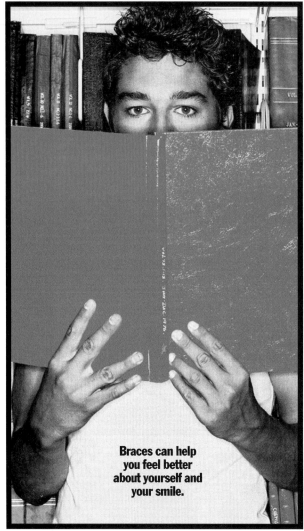

Braces can help you feel better about yourself and your smile.

good news is that braces can help them feel better about their smile and their whole face.

If a dentist suspects that a kid or teen needs braces or other corrective devices, he or she will refer the patient to an orthodontist. Orthodontists are dentists who have special training in the diagnosis and treatment of misaligned teeth and jaws. Most regular dentists can tell if teeth will be misaligned once a patient's adult teeth begin to come in – sometimes as early as age 6 or 7. But in many cases, the patient won't be referred to an orthodontist until he's closer to his teen years – the orthodontist wants to devote his or her time to straightening adult teeth, the ones that will be sticking around and not falling out.

Diagnosis

First the orthodontist will need to reach a diagnosis before deciding on treatment. Reaching the diagnosis means making use of several different tools, including X-rays, photographs and impressions.

The X-rays give the orthodontist a good idea of where the teeth are positioned and if any more teeth have yet to come through the gums. Special X-rays that are taken from 360 degrees around the head may also be ordered; this type of X-ray shows the relationships of the teeth to the jaws and the jaws to the head.

The orthodontist may also take regular photographs of the patient's face to help him or her understand these relationships better. And finally, the orthodontist may need to make an impression of the patient's teeth. This is done by having the patient bite down on a mushy material that is used later to form an exact copy of the teeth.

Treatment

Once a diagnosis is made, the orthodontist can then decide on the right kind of treatment. In some cases, a removable retainer will be all that's necessary. In other rare cases (especially when there is an extreme overbite or underbite), an operation will be necessary. But in most cases, the answer is braces.

Braces straighten teeth because they do two very important things: stay in place for an extended amount of time, and exert steady pressure. It's this combination that allows braces to successfully change the arrangement of teeth in a patient's mouth, periodically adjusted by the orthodontist.

An orthodontist can outfit patients with a few different kinds of braces. Some braces are made of a lightweight metal and go around each tooth, while other metal ones are attached to the outside surfaces of the teeth with special glue. Clear braces can be attached to the outside surfaces of the teeth, as can ceramic ones that are the same color as teeth. Some patients can get newer "mini-braces," which are much smaller, or "invisible braces," which are affixed to the inside surfaces of the teeth. In many cases, the patient can choose which kind he or she wants.

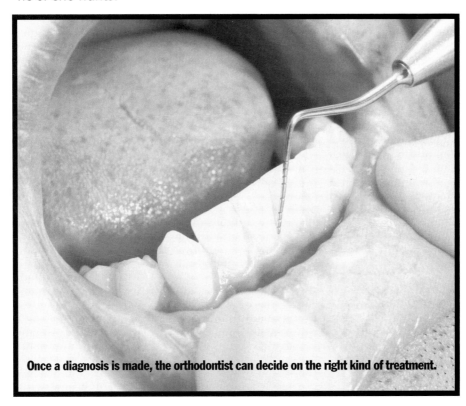

Once a diagnosis is made, the orthodontist can decide on the right kind of treatment.

Once the orthodontist puts the braces on, they will usually remain on the patient's teeth for anywhere from 6 months to 2 years. In some cases, the braces may need to remain on for longer.

After the length of time needed for correction has been established for the patient, the orthodontist must work on the other part of the treatment: making sure the braces exert steady pressure. To achieve this, the patient must come for regular visits, usually once a month or so. During these visits, the orthodontist will attach wires, springs, or rubber bands to the braces in order to create more tension and pressure on the teeth. Sometimes the rubber bands will connect certain teeth to one another to create a kind of opposing tension.

For some teens, the orthodontist may decide that extra tension is needed outside the mouth – when braces alone aren't enough to straighten the teeth or shift the jaw. In cases like these, a patient may need to wear head or neck gear with wires that attach inside the mouth, and elastic that attaches the gear to the head. Many times, they will need to wear this type of gear only at night or in the evening when at home.

It may take a while, but with the right combination and timing of wires, springs, rubber bands, and sometimes head gear, the teeth will slowly but surely move into their correct positions. During this period of time, it can help to know that you're not alone when you go for your adjustments – but that won't necessarily make you feel any better if your teeth hurt! Some of the adjustments can make your mouth feel a bit sore or uncomfortable because the tension tends to make itself felt in more places than your teeth. Most of the time, taking ibuprofen (such as Motrin) or acetaminophen (such as Tylenol) can help relieve the pain. If you always have a lot of pain after your braces are adjusted, talk to your orthodontist about it; he or she may be able to make the adjustments a bit differently.

Caring for Teeth With Braces

Your orthodontist will also make sure you know how to take special care of your teeth while your braces are on. Braces, wires, springs, rubber bands, and other appliances can act like magnets for food and plaque, which can leave permanent stains on the teeth if not brushed away. Most orthodontists recommend brushing after meals with fluoride toothpaste and taking special care to remove food stuck in braces. Some orthodontists will also prescribe or recommend a fluoride mouthwash, which can get into places in a mouth with braces that a toothbrush can't.

Some people with braces are more prone to canker sores (from the braces hitting the inside surface of the mouth). If this happens, an orthodontist may recommend an over-the-counter medicine that can be placed directly on the canker sore to help heal it.

Faces After Braces

After what can seem like an eternity to someone who has braces, the magic day finally comes: the orthodontist takes the braces off! After your teeth are cleaned thoroughly, the orthodontist may actually want to repeat the process of taking X-rays and impressions of your teeth. This allows him or her to carefully check the work, and in the case of X-rays, see if wisdom teeth are now visible.

In some cases, the orthodontist will recommend extraction of the wisdom teeth if they are starting to come in after the braces have been removed. The reason? The wisdom teeth can cause the newly straightened teeth to shift and move in the mouth.

And speaking of teeth shifting and moving, a very important part of a person's post-braces treatment is retention, or keeping the teeth in their new place. The truth is that most teens, after wearing braces and going for adjustments for up to 2 years or longer, don't want anything to do with the orthodontist or having appliances in their mouths. But even though the teeth have been successfully moved with braces, they are still not completely stable. They need to settle in their corrected positions until the bones, gums and muscles adapt to the change. This is usually accomplished with the use of retainers, which work by retaining the straight position of the teeth.

Some retainers are made of clear plastic and metal wires that cover the outside surface of the teeth, whereas others are made of rubber. Most retainers need to be worn all the time for the first 6 months, then usually only during sleeping. How long a retainer must be worn depends on the patient – one person might wear it for a few months, while another might have to wear it for several years. Whatever the time frame, retainers are very important; without them, the teeth could shift back into their crooked old positions, making all the orthodontist's work and your years of patience useless!

What's the most important thing to remember when you're feeling frustrated about having a face full of braces? You must not forget that during every school photo where you can't be persuaded to open your mouth because of your braces, there are millions of other people experiencing the same thing. And that no matter what, your braces will come off eventually – and you'll be left with a wonderful, straight smile.

[Ref: www.kidshealth.org/teen/body_basics/braces_p3.html]

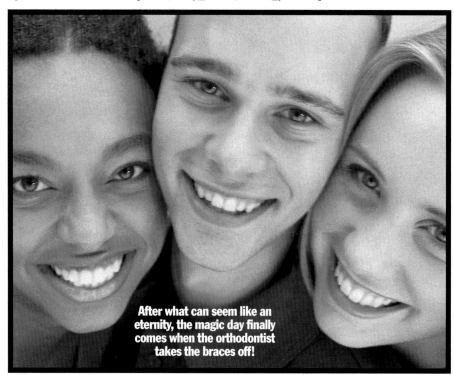

After what can seem like an eternity, the magic day finally comes when the orthodontist takes the braces off!

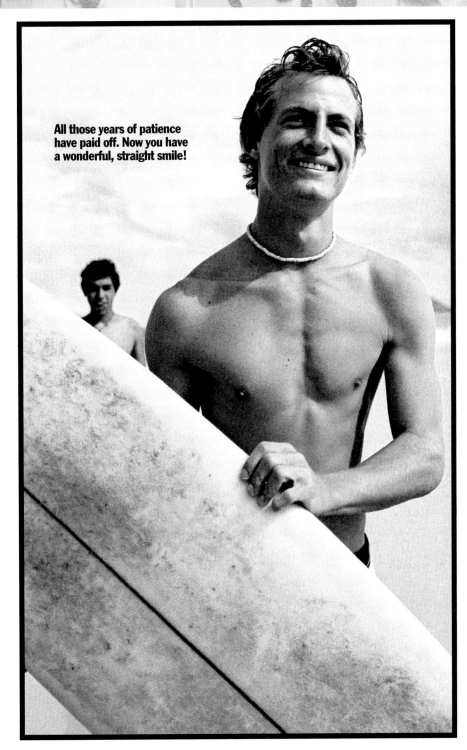

All those years of patience have paid off. Now you have a wonderful, straight smile!

CHAPTER ELEVEN

Cigarettes: Giving Up On Smoke

First, *congratulate yourself!* Just deciding to read this chapter is a great first step toward becoming tobacco-free. Many teens won't admit to themselves that they can't quit any time they want to – and they keep right on smoking. And there are lots of reasons to quit. Nearly one in five deaths in the United States is related to tobacco – which is more than 400,000 lives lost per year. Need a few more reasons?

• It's expensive – if you smoke a pack a day, it can cost you more than $1000 a year. (That could buy you about 75 CDs, a top-quality mountain bike, or a down payment on a car, just to name a few things!)

• It makes your teeth yellow and your breath, hair and clothes stink.

• You're less of a sports competitor if you smoke – you get short of breath more easily.

But beyond all these scary statistics and smelly breath, the first part of quitting is realizing that you're most likely addicted to nicotine, one of the chemicals in cigarettes and smokeless tobacco. According to many experts, the nicotine in tobacco is as addictive as cocaine, heroine or opium. In fact, it's so addictive that 40 percent of teens who smoke have tried to quit at one point and failed. But don't let this discourage you. There are some things you can do to help you quit smoking for good.

Get support.
Teens who have friends and family who will help them quit are much more likely to succeed. If you don't want to tell your parents or family that you smoke, make sure your friends know, and consider confiding in a counselor or other adult you trust. And if you're having a hard time finding any-one to support you (if, say, all your friends smoke and none of them is interested in quitting), you might consider joining a support group, either in person or online.

Set a quit date.
You should pick the day to stop smoking. Tell your friends (and if they know you smoke, tell your family) that you're going to quit smoking and when. Try to think of that day as the dividing line between the smoking you and the "new and improved" nonsmoker you. Mark it on your calendar.

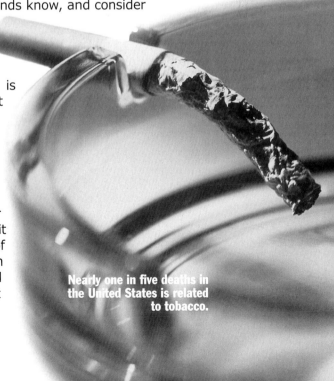

Nearly one in five deaths in the United States is related to tobacco.

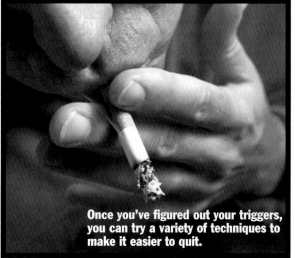

Once you've figured out your triggers, you can try a variety of techniques to make it easier to quit.

Throw away your cigarettes!

That means *all your cigarettes* – even that emergency pack you have stashed in the secret pocket of your backpack. Get rid of your ashtrays and lighters, too. That way you'll make it a little bit harder to smoke.

Wash all your clothes.

Get rid of the smell of cigarettes as much as you can by washing all your clothes and having your coats or sweaters dry-cleaned. If you smoked in your car, clean that out, too.

Think about your triggers.

You've probably smoked a lot of cigarettes since you started, and you're probably aware of certain situations when you particularly tend to smoke – when you're at your best friend's house, drinking coffee after the movies, or just driving around. These situations are your triggers for smoking – it feels automatic to reach for a cigarette at those times. Once you've figured out your triggers, you can try a variety of techniques to make it easier to quit.

• Avoid these trigger situations (if you smoke when you drive, get a ride to school, or take the bus for a couple of weeks).

• Change the situation (suggest you sit in the nonsmoking section the next time you go out to eat).

• Substitute something else for cigarettes (cinnamon sticks, carrots, gum, straws, toothpicks, and even pacifiers all make good substitutes).

Physical Symptoms

Expect some physical symptoms. If you smoke regularly, you're probably physically addicted to nicotine and your body may experience some symptoms of withdrawal when you quit. These symptoms may include:

• headaches or stomachaches
• crabbiness, jumpiness or depression
• lack of energy
• dry mouth or sore throat
• desire to pig out

The good news is, these withdrawal symptoms will pass – so be patient and don't give in and sneak a smoke, or you'll just have to deal with the symptoms longer.

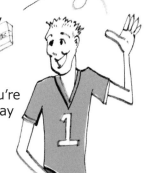

Keep yourself busy.

Many people find it's best to quit on a Monday, when they have school or work to keep them busy. The more distracted you are, the less likely you are to crave cigarettes. Staying active is also a good way to make sure you keep your weight down and your energy up, even as you experience the symptoms of nicotine withdrawal.

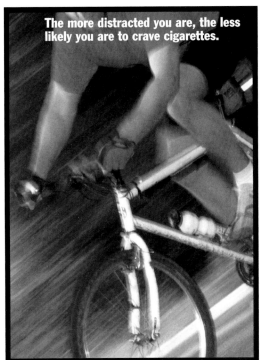

The more distracted you are, the less likely you are to crave cigarettes.

Drink lots of water.

Liquid will help flush the nicotine out of your system and will help you to feel better as the withdrawal symptoms set in. And while you're at it, stay away from caffeine, which can make you even more jumpy.

Quit gradually!

Some people find that switching to cigarettes that have a lower nicotine level and then gradually decreasing the number that they smoke each day is an effective way to quit. (This strategy doesn't work for everyone – you may find you've got to quit cold turkey.)

Use a nicotine replacement.

If you find that none of these strategies is working, you might consider a nicotine replacement. These include gum, patches, inhalers and nasal sprays. Sprays and inhalers are available by prescription only, and although you can buy the patch and gum without a prescription, you should see your doctor before you do so. That way you can find out which is best for you based on your type of addiction. For example, the patch requires the least effort on your part, but it also doesn't provide the almost instantaneous nicotine "kick" you'll get from the gum.

Reward yourself!

Set aside the money you usually spend on cigarettes. When you've stayed tobacco-free for a week, 2 weeks, or a month, buy yourself a new CD, some clothes, or a book – anything you really like. *What if you slip up?* If you're like many people, you may quit successfully for weeks or even months, and then suddenly have a craving that's so strong you feel like you must give in. Or maybe you accidentally find yourself in one of your trigger situations and give in to temptation. It may be tempting to give up and decide that you've blown it – and to start smoking again. What should you do?

• Think about your slip as one mistake, not a sign that you've failed. Take notice of when and why it happened and move on.

• Did you become a heavy smoker after one cigarette? We didn't think so – it happened more gradually, over time. Keep in mind that one cigarette didn't make you a smoker to start with, so smoking one cigarette (or even two or three) after you've quit doesn't make you a smoker again.

• Remind yourself why you quit and how well you've done – or have someone in your support group do this for you.

Remember this: It's hard to quit smoking. If you don't succeed the first time, don't give up. Some people have to quit two or three times before they're successful.

[Ref: www.kidshealth.org/teen/body_basics/quit_smoking_p3.html]

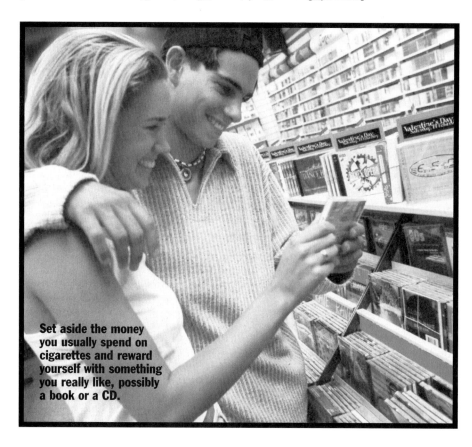

Set aside the money you usually spend on cigarettes and reward yourself with something you really like, possibly a book or a CD.

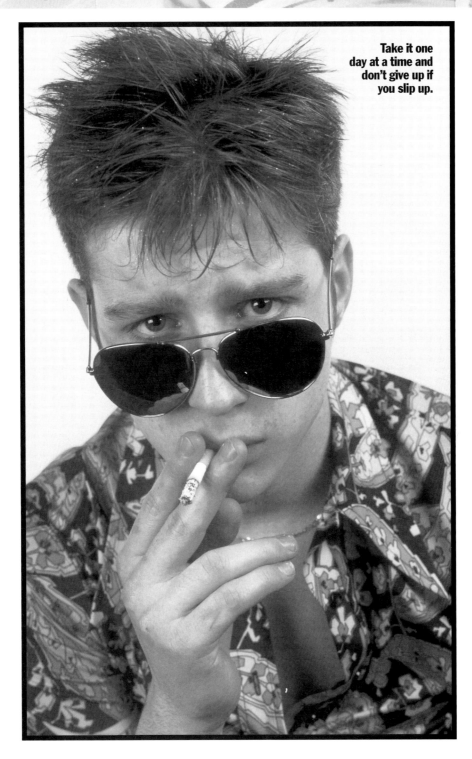

Take it one
day at a time and
don't give up if
you slip up.

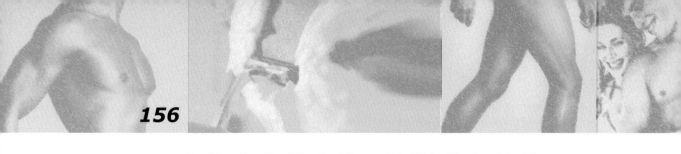

CHAPTER TWELVE

Hair Removal

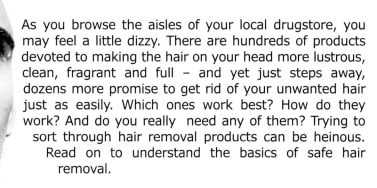

As you browse the aisles of your local drugstore, you may feel a little dizzy. There are hundreds of products devoted to making the hair on your head more lustrous, clean, fragrant and full – and yet just steps away, dozens more promise to get rid of your unwanted hair just as easily. Which ones work best? How do they work? And do you really need any of them? Trying to sort through hair removal products can be heinous. Read on to understand the basics of safe hair removal.

The Hair You Wear

Before you start getting rid of it, you should understand hair basics. Hair is made of keratin, a hard protein that's also found in your fingernails and toenails. You have hair, even if it's difficult to see, all over your body, with the exception of the pink part of your lips, the palms of your hands, and the soles of your feet. Hair growth begins beneath the surface of your skin at a hair root inside a hair follicle, a small tube in the skin.

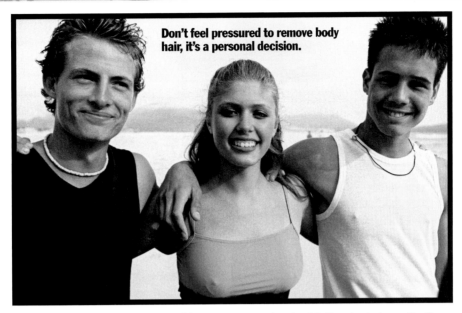

Don't feel pressured to remove body hair, it's a personal decision.

You have two types of hair on your body. Vellus hair is soft, fine, short, and is usually colorless, and in most people, grows on the chest, back and face. This hair is normally darker and more noticeable in some people, especially those with darker complexions and those of certain ethnic groups. Vellus hair helps your body maintain a steady temperature by providing insulation – kind of like having your own thin coating of fur.

Terminal hair is coarser, darker, and longer than vellus hair and is the type of hair that grows on your head. When a teen reaches puberty, terminal hair starts to grow in the armpits and pubic region. On guys, terminal hair begins to grow on the face and other parts of the body such as the chest, legs and back. Terminal hair provides cushioning and protection.

In some cases, excess hair growth, called hirsutism (pronounced: her-suit-iz-um), may be the result of certain medical conditions. In girls, ovary problems and other hormonal disorders can cause dark, coarse hair to grow on the face, especially the upper lip, and on the arms, chest and legs. Some medications such as birth control pills and other hormone-containing medications (like the anabolic steroids that some athletes and bodybuilders take) can also cause hirsutism.

Although about 81 percent of American women remove hair from their underarms and legs, only about 51 percent of European women do. Many cultures view body hair as beautiful and natural. If a girl or guy chooses to remove body hair, that's okay. It's a personal decision. Getting rid of hair doesn't make you healthier or a better person, and you shouldn't feel pressured to do so if you don't want to.

Getting Rid of Hair

Shaving

How it works: Using a razor, you remove the tip of the hair shaft that has penetrated the skin. Some razors are completely disposable, some have a disposable blade, and some are electric. Guys often shave their face, and women often shave underarms, legs and bikini areas.

How long it lasts: 1 to 3 days.

Pros: Shaving is fairly inexpensive. All you need is some warm water, a razor, and if you choose, shaving gel or cream. You don't need an appointment – shaving is a do-it-yourself endeavor, resulting in smooth, hairless skin.

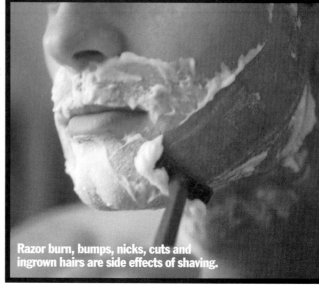

Razor burn, bumps, nicks, cuts and ingrown hairs are side effects of shaving.

Cons: Razor burn, bumps, nicks, cuts and ingrown hairs are side effects of shaving. Ingrown hairs occur when hairs are cut below the level of the skin. As the hair begins to grow back, it grows within the surrounding tissue rather than growing out of the follicle. The hair curls around and starts growing into the skin. Irritation, redness and swelling can occur at the hair follicle.

Tips: Look for blades that have safety guard wires – they minimize nicks and cuts. Also, you'll get a closer shave if you do it in the shower after your skin has been softened by warm water. Go slowly, change your blades often to avoid nicks, and use a moisturizing cream to soften the hair. Shave in the direction your hair grows to avoid ingrown hairs. If you have an ingrown hair, try exfoliating (removing dead skin cells) with a loofah, then sterilize a pointed pair of tweezers with rubbing alcohol, and attempt to pluck out the ingrown hair.

Plucking

How it works: Using tweezers, a person stretches the skin tightly, grips a single hair close to the root, and pulls it out.

How long it lasts: 3 to 8 weeks

Pros: Plucking is time-consuming because you can remove only one hair at a time. However, it's inexpensive because all you need are tweezers.

Cons: Plucking can be painful, so it's best to do it only on small areas, such as the eyebrows. Ingrown hairs can result if the hair breaks off below the skin. Temporary red bumps may appear because the hair follicle is swollen and irritated.

Tips: Make sure you sterilize your tweezers with rubbing alcohol before and after use to reduce the chance of infection.

Depilatories

How they work: A depilatory is a cream or liquid that removes hair from the skin's surface. It works by reacting with the protein structure of the hair, so the hair dissolves and can be washed or wiped away. A common brand of depilatory is Nair.

How long it lasts: Several days to 2 weeks.

Pros: Depilatories work quickly, are readily available at drug and grocery stores, and are inexpensive. They're best on the leg, underarm and bikini areas; special formulations are available for other areas of the body.

Cons: Applying depilatories can be messy and many people dislike the odor. If you have sensitive skin, you might have an allergic reaction to the chemicals in the depilatory, which may cause a rash or inflammation. For people with coarse hair, a depilatory may not be as effective.

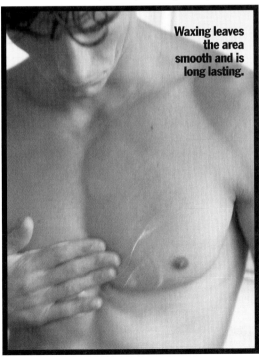

Waxing leaves the area smooth and is long lasting.

Tips: Read product directions carefully and be sure to apply the product only for the recommended amount of time for best results.

Waxing

How it works: A sticky wax is spread on the skin area with the unwanted hair, and then a cloth strip is applied over the wax and quickly pulled off, taking the hair root and dead skin cells with it. The wax can be warmed or may be applied cold. Waxing can be done at a salon or at home.

How long it lasts: 3 to 6 weeks.

Pros: Waxing leaves the area smooth and is long lasting. Waxing kits are readily available in drug and grocery stores.

160

Cons: Many people mention that the biggest drawback to waxing is the pain when the hair is ripped out by the root. Redness, inflammation, and bumps may occur after a waxing. Professional waxing is also expensive compared to other hair-removal methods. People with diabetes should avoid waxing because they are more susceptible to infection. Also, teens who use acne medications such as Retin-A and Accutane may want to skip the wax because those medicines make the skin more sensitive. Teens with moles or skin irritation from sunburn should also avoid waxing.

Tips: Hair should be at least 1/4 inch long before waxing, so wait at least a few weeks before making your next waxing appointment.

Electrolysis

How it works: A professional electrologist inserts a needle into the follicle and sends an electric current through the hair root, killing it.

How long it takes: A small area such as the brow line may take 4 to 10 hours and a larger area such as the chest may take 8 to 16 hours.

Pros: Electrolysis is the only type of hair removal that is permanent.

Cons: Electrolysis costs big bucks and takes lots of time, so it's usually only used on smaller areas such as eyebrows and underarms. Many people describe the process as painful, and dry skin, scabs, scarring and inflammation may result after treatment. Infection may be a risk if the needles and other instruments aren't properly sterilized.

Tips: Talk to your doctor if you're interested in this method. He or she may be able to recommend an electrologist with the proper credentials.

Read product directions carefully and be sure to apply the product only for the recommended amount of time for best results.

Laser Hair Removal

How it works: A laser is directed through the skin to the hair follicle, where it stops growth. This treatment works best on light-skinned people with dark hair because the melanin (colored pigment) in the hair absorbs more of the light, making it more effective.

How long it lasts: 6 months

Pros: This type of hair removal is long lasting and large areas of skin can be treated at the same time.

Cons: A treatment session may cost $500 or more. Side effects of laser hair removal may include inflammation and redness.

Tips: The use of cold packs may help diminish any inflammation after treatment. Avoiding the sun before a treatment may make results more effective.

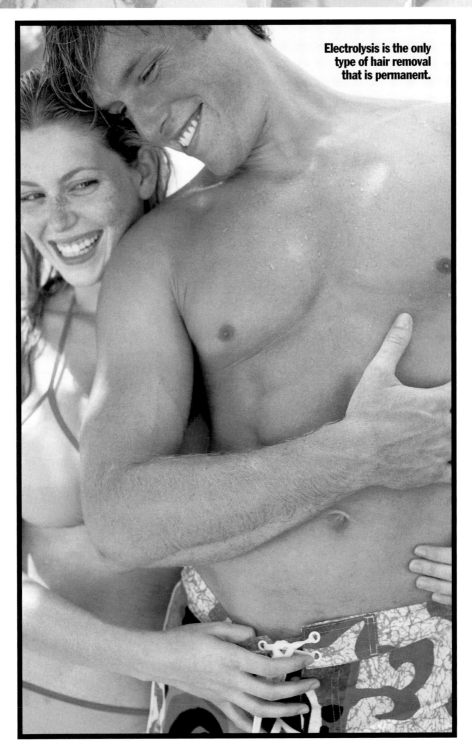

Electrolysis is the only type of hair removal that is permanent.

CHAPTER THIRTEEN

Supplements

You've seen the headlines: "Natural herbs melt pounds away – without diet or exercise!" and "Amazing new discovery boosts athletic performance!" The ads usually claim that a doctor has discovered a new dietary supplement, a miracle substance that will make you thinner, stronger, smarter or better at whatever you do. Best of all, this supplement works without any real effort – all you have to do is send in your money and swallow what they send you.

What are dietary supplements?

Dietary supplements are products that include vitamins, minerals, amino acids, herbs or botanicals (plants) – or any concentration, extract or combination of these – as part of their ingredients. You can purchase dietary supplements in pill, gel capsule, liquid or powder form. We should also tell you that the supplement industry brings in billions of dollars yearly. Now you'd think that an industry this large would be safe and properly regulated, but it's not. Every month some new supplement company comes on the market claiming their product is the safest and most effective. Unfortunately most of them have one goal in mind – to separate you from those few dollars you earned at your part-time job. We could write a whole book on the shady characters who hang out in the supplement world. Let's just say – *buyer beware!*

Do I need to take supplements?

This is one of the hardest questions to answer. In fact there is really more than one answer. In simple terms no supplement can take the place of good nutritious food. Your body needs a certain amount of nutrients each day. If you are getting this amount in your diet (i.e. through food), you don't need to take most supplements. The problem contained within the previous sentence is – many people *do not* consume adequate amounts of nutrients in their diet. Either they don't consume enough food, or they are eating the wrong kinds of food. Skipping breakfast, having a small lunch and then a large supper is not the most efficient way to eat. But given the lifestyle many people lead, the previous is the typical eating profile that many people follow. In this case a multivitamin, and perhaps a meal-replacement or protein-powder supplement makes good sense. But you don't take a

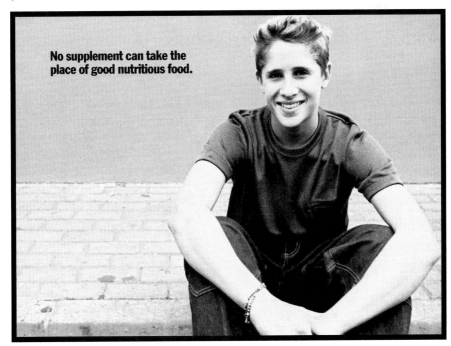

No supplement can take the place of good nutritious food.

supplement in place of a meal. Besides the known nutrients, food contains many things that biochemists have yet to identify.

Before we leave this topic we will admit there are a few supplements that can be considered more than just nutrients. They are in fact performance boosters. They are found naturally in food but in such low concentrations that they don't do much. However, when taken in supplement form they make a big difference. Most are safe, but a few carry risks. The following are some of the most popular supplements you'll hear about these days. We are quite sure that you or many of your classmates are using them.

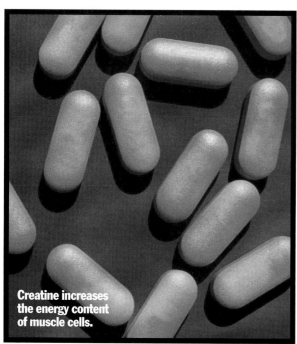

Creatine increases the energy content of muscle cells.

Creatine

Creatine is without doubt the most popular over-the-counter (from now on abbreviated OTC) supplement available. There are a number of reasons why creatine has reached such a lofty status. For one thing, it works. Numerous studies have shown that creatine does increase athletic performance. Another reason is cost. Creatine is relatively inexpensive. A third reason is safety. If used properly, creatine has few if any side effects. Let's take a look at this supplement that has taken the athletic community by storm.

What is creatine?

Creatine is a compound that can be consumed in the diet or manufactured from amino acids. The average body goes through about 2 grams of creatine per day. Most of our body's creatine is contained within skeletal muscle, although some is also present in the heart, brain and testes (in males). Following ingestion (or synthesis) creatine is transported into our muscles where it serves to increase muscle energy levels. Creatine does so by increasing the availability of the cell's energy molecule, ATP.

Recently it has become popular to supplement one's diet with synthetically produced creatine with hopes of enhancing athletic performance. Exercise performance usually improves when muscle creatine levels increase by at least 20 percent as a result of creatine supplementation.

How does creatine work?

Simply speaking, creatine increases the energy content of muscle cells. Creatine does this by increasing the availability of ATP, the energy molecule of cells. Since our strength depends on how quickly ATP can be made available during exercise, increasing muscle creatine increases our strength.

How can I get creatine naturally?

In one form or another, creatine is normally obtained from the foods we eat. Creatine can be directly obtained by eating sources of skeletal muscle, that is, meat and fish. During the digestive process the creatine contained within meat and fish is directly absorbed into the blood stream, where it is transported to skeletal muscle. For reference, approximately 2-3 pounds of raw meat or fish contains about the same amount of creatine as 5 grams of pure creatine monohydrate. However, since heat degrades creatine, cooking reduces the creatine content of meat and fish. Therefore, you'll need to eat more cooked meat to get the same amount of creatine as from uncooked sources.

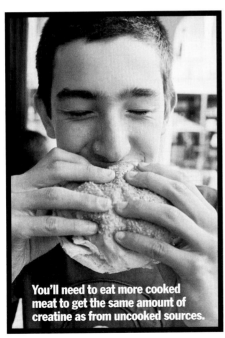

You'll need to eat more cooked meat to get the same amount of creatine as from uncooked sources.

What is the process of creatine synthesis?

When dietary creatine intake doesn't meet the body's needs, new creatine can also be synthesized from three amino acids: arginine, glycine and methionine. These amino acids are made available during the digestion of foods. Importantly, methionine availability sets an upper limit on creatine synthesis, since the body cannot produce it on its own. Methionine must, therefore, be provided in our diets. Since fish is one of the richest natural sources of methionine, eating fish provides both a direct source of creatine as well as an adequate supply of dietary methionine for new creatine synthesis. It should now be obvious

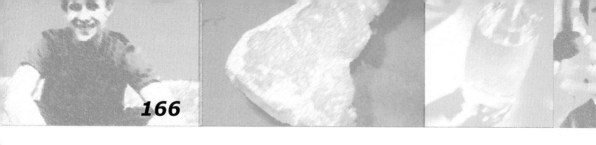

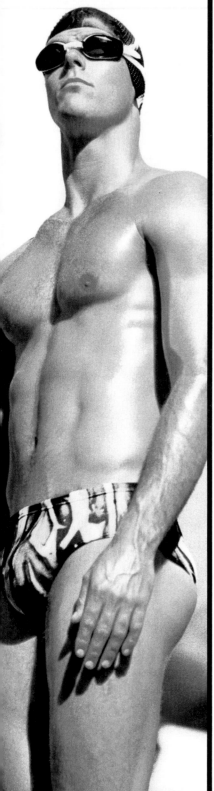

why vegetarians typically express lower than "normal" creatine levels. Creatine might therefore be advisable for athletes who purposefully restrict their animal protein intake.

How does creatine get into muscle?

After a meal, creatine is transported from the blood into skeletal muscle by special transporter molecules on the muscle surface. It has been previously shown in animal studies that the activity of these creatine transporters is influenced by the presence of creatine in the blood stream. For example, prolonged exposure to elevated plasma creatine interrupts creatine uptake into skeletal muscle via these transporters. The new production of creatine from amino acids is also stopped by elevated plasma creatine. These are examples of feedback regulatory processes that are common in animals. However, how exogenous creatine supplementation influences these processes in humans is still an open issue. That's why it is often recommended to periodically stop taking creatine to let the body recuperate.

Transporter function is also regulated by other physiological processes. For example, creatine transporter activity is enhanced by co-ingestion of highly glycemic foods, an effect mediated by insulin release. Therefore, some experts take measures to improve insulin sensitivity in hopes of enhancing creatine uptake into skeletal muscle.

Do all muscles respond the same to creatine?

Not all muscle types rely to the same extent on creatine energy production. Muscles can be broadly categorized as either being fast muscle or slow muscle. As the name implies, fast muscle fibers mediate abrupt movements. Fast muscle fibers are also those that predominantly utilize creatine energy production. That's why explosive movements respond best to creatine supplementation.

By contrast, slow muscle fibers do not rely that heavily on creatine energy production. Slow muscle fibers are also those that play an important role during endurance exercise. It follows that endurance tasks are influenced less by creatine supplementation. In addition, many endurance sports may be adversely affected by the increase in weight associated with creatine supplementation.

How much creatine and when should I take it?

First, you should not *oversupplement* with creatine! Secondly, there is *no specific dose* that is right for everyone. The creatine dose you take depends on your weight, percent bodyfat, fitness goals, and the type and intensity of training. As of yet, creatine doses have not been independently optimized for women.

Typical doses for pure creatine monohydrate cited in scientific studies range between 2 and 25 grams per day for an average size male (70 kilograms/154 pounds). However, if that particular creatine product contains additives, i.e. highly glycemic sugars, the recommended serving size would be accordingly greater. Read the label carefully. Nevertheless, the amount of creatine monohydrate taken in a single day should not exceed 25 grams for an average-framed male.

Loading

For the first few days of creatine supplementation no more than 0.3 grams of creatine per kilogram (2.2 pounds) of body weight should be taken. Divide this amount into four equal parts. Take one part every four hours. This period has been termed the loading phase and shouldn't exceed the time it takes your muscle stores to fill, usually five days.

Maintenance

After the loading phase the creatine dose can be reduced to just a few grams (0.03 grams/kilogram body weight) a day for no longer than one month. This is known as the maintenance phase. The maintenance amount is just what is needed to replace the amount of creatine degraded on a daily basis.

Dosages

Translating these formulas into practical terms: a 154-pound male would take 21 grams of creatine per day during the loading phase and 2 grams per day during the maintenance phase. *[Refer to table below.]*

Daily Dosages of Creatine for Males

Bodyweight:

Pounds	100	110	120	130	140	150	160	170	180	190	200
Kilograms	45.4	50.0	54.5	59.0	63.6	68.2	72.7	77.2	81.8	86.3	90.9

Dosage:

Loading Phase	14	15	16	18	19	20	22	23	25	26	27
Maintenance	1.4	1.5	1.6	1.8	1.9	2.0	2.2	2.3	2.5	2.6	2.7

[Below your bodyweight is the approximate creatine dose in grams.]

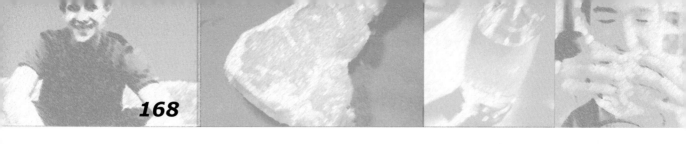

When to Supplement

During both the loading and maintenance phases, one serving should be taken immediately following your workout. This is when the metabolic state of muscle is most receptive to creatine uptake and appears to be associated with insulin sensitivity.

Washout

Remember, as far as creatine is concerned, more isn't necessarily better. Following the loading and maintenance phases, a washout period is advised to allow the body to recover from the abnormally high creatine levels that normally would not be encountered. One month is typically advised for complete washout.

Is loading necessary?

Even though the volume of anecdotal evidence suggests that the loading phase is necessary, it should be noted that a loading period may not be an absolute requirement for physical performance to be enhanced. As little as 3 grams of creatine a day for a few weeks has been shown to increase muscle creatine levels sufficiently to show a difference in physical performance.

As far as creatine is concerned, more isn't necessarily better.

How does creatine cause muscle growth?

Creatine may enhance muscle growth through two possible mechanisms. These are outlined below.

1. Muscle Volumizing

The first involves the movement of fluids from the blood stream into skeletal muscle, causing our muscles to swell. This process has been termed *volumizing* in the scientific literature. This phase of muscle growth can account for as much as 1 to 2 kilograms of additional body mass within the first few weeks of supplementation.

2. Protein Synthesis

The second form of muscle growth that might be attributed to *creatine* involves its ability to increase muscle energy capacity. Since creatine would allow us to exercise more intensely, our gains in muscle mass should be greater. It has been shown that biochemical markers for new muscle production (protein synthesis) increase following creatine use.

Furthermore, some studies suggest that muscle volumizing *per se* may stimulate muscle protein synthesis.

Is it necessary to continue taking creatine to stay strong?

Unfortunately, some of the gains in strength will disappear after you stop taking creatine. This is inevitable and will take about one month; the time for your muscle creatine levels to return to normal. However, since creatine supplementation allows one to exercise harder, which is the best stimulus for muscle growth, some gains in strength may persist after you stop taking creatine. In support of this notion, biochemical indicators of protein synthesis increase in response to creatine use, possibly indicating more muscle proteins are being produced.

Protein Supplements

Nutritional supplements are gaining popularity and acceptance rapidly in America but many people don't really know why they use these items, other than the fact that they are convenient and that everyone else seems to be using them too. Grabbing a quick protein bar or shake will fill your needs if you're looking for a meal on the go. But, supplements can do so much more for you when you understand how they can help the body function better.

The fact is, it's almost impossible to give your body all the beneficial proteins, vitamins and necessary nutrients it needs through simple food consumption. It is certainly important to eat balanced meals daily. However, high-quality supplements can provide a concentration of the nutrients you are seeking without a lot of added calories or fats that can be contained in basic foods.

Many schools of thought exist regarding the amount of protein your body needs every day in order to be at healthiest and most productive best. Some of the food guidelines provided by the Heart Association or Diabetic Association call for approximately 6 to 10 ounces, which equates to 50 to 70 grams daily. Most fitness diets tell us we need to eat 1 to 1-1/2 grams of protein daily for every pound of bodyweight. For example, if you weigh 160 pounds and exercise regularly, you should eat 160 to 240 grams of protein every day. That equates to 20 to 35 ounces of some sort of protein daily. Obviously, many people would find it almost impossible to eat 35 ounces of meat daily. Not only is the volume tremendous, but the amount of extra fat associated with meat products can be very high at this volume as well. That's when supplements become important.

Using protein supplements with very low fat, carbohydrate and sugar content will boost protein levels in a very concentrated form. At least half of the protein you eat is burned up in the digestive process so you should always eat more and not less whenever you can. Protein has the ability to stimulate the metabolism through it's thermogenic effect, and stabilizes insulin levels – which is necessary to metabolize fat properly.

Types of Protein Supplements
There seems to be a bewildering array of protein supplements on the market, but thankfully they can be split into the following three categories:
1. Whey proteins
2. Milk and egg proteins
3. Soy proteins/other vegetable proteins

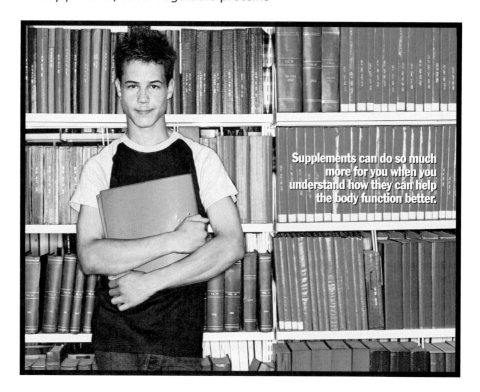

Supplements can do so much more for you when you understand how they can help the body function better.

Consistent whey protein intake coupled with exercise will result in consistent musclebuilding.

Whey Protein

Of the many protein sources out there, whey protein is the ultimate. It comes from milk. During the process of turning milk into cheese, whey protein is separated out. Protein can be found in a variety of foods – mainly meats such as beef, chicken and fish. Dairy products as well as eggs, cottage cheese, soy and vegetable protein also contain good amounts of protein.

Whey protein (the highest quality and best form of protein) is incredible stuff. It provides the body with the necessary building blocks to produce amino acids that are used for building muscle tissue. Studies have been conducted to compare whey protein with other sources. They have found that whey protein contains the perfect combination of overall amino acid makeup ... and in just the right concentrations for optimal performance in the body. Both hormonal and cellular responses seem to be greatly enhanced with supplementation of whey protein, too! Not to mention the benefits whey protein has on the body's immune system according to documented scientific research. Whey protein also plays a role as an antioxidant and an immune system builder. Most importantly, consistent whey protein intake coupled with exercise will result in consistent musclebuilding.

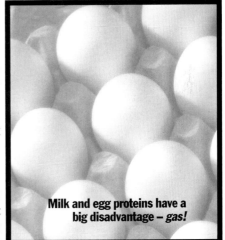

Milk and egg proteins have a big disadvantage – *gas!*

Milk and Egg Protein

As the name implies, milk and egg proteins are made from these two basic food sources. Milk and eggs are among the purest sources for protein and these protein supplements have been around for decades. From a quality point of view milk and egg protein supplements are nearly as good as whey protein supplements. But they do have one big disadvantage – *gas!*

Many people report that milk and egg supplements leave them feeling bloated and nauseous. Others report intestinal cramping leading to gas passing. Another drawback is that they don't mix as well as whey protein. To mix whey protein all you really need is a glass and spoon. A few stirs with the spoon and it's ready to drink. Most milk and egg proteins require a blender. Now if you are home this is no big deal, but you're limited to the number of places you can prepare a drink.

Soy Protein

Soy protein is one of those supplements that seem to have had their day, were then replaced by newer products, and are now making a partial comeback. Soybeans are the only plant food that has all of the essential amino acids our body requires, making it a "complete protein." Soy foods do not have any cholesterol, and most are high in fiber. Soy also has many vitamins, minerals and phytochemical compounds (like isoflavones) that work together to create numerous health benefits (including anti-cancer and anti-heart disease properties). Research shows that a daily intake of at least 25 grams of soy protein and 30 to 50 milligrams of isoflavones can improve and safeguard your health. This is the equivalent of 1 or 2 servings of soy foods a day. Like milk and egg protein supplements, soy protein supplements are not as easily digested as whey protein sources. And similarly they need to be blended.

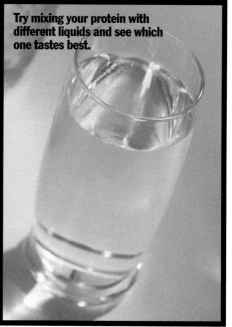

Try mixing your protein with different liquids and see which one tastes best.

And the winner is ...

Even though whey protein is considered the best protein source available, it doesn't rank that much higher than milk and egg sources. Either would be a good source of extra protein. Given the health-promoting benefits of soy protein, it's probably a good idea to mix a small amount of soy protein with one of the other two sources. That way you'll be getting the best of both worlds.

Do I mix it with milk or water?

As a final comment on protein supplements we should touch on the issue of mixing mediums. Some fitness experts make a big deal out of what you should mix your protein powder with. In our view the best liquid to use is the one you prefer. It's that simple. Milk is probably the most popular, but for those who can't handle milk, a perfectly good substitute would be juice or water. Our advice is to try mixing your protein with different liquids and see which one tastes best.

Fat-Burners

Ephedrine

By the time you read this, ephedrine will possibly have been banned in the US and Canada. That's too bad as ephedrine is probably the most effective OTC supplement available.

Unfortunately, thanks to a few idiots who abused the drug, and a few determined legislators, ephedrine may soon be placed in the same category as heroine and cocaine. What's all the fuss about? Read on! *Ephedrine, ephedra* and *ma huang* are all terms used to refer to the same substance derived from the plant ephedra. (There are many common names for these evergreen plants, including squaw tea and Mormon tea.) Ephedra is a shrub-like plant that is found in desert regions of central Asia and other parts of the world. The dried greens of the plant are used medicinally. Ephedra is a stimulant containing the herbal form of ephedrine, an FDA-regulated drug found in over-the-counter asthma medications.

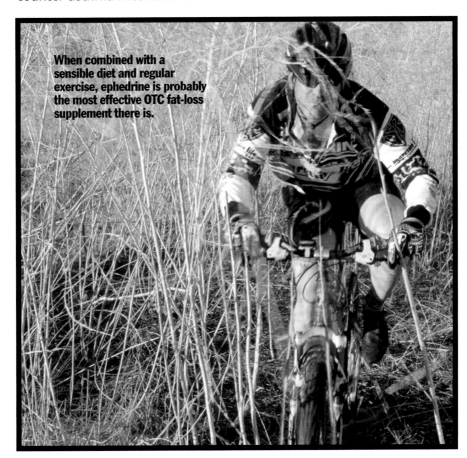

When combined with a sensible diet and regular exercise, ephedrine is probably the most effective OTC fat-loss supplement there is.

In the United States, ephedra and ephedrine are sold in health-food stores under a number of brand names. Ephedrine is widely used for weight loss, as an energy booster, and to enhance athletic performance. Let's look at fat loss first.

Ephedrine is an example of a thermogenic drug. This means it raises body temperature slightly, thus making fat deposits more susceptible for burning as an energy source. When combined with a sensible diet and regular exercise, ephedrine is probably the most effective OTC fat-loss supplement there is.

If all ephedrine did was speed up fat loss, there probably wouldn't be much fuss. Unfortunately ephedrine is also a stimulant, ranking somewhere between caffeine and amphetamine in this regard. Now while some individuals obtain their "kick" from common cold medications, others opt for pure ephedrine tablets (usually containing 25 mg per tablet). We'll be the first to admit that while one or two ephedrine tablets will probably not harm a healthy person, more than this could lead to major health issues.

A few people mistakenly subscribe to the "some is good, more is better" philosophy when it comes to stimulant usage. What's worse, many teens combine ephedrine with alcohol as a party mixture. *Deaths* have been linked to this dangerous concoction, but on the other hand the media usually neglects to report on the alcohol factor or the dosage of ephedrine involved. It's made to sound as if the teenager died from taking just one or two ephedrine tablets.

Is it any wonder, then, that the FDA (US) and Health and Welfare Canada are attempting to ban ephedrine products containing more than 8 mg per serving? (Perhaps they already have done by now.)

Should teens use ephedrine?

Despite our view that ephedrine is relatively safe – provided it's not abused (or used by someone with a heart condition) – it's prob-

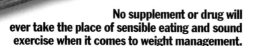

No supplement or drug will ever take the place of sensible eating and sound exercise when it comes to weight management.

ably a good idea for teens to avoid ephedrine. For one thing it's very easy to build tolerance to ephedrine. By that we mean, a point will be reached where one tablet is not enough. You'll need to take two. After a period of time, two becomes three, which in turn becomes four. Another reason to avoid ephedrine is that you may start to rely on it to replace regular exercise and diet. No drug or supplement will ever take the place of sensible eating and sound exercise when it comes to weight management.

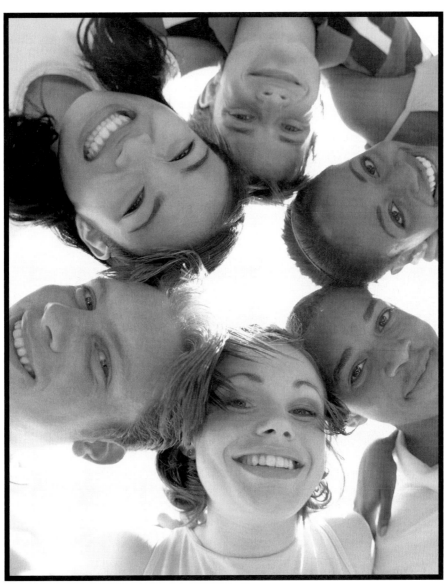

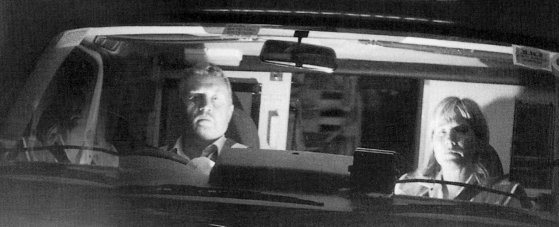

CHAPTER FOURTEEN

The Dangers
of Recreational
Drugs

Although tobacco and alcohol are the most common substances found in high schools, other substances such as Ecstasy, Herbal Ecstasy, Rohypnol, GHB, Ketamine and LSD have gained popularity with teens in recent years. Nightclubs, bars, parties and raves typically attract teenagers, college students and young adults who may risk their health in the interest of a good time. Raves are a form of dance and recreation that is held in a clandestine location with fast-paced high-volume music, a variety of high-tech entertainment, and often the use of drugs.

Young people are attracted to these club drugs for their cheap, intoxicating highs, mistakenly believing them to be safe. Unfortunately, most partygoers do not realize the dangers of using club drugs. Once more, combinations of any of these drugs with alcohol can lead to unexpected adverse reactions – and death!

Ecstasy

Ecstasy or MDMA (methylene dioxymethamphetamine) is a stimulant that combines the properties of methamphetamine or "speed" with mind-altering or hallucinogenic properties. Considered the most commonly used "designer drug," Ecstasy is a close derivative of methamphetamine, and can be described as a *hallucinogenic stimulant.* Designer drugs are illicit variations of other drugs. Because of many different recipes used to manufacture Ecstasy, deaths have been caused by some other substances inadvertently created during production, such as PMA (paramethamphetamine).

Ecstasy is illegal, and is known on the street as Adam, X-TC, Clarity, Essence, Stacy, Lover's Speed, Eve, etc. Ecstasy is most often found in tablet, capsule or powder form and is usually consumed orally, although it can also be injected. Ecstasy is sometimes packaged in capsules or generic tablets to imitate prescription drugs, with the average "dose" costing anywhere from $7 to $30 per pill. Ecstasy can also contain methadone, LSD, opiates such as heroin or Fentanyl, or strong anesthetics such as ketamine.

What are the effects of Ecstasy?

An Ecstasy high can last from 6 to 24 hours, with the average "trip" lasting only about 3 to 4 hours. At moderate doses, Ecstasy is reported to cause euphoria, feelings of well-being, enhanced mental or emotional clarity, anxiety or paranoia. Heavier doses can cause hallucinations, sensations of lightness and floating, depression, paranoid thinking, and violent, irrational behavior.

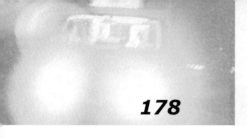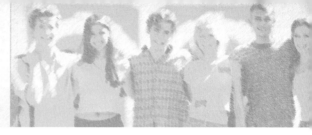

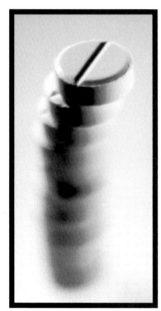

Physical reactions can include the following symptoms: loss of appetite, nausea, vomiting, blurred vision, increased heart rate and blood pressure, muscle tension, faintness, chills, sweating, tremors, reduced appetite, insomnia, convulsions, and a loss of control over voluntary body movements. Some reactions have been reported to persist from one to 14 days after taking Ecstasy.

Individuals who are pregnant, have a heart condition, are epileptic, or have high blood pressure are at high risk of adverse reactions. In addition, users are at particular risk of heat exhaustion and dehydration with physical exertion, particularly when Ecstasy is taken in a dance-party setting. Deaths have occurred because users don't drink enough water and become overheated.

What is Rohypnol?

Rohypnol (flunitrazepam) is a strong sedative, which is manufactured and distributed by Hoffman-La Roche. It is illegal in the US. A member of the benzodiazepine family, which includes drugs such as Librium, Xanax and Valium, Rohypnol is about ten times the strength of Valium. Typically, black-market Rohypnol is smuggled into Texas from the Mexican pharmacias; supplies in Florida come from Latin America. Street prices in Texas range from $1 to $5 per pill. Slang terms for Rohypnol include Roach, Roche (ro-shay), Roofies, Run-Trip-and-Fall, R-2, Mexican Valium, Ropynol, Rib and Rope. In Texas, to go under the influence of Rohypnol is "to get roached."

How is Rohypnol used?

Rohypnol is manufactured as small, white tablets with "Roche" inscribed on one side with an encircled "1" or "2" indicating a 1 mg or 2 mg dose. These tablet markings are commonly found on other Roche pharmaceuticals, and a pattern of abusing any drug made by Roche (Valium, Klonopin/Clonopin, Rivotril) has also developed. Rohypnol is usually taken orally, although there are reports that it has been ground up and snorted. Rohypnol is illegal in the United States, and it can draw significant penalties for the possession and sale of the drug.

What are the effects of Rohypnol?

After taking Rohypnol, the user may feel intoxicated, then sleepy – a feeling that may last up to 8 hours. Users under the influence may exhibit slurred speech, impaired judgment, and difficulty walking. Rohypnol can cause deep sedation, respiratory distress, blackouts that can last up to 24 hours, and amnesia where users forget events experienced while under the influence. In some cases, the drug has paradoxical effects and causes users to become aggressive. The potential for overdose or death can occur, especially when mixed with other drugs like alcohol.

What is GHB?

GHB (gamma-hydroxybutyrate) was once sold in health-food stores as a performance-enhancing additive to bodybuilding formulas. Although rumored that GHB stimulates muscle growth, this claim has never been proven. GHB is a central nervous system depressant that is abused for its intoxicating effects. In 1990 the FDA banned the used of GHB except under the supervision of a physician because of many reports of severe, uncontrollable side effects. Slang terms for GHB include Grievous Bodily Harm, Easy Lay, Gook, Gamma 10, Liquid X, Liquid E, Liquid G, Georgia Home Boy, Soap, Scoop, Salty Water, Somatomax, G-riffick, Cherry Meth, Fantasy, Organic Quaalude, Nature's Quaalude and Zonked.

How is GHB used?

GHB is consumed orally in capsule form or as a grainy, white to sandy-colored powder. Powdered GHB is often dissolved in liquids like water or alcoholic beverages and then consumed. However, it is most frequently sold as a slightly salty, clear liquid in small bottles where users pay by the capful or by the teaspoonful. Most GHB is created in clandestine laboratories where purity and quality cannot be guaranteed. Often substituted for Ecstasy, another club drug, a capful may cost the user $3 to $5 per dose. GHB is also used as a sedative to come down off stimulants like ephedrine, Ecstasy, speed or cocaine.

What are the effects of GHB?

GHB produces intoxication followed by deep sedation. Once ingested, the drug will begin to take effect within 15 minutes to an hour, lasting 1 to 3 hours. GHB can cause nausea, vomiting, delusions, depression, vertigo, visual disturbances, seizures, respiratory distress, loss of consciousness, amnesia and coma. When combined with alcohol and other drugs, the potential for deadly overdoses escalates rapidly. Numerous cases of overdose in Texas and nationwide have required emergency room treatment and mechanical assistance to breathe.

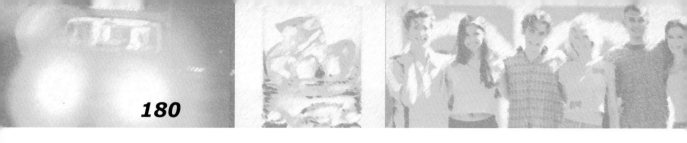

What is Special K or ketamine?

Ketamine (ketamine hydrochloride) is primarily used in veterinary medicine. Its use as a surgical anesthetic for humans is limited. Most supplies found on the street are diverted from legitimate sources. On the club scene, ketamine can be found in liquid form or as a white powder that is snorted, or smoked with marijuana or tobacco products. A combination of ketamine and cocaine is called "CK." Other slang terms are Special K, Vitamin K, New Ecstasy, Psychedelic Heroin, Ketalar, Ketaject and Super-K.

What are the effects of ketamine?

Users experience profound hallucinations and visual distortions similar to the effects of PCP. They call these effects "K-Land." A larger dose can produce a more frightening experience called a "K-hole" or an "out-of-body, near-death experience." They may also experience a loss of senses, sense of time, and identity which can last anywhere from 30 minutes to 2 hours. Ketamine can cause delirium, amnesia, impaired motor function, high blood pressure, depression, recurrent flashbacks, and potentially fatal respiratory problems.

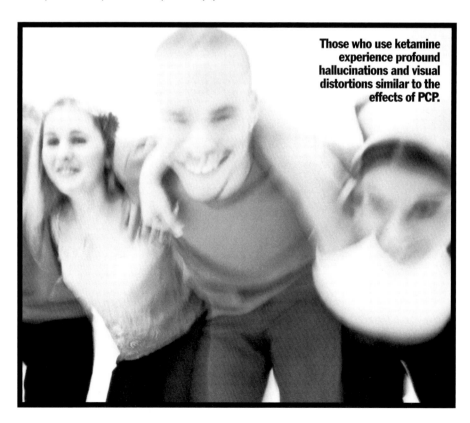

Those who use ketamine experience profound hallucinations and visual distortions similar to the effects of PCP.

What is LSD?

LSD (lysergic acid diethylamid) is a potent hallucinogen derived from lysergic acid. Lysergic acid can be found on ergot, a fungus that grows on rye and other grains. Commonly referred to as "acid" on the club scene, a "hit" or dose can be found as tablets, capsules, liquid form, thin squares of gelatin, or absorbed on colorful paper to be licked. Although colorless and odorless, LSD has a slight bitter taste. "Blotter acid," which is absorbent paper soaked in LSD and sold as squares, can be obtained for $4 to $5 for a "high" or "trip" that lasts 3 to 12 hours. Other slang terms for LSD include Microdot, White Lightning, Blue Heaven, Windowpane, and Sugar Cubes. *And it's illegal.* LSD is a Schedule 1 Controlled Substance with severe penalties for possession and use.

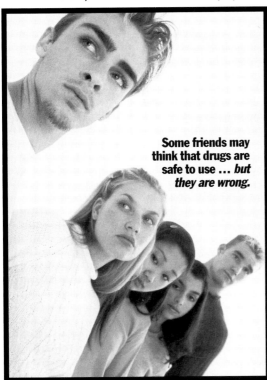

Some friends may think that drugs are safe to use ... *but they are wrong.*

What does LSD do?

The effects of LSD are wildly unpredictable depending on a number of factors. The user will begin to feel the effects within 30 to 90 minutes of ingestion and the "high" may last up to 12 hours. Users under the influence will have dilated pupils, increased body temperature, increased heart and blood pressure rates, loss of appetite, sleeplessness, dry mouth, tremors, and increased perspiration. A "bad trip" could include terrifying thoughts and feelings, fear of losing control, fear of insanity and death, as well as flashbacks after the fact. Moreover, LSD may reveal long lasting psychological problems, including schizophrenia and severe depression. Chronic users can develop a tolerance to LSD, meaning they must take more of the drug to feel the same effects.

How are teens usually introduced to club drugs?

Many young people are introduced to club drugs by their peers on the nightclub or rave scene. People often try drugs like Ecstasy, Herbal Ecstasy, Rohypnol, GHB, Ketamine, and LSD because their friends are using them, and they think that drugs are safe to use ... *but they are wrong.*

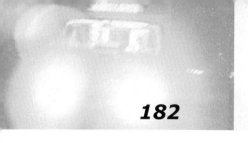
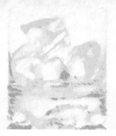
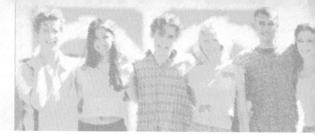

Are adolescents and young adults at risk?

One major concern about these club drugs is their widespread use among high school youths, college students, and young adults who frequent nightclubs and all-night rave parties. Lured by the availability and intoxicating effects of these drugs, many youths are unaware of the dangers. Rohypnol and GHB, in particular, can cause blackouts and amnesia – and that places individuals under the influence at risk of sexual assault or other criminal acts. In addition, when young people start using drugs regularly, they often lose interest in school work, which of course affects academic success as well. Chronic drug use can place students and young adults at risk of dropping out of school or college, loss of employment, and possible encounters with law enforcement.

Marijuana

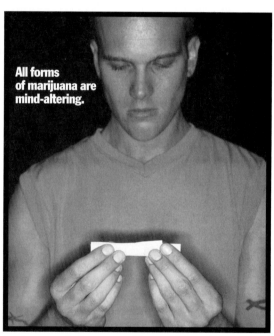

All forms of marijuana are mind-altering.

Marijuana is a green, brown, or gray mixture of dried, shredded leaves, stems, seeds and flowers of the hemp plant. You may hear marijuana called by street names such as pot, herb, weed, grass, boom, Mary Jane, gangster or chronic. There are more than 200 slang terms for marijuana. Sinsemilla (sin-seh-me-yah; it's a Spanish word), hashish ("hash" for short), and hash oil are stronger forms of marijuana.

All forms of marijuana are mind-altering. In other words, they change how the brain works. They all contain THC (delta-9-tetrahydrocannabinol), the main active chemical in marijuana. They also contain more than 400 other chemicals. Marijuana's effects on the user depend on the strength or potency of the THC it contains. THC potency of marijuana has increased since the 1970s, but has been about the same since the mid-1980s.

Q: How is marijuana used?
A: Marijuana is usually smoked as a cigarette (called a joint or a nail), or in a pipe or a bong. Recently, it has appeared in cigars called blunts.

Q: How long does marijuana stay in the user's body?
A: THC in marijuana is strongly absorbed by fatty tissues in various organs. Generally, traces (metabolites) of THC can be detected by

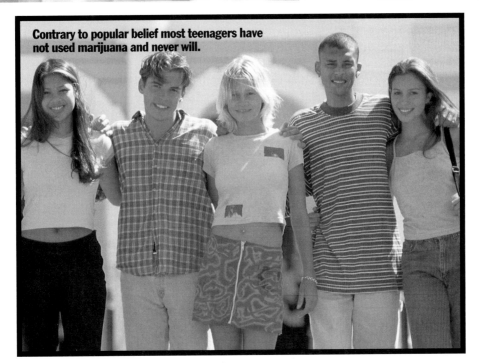

Contrary to popular belief most teenagers have not used marijuana and never will.

standard urine-testing methods several days after a smoking session. However, in heavy chronic users, traces can sometimes be detected for weeks after they have stopped using marijuana.

Q: How many teens smoke marijuana?
A: Contrary to popular belief most teenagers have not used marijuana and never will. Among students surveyed in a yearly national survey, only about one in five 10th-graders report they are current marijuana users (that is, used marijuana within the past month). Fewer than one in four high school seniors are current marijuana users.

Q: Why do young people use marijuana?
A: There are many reasons why some children and young teens start smoking marijuana. Most young people smoke marijuana because their friends or brothers and sisters use marijuana and pressure them to try it. Some young people use it because they see older people in the family using it. Others may think it's cool to use marijuana because they hear songs about it and see it on TV and in movies.

Some teens may feel they need marijuana and other drugs to help them escape from problems at home, at school, or with friends. No matter how many shirts and caps you see printed with the marijuana leaf, or how many groups sing about it, remember this: You don't have to use marijuana just because you think everybody else is doing it. *Most teens do not use marijuana!*

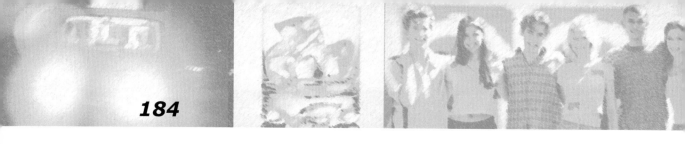

Q: *What happens if you smoke marijuana?*
A: The effects of the drug on each person depend on the user's experience, as well as:
• how strong the marijuana is (how much THC it has)
• what the user expects to happen
• where (the place) the drug is used
• how it is taken
• whether the user is drinking alcohol or using other drugs

Some people feel nothing at all when they smoke marijuana. Others may feel relaxed or high. Sometimes marijuana makes users feel thirsty and very hungry – an effect called "the munchies." Some get bad effects from marijuana. They may suffer sudden feelings of anxiety and have paranoid thoughts. This is more likely to happen when a more potent variety of marijuana is used.

Q: *What are the short-term effects of marijuana use?*
A: The short-term effects of marijuana include:
• problems with memory and learning
• distorted perception (sights, sounds, time, touch)
• trouble with thinking and problem-solving
• loss of coordination
• increased heart rate, anxiety

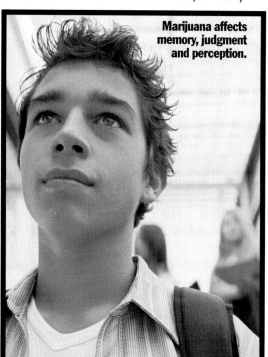

Marijuana affects memory, judgment and perception.

These effects are even greater when other drugs are mixed with the marijuana – and users do not always know what drugs are given to them.

Q: *Does marijuana affect school, sports or other activities?*
A: It can. Marijuana affects memory, judgment and perception. The drug can make you mess up in school, in sports or clubs, or with your friends. If you're high on marijuana, you are more likely to make stupid mistakes that could embarrass or even hurt you. If you use marijuana a lot, you could start to lose interest in how you look and how you're getting along at school or work.

Athletes could find their performance is off. Timing, movements and coordination are all affected by THC. Also, since marijuana use can affect thinking and judgment, users can forget to have safe sex and possibly expose themselves to HIV, the virus that causes AIDS.

Q: What are the long-term effects of marijuana use?
A: Findings so far show that regular use of marijuana or THC may play a role in some kinds of cancer and in problems with the respiratory and immune systems.
• *Cancer* – It's hard to know for sure whether or not regular marijuana use causes cancer. But it is known that marijuana contains some of the same, and sometimes even more, of the cancer-causing chemicals found in tobacco smoke. Studies show that someone who smokes five joints per week may be taking in as many cancer-causing chemicals as someone who smokes a full pack of cigarettes every day.
• *Lungs and airways* – People who smoke marijuana often develop the same kinds of breathing problems that cigarette smokers have: coughing and wheezing. They tend to have more chest colds than nonusers. They are also at greater risk of getting lung infections like pneumonia.
• *Immune system* – Animal studies have found that THC can damage the cells and tissues in the body that help protect people from disease. When the immune cells are weakened, you are more likely to get sick.

Q: Does marijuana lead to the use of other drugs?
A: It could. Long-term studies of high school students and their patterns of drug use show that very few young people use other illegal drugs without first trying marijuana. For example, the risk of using cocaine is 104 times greater for those who have tried marijuana than for those who have never tried it. Using marijuana puts children and teens in contact with people who are users and sellers of other drugs. So there is more of a risk that a marijuana user will be exposed to and urged to try more drugs.

Using marijuana puts teens in contact with people who are users and sellers of other drugs.

To better determine this risk, scientists are examining the possibility that long-term marijuana use may create changes in the brain that make a person more at risk of becoming addicted to other drugs, such as alcohol or cocaine. While not all young people who use marijuana go on to use other drugs, further research is needed to predict who will be at greatest risk.

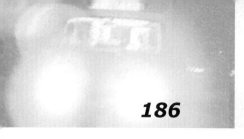

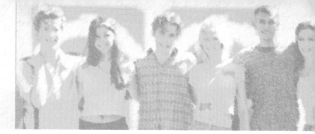
Q: How can you tell if someone has been using marijuana?
A: If someone is high on marijuana, he or she might ...
• seem dizzy and have trouble walking
• seem silly and giggly for no reason
• have very red, bloodshot eyes
• have a hard time remembering things that just happened
When the early effects fade, over a few hours the user can become very sleepy.

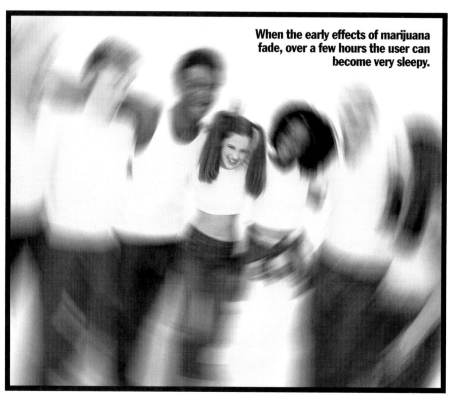

When the early effects of marijuana fade, over a few hours the user can become very sleepy.

Q: Is marijuana sometimes used as a medicine?
A: There has been much talk about the possible medical use of marijuana. Under US law since 1970, marijuana has been a Schedule I controlled substance. This means that the drug, at least in its smoked form, has no commonly accepted medical use.

THC, the active chemical in marijuana, is manufactured into a pill available by prescription that can be used to treat the nausea and vomiting that occur with certain cancer treatments and to help AIDS patients eat more to keep up their weight. According to scientists, more research needs to be done on side effects and potential benefits of marijuana before it is used medically with any regularity.

Q: How does marijuana affect driving?
A: Marijuana has serious harmful effects on the skills required to drive safely: alertness, the ability to concentrate, coordination, and the ability to react quickly. These effects can last up to 24 hours after smoking marijuana. Marijuana use can make it difficult to judge distances and react to signals and sounds on the road.

Marijuana may play a role in car accidents. In one study conducted in Memphis, Tennessee, researchers found that, of 150 reckless drivers who were tested for drugs at the arrest scene, 33 percent tested positive for marijuana, and 12 percent tested positive for both marijuana and cocaine. Data have also shown that while smoking marijuana, people show the same lack of coordination on standard "drunk driver" tests as do people who have had too much to drink.

Q: If a girl is pregnant and smokes marijuana, will the baby be hurt?
A: Doctors advise pregnant women not to use any drugs because they could harm the growing fetus. One animal study has linked marijuana use to loss of the fetus very early in pregnancy.

Some scientific studies have found that babies born to marijuana users were shorter, weighed less, and had smaller head sizes than those born to mothers who did not use the drug. Smaller babies are more likely to develop health problems. There are also research data showing nervous system problems in children of mothers who smoked marijuana.

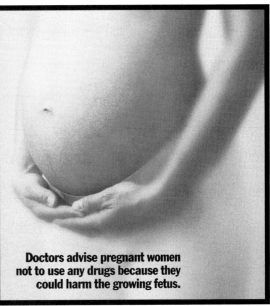

Doctors advise pregnant women not to use any drugs because they could harm the growing fetus.

Researchers cannot be certain whether a newborn baby's health problems, if they are caused by marijuana, will continue as the child grows. Preliminary research shows that children born to mothers who used marijuana regularly during pregnancy may have trouble concentrating.

Q: What does marijuana do to the brain?
A: Some studies show that when people have smoked large amounts of marijuana for years, the drug takes its toll on mental functions. Heavy or daily use of marijuana affects the parts of the brain that control memory, attention and learning. A working short-term memory is needed to learn and to perform tasks that call for more than one or two steps.

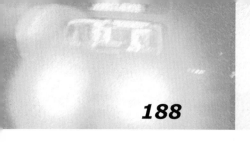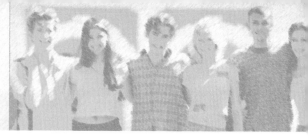

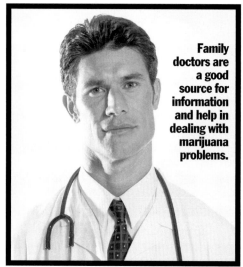

Family doctors are a good source for information and help in dealing with marijuana problems.

Smoking marijuana causes some changes in the brain that are like those caused by cocaine, heroin and alcohol. Some researchers believe that these changes may put a person more at risk of becoming addicted to other drugs, such as cocaine or heroin. Scientists are still learning about the many ways that marijuana could affect the brain.

Q: Can people become addicted to marijuana?
A: Yes. While not everyone who uses marijuana becomes addicted, when a user begins to seek out and take the drug compulsively, that person is said to be dependent or addicted to the drug. In 1995 165,000 people entering drug treatment programs reported marijuana as their primary drug of abuse, showing they need help to stop using the drug.

According to one study, marijuana use by teenagers who have prior serious antisocial problems can quickly lead to dependence on the drug. Some frequent, heavy users of marijuana develop a tolerance for it. "Tolerance" means that the user needs larger doses of the drug to get the same desired results that he or she once got from smaller amounts.

Q: What if a person wants to quit using the drug?
A: Up until a few years ago, it was hard to find treatment programs specifically for marijuana users. Now researchers are testing different ways to help marijuana users abstain. There are currently no medications for treating marijuana addiction. Treatment programs focus on counseling and group support systems. There are also a number of programs designed especially to help teenagers who are abusers. Family doctors are also a good source for information and help in dealing with adolescent marijuana problems.

Cocaine

Slang terms include: *coke, dust, toot, snow, blow, sneeze, powder, lines, rock (crack).*

Cocaine affects your brain. The word *cocaine* refers to the drug in both powder (cocaine) and crystal (crack) form. It is made from the coca plant and causes a short-lived high that is immediately followed by the opposite – intense feelings of depression, edginess, and a craving for more of the drug. Cocaine may be snorted as a powder, converted to a liquid form for injection with a needle, or processed into a crystal form to be smoked.

Cocaine affects your body. People who use cocaine often don't eat or sleep regularly. They can experience increased heart rate, muscle spasms and convulsions. If they snort cocaine, they can also permanently damage their nasal tissue.

Cocaine affects your emotions. Using cocaine can make you feel paranoid, angry, hostile and anxious, even when you're not high.

Cocaine is addictive. Cocaine interferes with the way your brain processes chemicals that create feelings of pleasure, so you need more and more of the drug just to feel normal. People who become addicted to cocaine start to lose interest in other areas of their lives, like school, friends and sports.

Cocaine can kill you! Cocaine use can cause heart attacks, seizures, strokes and respiratory failure. People who share needles can also contract hepatitis, HIV/AIDS and other diseases.

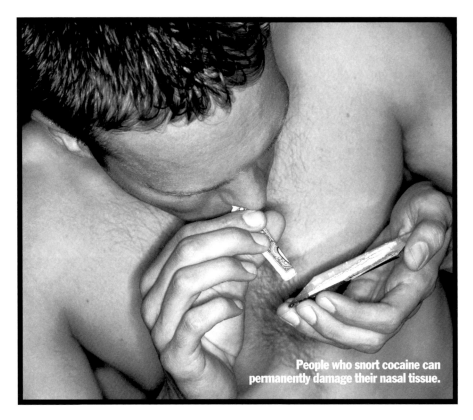

People who snort cocaine can permanently damage their nasal tissue.

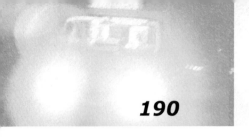

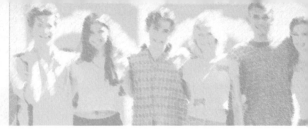

Know the Law
Cocaine *in any form* is illegal. Stay informed. Even first-time cocaine users can have a seizure or fatal heart attack.

Know the Risks
Combining cocaine with other drugs or alcohol is extremely dangerous. The effects of one drug can magnify the effects of another, and mixing substances can be deadly.

Cocaine is Expensive
Regular users can spend hundreds and even thousands of dollars on cocaine each week and some will do anything to support their addiction.

Stay in Control
Cocaine impairs your judgment which may lead to unwise decisions relating to sexual activity. This can increase your risk for HIV/AIDS and other diseases, as well as rape and unplanned pregnancy.

Look Around You
The vast majority of teens *are not* using cocaine. According to a 1998 study, less than 1 percent of teens are regular cocaine users. In fact, 98 percent of teens have never even tried cocaine.

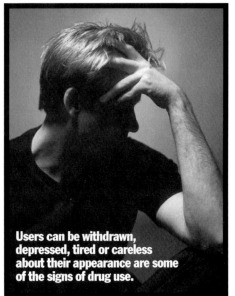

Users can be withdrawn, depressed, tired or careless about their appearance are some of the signs of drug use.

How can you tell if a friend is using cocaine? Sometimes it's tough to tell. But there are signs you can look for. If your friend has one or more of the following warning signs, he or she may be using cocaine or other illicit drugs:
- red, bloodshot eyes
- a runny nose or frequently sniffing
- a change in eating or sleeping patterns
- a change in groups of friends
- a change in school grades or behavior
- withdrawn, depressed, tired or careless about his or her personal appearance
- loss of interest in school, family or activities he or she used to enjoy
- frequently needing money

What can you do to help someone who is using cocaine? Be a real friend. Save a life. Encourage your friend to stop or seek professional help.

Alcohol

Slang terms include: *booze, sauce, brews, brewskis, hooch, hard stuff, juice ...*

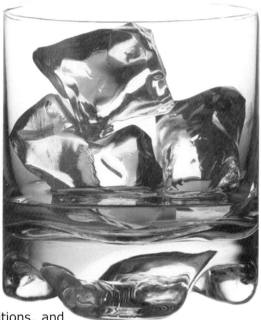

Alcohol affects your brain. Drinking alcohol leads to a loss of coordination, poor judgment, slowed reflexes, distorted vision, memory lapses, and even blackouts.

Alcohol affects your body. Alcohol can damage every organ in your body. It is absorbed directly into your bloodstream and can increase your risk for a variety of life-threatening diseases, including cancer.

Alcohol affects your self-control. Alcohol depresses your central nervous system, lowers your inhibitions, and impairs your judgment. Drinking can lead to risky behaviors, including having unprotected sex. This may expose you to HIV/AIDS and other sexually transmitted diseases or cause unwanted pregnancy.

Alcohol can kill you! Drinking large amounts of alcohol can lead to coma or even death. Also, in 1998, 35.8 percent of traffic deaths of 15-to-20-year-olds were alcohol-related.

Alcohol can hurt you, even if you're not the one drinking. If you're around people who are drinking, you have an increased risk of being seriously injured, involved in a car crash, or affected by violence. At the very least, you may have to deal with people who are sick, out of control, or unable to take care of themselves.

Know the Law

It is illegal to buy or possess alcohol if you are a minor. Regional laws vary, but in most places in North America, the legal age is 21.

Get the Facts

One drink can make you fail a breath test. In some states people under the age of 21 who are found to have any amount of alcohol in their system can lose their driver's license, be subject to a heavy fine, or have their car permanently taken away.

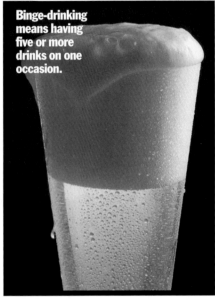

Binge-drinking means having five or more drinks on one occasion.

Stay Informed

Binge-drinking means having five or more drinks on one occasion. About 15 percent of teens are binge-drinkers in any given month.

Know the Risks

Mixing alcohol with medications or illicit drugs is extremely dangerous and can lead to accidental death. For example, alcohol-medication interactions may have been a factor in at least 25 percent of emergency room admissions.

Keep Your Edge

Alcohol can make you gain weight and give you bad breath.

Look Around You

Most teens aren't drinking alcohol. Research shows that 70 percent of people 12 to 20 haven't had a drink in the past month.

How can you tell if a friend has a drinking problem? Sometimes it's tough to tell. But there are signs you can look for. If your friend has one or more of the following warning signs, he or she may have a problem with alcohol:

- getting drunk on a regular basis
- lying about how much alcohol he or she is using
- believing that alcohol is necessary to have fun
- having frequent hangovers
- feeling run down, depressed, or even suicidal
- having "blackouts" – forgetting what he or she did while drinking
- having problems at school or getting in trouble with the law

What can you do to help someone who has a drinking problem? Be a real friend. You might even save a life. Encourage your friend to stop or seek professional help.

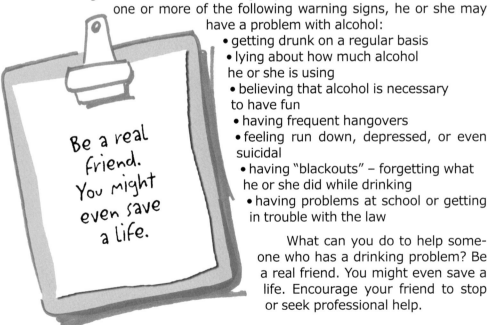

Be a real friend. You might even save a life.

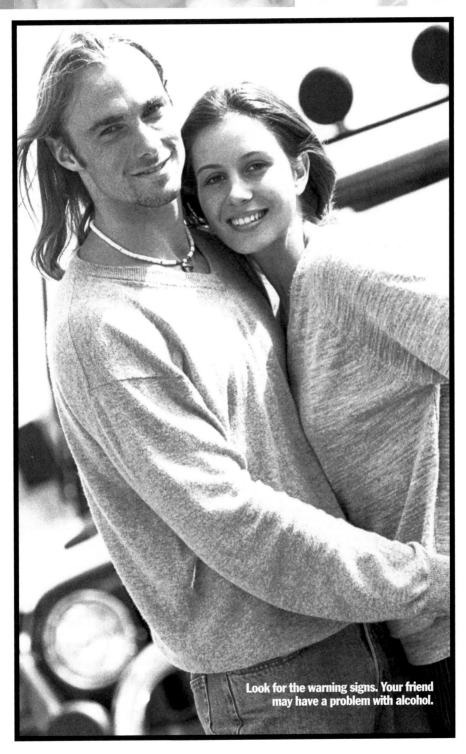

Look for the warning signs. Your friend may have a problem with alcohol.

CHAPTER FIFTEEN

Anabolic Steroids

What are steroids?

Steroids, sometimes referred to as *roids* or *juice,* are very closely related to certain hormones. The body produces steroids to support certain functions such as fighting disease and promoting growth. Anabolic steroids are artificially produced hormones that are similar to testosterone. Testosterone (pronounced: teh-stoss-tuh-rone) is a natural male sex hormone produced in the human body. Although testosterone is a male hormone, girls' bodies produce smaller amounts of it as well. Testosterone promotes masculine traits that guys develop during puberty, such as deepening of the voice and the growth of body hair. Testosterone levels also affect how aggressive a person is and how much sex drive he or she has. Athletes sometimes take anabolic steroids to help increase muscle mass and body strength.

Steroids can be taken in the form of pills, powders or injections. Some types of steroids have medical uses and are available by prescription, or in the form of dietary supplements. Dietary supplements that contain steroids often make *false claims* and very little is known about the long-term effects on the body of some of these substances.

How do anabolic steroids work?
Anabolic steroids stimulate muscle tissue to grow and "bulk up" by mimicking the effect of testosterone on the body. Steroids have become popular because they may improve endurance, strength, and muscle mass. But research has not shown that they improve skill, agility or performance.

Dangers of Steroids
Anabolic steroids cause many different types of problems. Less serious side effects include acne, purple or red spots on the body, swelling of legs and feet, persistent bad breath, and less commonly jaundice, or yellowing of the skin. Other side effects are:
• premature balding
• dizziness
• mood swings, including anger, aggression and depression
• nausea
• vomiting
• trembling
• high blood pressure that can damage the heart or blood vessels
• aching joints
• greater chance of injuring muscles
• liver damage
• shortening of final adult height

Risk for guys include:
• testicular shrinkage
• pain when urinating
• breast development
• impotence (inability to get an erection)
• sterility (inability to have children)

Risk for girls include:
• facial hair growth
• masculine trait development and loss of feminine body characteristics, such as shrinking of the breasts
• menstrual cycle changes

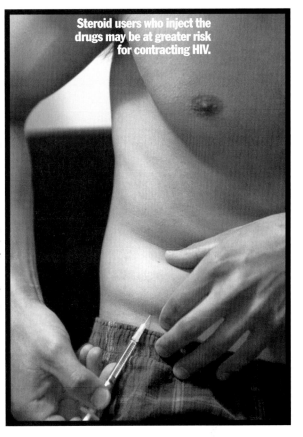

Steroid users who inject the drugs may be at greater risk for contracting HIV.

Steroid users who inject the drugs may be at greater risk for contracting HIV (human immunodeficiency virus), the virus that causes AIDS, if they share needles with other users. They are also at greater risk for contracting hepatitis, a disease of the liver. This is particularly scary because it's not always possible to tell if your friend or teammate is sick. It's not enough to take their word for it; sharing needles is never safe.

Anabolic steroids are so controversial because of all the health risks associated with them. Most are illegal and are banned by professional sports organizations and medical associations. If an athlete is caught using steroids, his or her career can be destroyed.

Despite the obvious dangers, some people combine or "stack" anabolic steroids with other drugs. Because it is difficult to understand how the drugs interact, there is the possibility of taking a deadly combination. Just as many medications should not be taken together, anabolic steroids have the same potential for negative interactions. Emergency departments have reported cases of vomiting, tremors, dizziness, and even coma (unconsciousness) in patients admitted after taking combinations of steroids.[1]

Steroids can also have serious psychological side effects. Some users become aggressive or combative, developing "roid rage," extreme uncontrolled bouts of anger caused by long-term steroid use. Others experience irritability, paranoia and severe depression when they try to stop taking steroids.

Alternatives to Steroids

Being a good athlete means training the healthy way: eating the right foods, practicing, and strength training without the use of drugs. Not only will you be improving your sports performance, you'll also be taking good care of your body.

[Ref. 1: www.kidshealth.org/teen/nutrition/move/steroids]

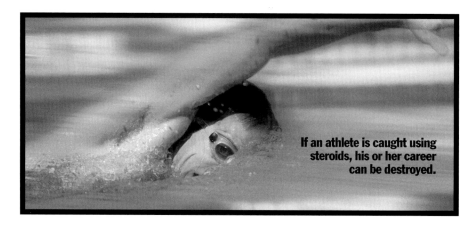

If an athlete is caught using steroids, his or her career can be destroyed.

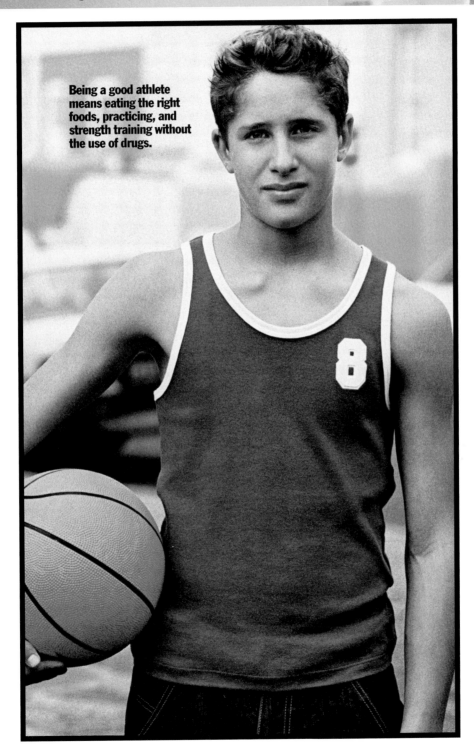

Being a good athlete means eating the right foods, practicing, and strength training without the use of drugs.

CHAPTER SIXTEEN

Birth Control

To do or not to do, that is the question ...

Few topics generate as much controversy as birth control for teens. On one side of the debate there are those who totally ignore the morality and dangers of sex (yes, unprotected sex can be dangerous!) and focus strictly on the prevention of pregnancy. On the other side are the "religious fanatics" who totally disagree with any form of birth control advice for teens. The authors sort of fall somewhere in the middle. We don't believe in unchecked promiscuous sex, but we also realize that no matter how often adults preach about not "doing it," some teens will still "do it." Therefore, in our view, it is better to be safe than sorry. The bottom line? If you are going to have sex, then it only makes sense to protect yourself from both STDs (sexually transmitted diseases) and an unwanted pregnancy. In short, you need to use some sort of birth control.

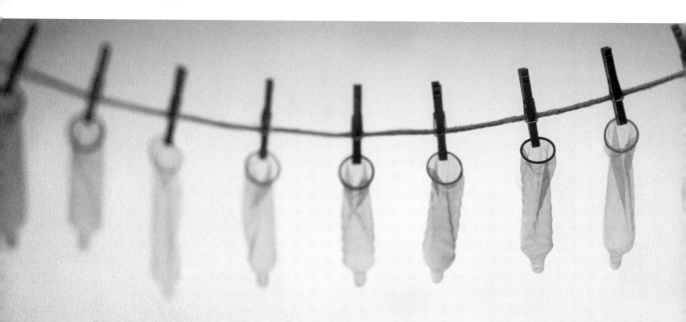

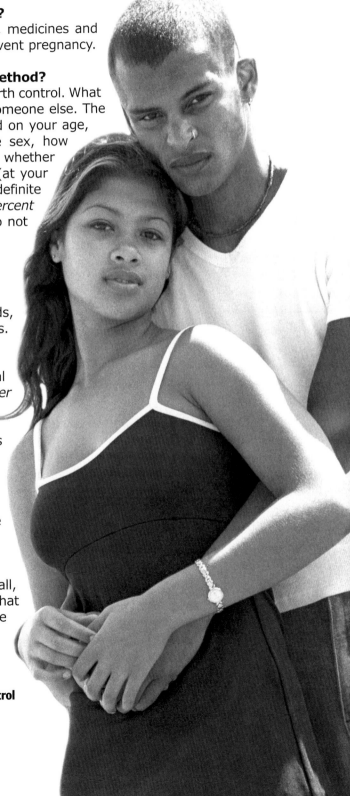

What are birth control methods?
Birth control methods are devices, medicines and approaches that people use to prevent pregnancy.

What is the best birth control method?
There is no one "best" method of birth control. What works for you may not work for someone else. The method you choose should depend on your age, your health, how often you have sex, how many sex partners you have, and whether or not you want to have children (at your age this last point should be a definite no!). However, the only *100 percent effective* birth control method is to not have sex.

Methods of Birth Control
Here is a list of birth control methods, how they work, and their side effects.

Barrier Methods
Cervical caps, condoms, dental dams, and diaphragms are *barrier methods* of birth control. They work by keeping the man's sperm from getting to the woman's egg. Condoms and dental dams can help keep STDs (including HIV/AIDS) from passing from person to person. Here is more information about each of the barrier methods.

Cervical Cap
What it is: The cervical cap is a small, soft rubber cup with a round rim that fits closely around the cervix. The doctor or nurse fits the girl for a cervical cap. You can only get the cap with a prescription.

The only 100 percent effective birth control method is to not have sex.

How it works: The cervical cap is used with a spermicide (a cream or jelly that kills sperm). Before having sex, the spermicide is squeezed from a tube into the cervical cap. Then the cap is put into the back of the vagina where it covers the cervix. This keeps the sperm from getting into the girl's cervix and uterus. Once in place, the cap can be left in for up to 48 hours. You may have sex more than once during that time as long as the cap is in place.

Side effects: There are no bad side effects from the cervical cap. Some women may have trouble putting the cap into their vagina and fitting it over the cervix. They must remember to take the cervical cap out, or risk infection if it is left in the vagina for over 48 hours.

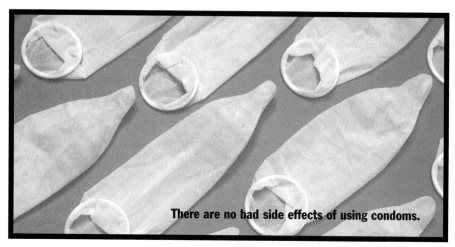

There are no bad side effects of using condoms.

Condom

What it is: A condom is a sheath (covering) that is put over an erect penis. Most condoms are made of latex rubber and some have spermicide (cream that kills sperm) on them. You do not need to see a doctor or have a prescription to get condoms. You can get them from the drug store. It's quite possible your school may have condom dispensers installed in the washrooms.

How it works: The condom is put over the erect penis before sex. There should be empty space at the tip of the condom to hold the sperm and keep it from going into a woman's vagina or cervix. You cannot use the same condom more than once, so be sure to use a new one each time you have sex. Do not put Vaseline jelly, hand lotion, massage oil or baby oil on condoms, because that will weaken the condom. Use condoms when you have sex – that's the best way to keep from getting and/or passing STDs, including HIV/AIDS.

Side effects: There are no bad side effects of using condoms.

Female Condom

What it is: The female condom looks a little like the male condom. It is a sheath (covering) that goes into the woman's vagina. Women do not need to see a doctor or have a prescription to get a female condom.

How it works: The closed end of the female condom is put into the vagina and the open end is left outside of the vagina, covering the vaginal lips (or labia). It should be put on before sex and used only once. Each time you have sex, she needs another condom. Do not use a female condom with a male condom. They may not stay in place together. The female condom helps protect against STDs, but it is not as effective as the male condom.

Side effects: There are no bad side effects from female condoms.

Dental Dam

What it is: The dental dam is a square piece of rubber that is put over the vaginal lips (labia).

How it works: The dental dam is put over the vaginal lips before having sex. It can help prevent STDs (including HIV/AIDS) from spreading.

Side effects: There are no bad side effects from the dental dam.

Diaphragm

What it is: The diaphragm is somewhat larger than the cervical cap, but works in the same way. It is a soft rubber cup with a round rim that fits inside the vagina and covers the cervix. The doctor or nurse fits the woman for a diaphragm and supplies the necessary prescription.

How it works: The diaphragm is used with a spermicide (a cream or jelly that kills sperm). Before sex, the woman squeezes spermicide from a tube into the diaphragm. Then she puts the diaphragm into the back of the vagina so that it covers the cervix. This keeps the sperm from getting into the cervix and uterus. She leaves the diaphragm in for 6 hours after she has sex. If she has more sex during the 6 hours, she must be sure to put more spermicide into the vagina.

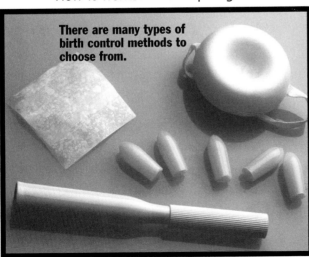

There are many types of birth control methods to choose from.

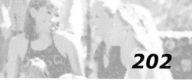

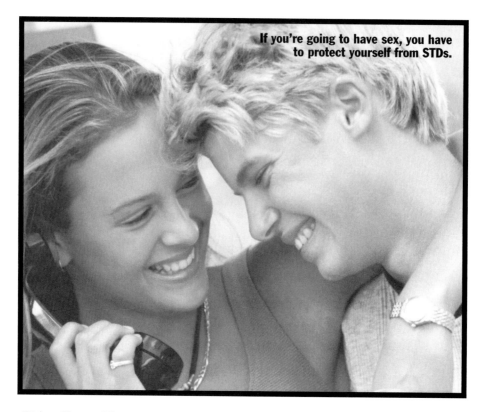

If you're going to have sex, you have to protect yourself from STDs.

Side effects: There are no bad side effects, as long as she remembers to take the diaphragm out after 6 hours. Some women may have trouble putting the diaphragm into their vagina and fitting it over the cervix.

Vaginal Spermicide

What it is: Spermicides kill sperm. Vaginal spermicides come in foam, cream, jelly, film, suppository and tablet forms.

How it works: The woman puts a spermicide into her vagina before sex to kill sperm and keep from getting pregnant. Doctors say spermicides work best when used with other methods of birth control such as a diaphragm, cervical cap or condom. Be sure to read the instructions on the spermicide. Some products tell you to wait 10 minutes or more after putting the spermicide in before you have sex. More spermicide must be put into the vagina each time you have sex. She should leave the spermicide in for 6 to 8 hours after sex.

Side effects: There are no bad side effects from vaginal spermicides. However, some women are allergic to the chemicals in spermicides.

The Pill

What it is: The birth control pill is made up of estrogen and progestin (female hormones). A woman must take her birth control pill every day to keep from getting pregnant. She needs to have a checkup and talk to her doctor before taking this medication. You need a prescription to get birth control pills.

How it works: The pill works by keeping the woman from ovulating (releasing an egg from her ovary each month).

Side effects: There are good and bad side effects from the birth control pill. Good side effects may include having more regular periods, and having less chance of getting ovarian and endometrial cancer and pelvic inflammatory disease (PID). Bad side effects may include more chance of getting heart disease, high blood pressure, blood clots and blocked arteries. Other more minor side effects include feeling sick to the stomach, headaches, sore breasts, weight gain, irregular bleeding and depression. Many of these minor side effects go away after a few months on the pill.

Women who smoke, are over 35, or have a history of blood clots or breast or endometrial cancer *should not* take the pill.

The pill works by keeping the woman from ovulating.

The Mini-Pill

What it is: The mini-pill is another kind of birth control pill. It has only one hormone in it, progestin. It must be taken every day. A woman needs to have a checkup and talk to her doctor before taking the mini-pill. You need a prescription to get the mini-pill.

How it works: The mini-pill works by changing a woman's cervical mucus, making it harder for the sperm to reach the egg, and by changing the lining of the uterus to keep the egg from implanting in the uterus.

Side effects: Because mini-pills do not have estrogen, they tend to have milder side effects than other birth control pills. The good side effects may include less bleeding and cramping during her period, and lower chances of getting endometrial and ovarian cancer, and pelvic inflammatory disease. Mild side effects of the mini-pill include changes in her period, missed periods, weight gain and sore breasts.

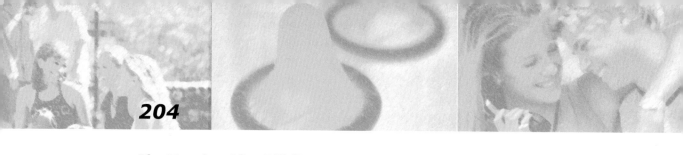

The Morning After Pill (Emergency Contraceptive)

What it is: Morning after pills are made up of female hormones, and are taken after a woman has unprotected sex (having sex without using a birth control method). Women must see their doctor to get a prescription for the morning after pill.

How it works: Morning after pills must be taken within 72 hours of having unprotected sex to keep the egg from reaching the uterus.

Side effects: Side effects may include nausea, vomiting, sore breasts, irregular bleeding, bloating and headaches. Frequent use of the morning after pill may cause periods to become irregular and unpredictable.

RU486 Pill

What it is: RU486 (also called "mifepristone") is different than emergency contraception. It is actually a series of pills that cause an abortion very early in pregnancy. RU486 is widely used in Europe, and was approved for use in the United States in September 2000. A woman must see her doctor to get a prescription for RU486. It is sometimes called the "abortion pill."

How it works: This pill causes the uterine lining to shed after the fertilized egg has planted itself there. RU486 can only be used up to six weeks after you become pregnant.

Side effects: Most women using RU486 will have side effects like cramping and bleeding. Bleeding and spotting usually last for 9 to 16 days. Women who have very heavy bleeding should see their doctor.

Frequent use of the morning after pill may cause periods to become irregular and unpredictable.

Depo-Provera

What it is: Depo-Provera is a birth control method that is injected (given as a shot) by a doctor into a woman's bottom or arm muscle every three months.

How it works: Depo-Provera uses the female hormone progestin to prevent ovulation; changes the cervical mucus to keep the sperm from reaching the egg; and changes the lining of the uterus to keep the egg from implanting in the uterus.

Side effects: Side effects may include irregular or missed periods, weight gain and sore breasts.

Norplant

What it is: Norplant is a birth control method that is put into a woman's arm. A doctor does an operation to put small, matchstick-sized rods under the skin of the upper arm.

How it works: Norplant works as the rods slowly release a hormone that keeps the woman from getting pregnant for three to five years. Norplant works like the mini-pill. It changes her cervical mucus, making it harder for the sperm to reach the egg, and by changing the lining of the uterus to keep the egg from implanting in the uterus.

Side effects: Side effects may include changes in her period, weight gain and sore breasts. Some women get infected at the site of the implant.

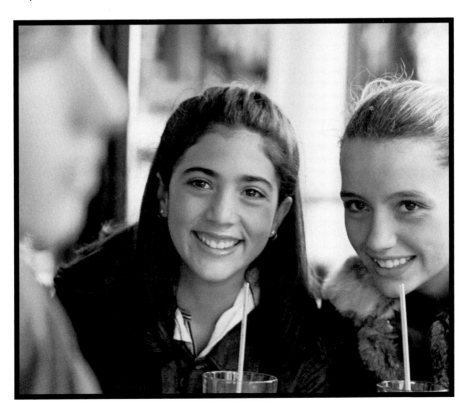

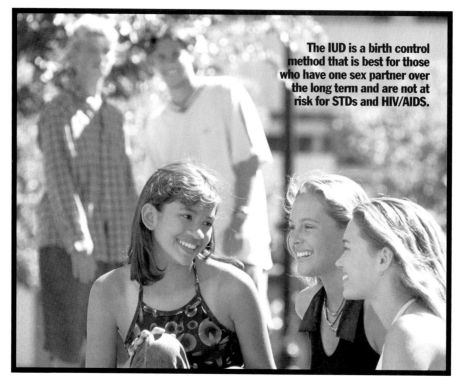

The IUD is a birth control method that is best for those who have one sex partner over the long term and are not at risk for STDs and HIV/AIDS.

Intrauterine Device (IUD)

What it is: An IUD is a T-shaped device that the doctor puts into a woman's uterus. Some IUDs must be replaced every year, while other IUDs can stay in her uterus for up to 10 years. The IUD is a birth control method that is best for those who have one sex partner over the long term and are not at risk for STDs and HIV/AIDS.

How it works: Doctors believe that IUDs work by keeping sperm and egg from meeting.

Side effects: Side effects may include more bleeding and cramping during her period, perforation of the uterus (the IUD pokes a hole in the uterus), and more chance of infections, including pelvic inflammatory disease (PID). The Dalkon Shield IUD was taken off the market in 1975 because it caused so many infections and problems for women. Today these serious problems from IUDs are rare.

Tubal Ligation

What it is: Tubal ligation ("getting the tubes tied") is a surgical method of birth control for women. This method of birth control is permanent, for women who do not want any or any more children. They must consult their doctor about tubal ligation. It is a serious decision.

How it works: A doctor operates on the woman's fallopian tubes to keep her eggs from going to her uterus.

Side effects: Side effects may include infection, bleeding, and problems from general anesthesia.

Vasectomy

What it is: Vasectomy is a surgical method of birth control for men. This is a permanent method of birth control and is for men who do not want any or any more children. Talk to your doctor about a vasectomy. It is a serious decision.

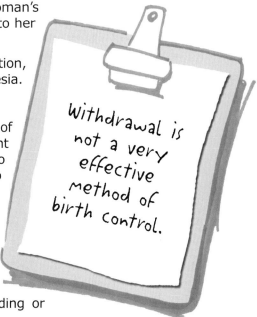

Withdrawal is not a very effective method of birth control.

How it works: A doctor operates on your *vas deferens* (tube which takes sperm from the testicle to the penis) to keep the sperm from going to your penis.

Side effects: Side effects may include bleeding or infection after the operation.

Natural Family Planning/Fertility Awareness

What it is: Natural family planning/fertility awareness are methods of birth control that rely on a woman's menstrual cycle to predict when she is likely to get pregnant and when she is not likely to get pregnant. Many couples use natural family planning as their method of birth control for health and/or religious reasons.

How it works: Natural family planning means that a man and woman do not have sex on days when she is most fertile (when she is most likely to get pregnant). Some people use a calendar to count the days before and after ovulation, others use a thermometer to track when she is most fertile, and others check changes in cervical mucus.

Side effects: There are no side effects from these methods.

Withdrawal

What it is: Withdrawal is a birth control method whereby the man pulls his penis out of the woman's vagina before he has an orgasm.

How it works: Withdrawal means "pulling out" before he releases his sperm. Some sperm can leak out of the penis before orgasm, so this is *not* a very effective method of birth control.

Side effects: There are no side effects from the withdrawal method.

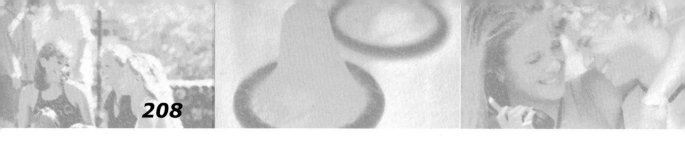

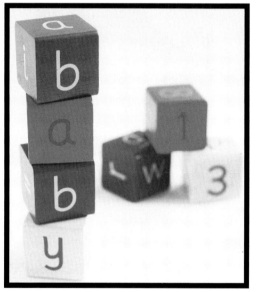

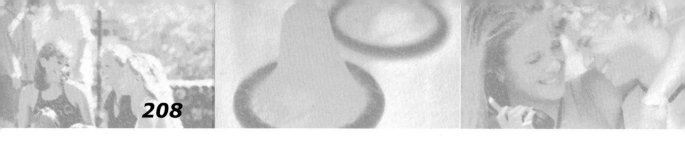

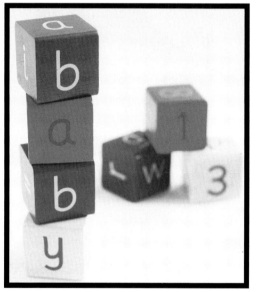

Does using birth control protect me from getting HIV/AIDS and other STDs?

The condom is the best birth control method for preventing HIV/AIDS and STDs. The cervical cap, dental dam, diaphragm, and female condom may give some protection, but they don't work as well as *the condom* in preventing STDs. Birth control pills, IUDs, Depo-Provera, Norplant, natural family planning, and the withdrawal method *do not* give you protection from STDs.

Five Common Causes of Pregnancy While Using Contraceptives

It would be great if birth control guaranteed against pregnancy, but unfortunately that's not the case. Believe it or not, 53 percent of unplanned pregnancies occur in women who are using contraceptives. The majority of unplanned pregnancies, 76 percent of them in 1994, occur in women over the age of 20 according to a 1999 article.[1] Why are so many women getting pregnant while practicing birth control? Here are five reasons why ...

1. Not following instructions for use correctly – If she takes "the pill," she should take it at the same time every day and make sure she follows all directions for her particular prescription. If you use condoms, make sure you are using them properly and that they are in good condition. If she uses a diaphragm or cervical cap, make sure it covers her cervix as directed by her clinician. Women who use the IUD should follow their clinician's instructions for checking that the IUD is in place each month.

2. Inconsistent use of the contraceptive – Contraceptives must be used regularly and according to instructions to achieve maximum effectiveness. If she forgets to take *just one* birth control pill, she is increasing the risk of pregnancy. Barrier methods of contraception such as condoms, cervical caps and diaphragms must be used consistently to be effective. Women who practice natural family planning must use it precisely and consistently for effective pregnancy prevention. Remember, all it takes is one unprotected act of sexual intercourse for her to get pregnant.

3. Condoms broken during sex – An estimated 2 to 5 percent of condoms *break or tear* during use. Most often this is caused by misuse; not using enough water-based lubrication can cause condom damage, as can creating tiny tears with jewelry or fingernails, among other objects. Condoms that are past the expiration date, that have been stored improperly, damaged during or after manufacture, or that are improperly used are other possible causes of condom failure (that three-year-old condom in your wallet is a pregnancy waiting to happen). Vaginal spermicides should always be used with condoms to help decrease the possibility of pregnancy should condom failure occur.

4. Relying on oral contraceptive birth control pills while taking antibiotics or other drugs or herbs – Antibiotics have been found to interfere with the effectiveness of combination oral contraceptives by decreasing steroid hormone plasma concentrations. Women who use combined oral contraceptives should use an alternative method of contraception during months that they take antibiotics.

5. Believing that you can't get your girlfriend pregnant while she's on her period – Pregnancy normally occurs midcycle; however, many women have become pregnant while on their period and at other times of the month that might normally be considered nonfertile. In simple terms there is no completely "safe" time during her cycle.

[Ref. 1: Journal of the American Medical Association, 1999;282:1359-1364]

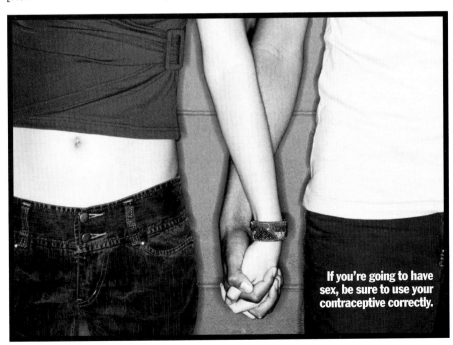

If you're going to have sex, be sure to use your contraceptive correctly.

CHAPTER SEVENTEEN

Sexually Transmitted Diseases: STDs

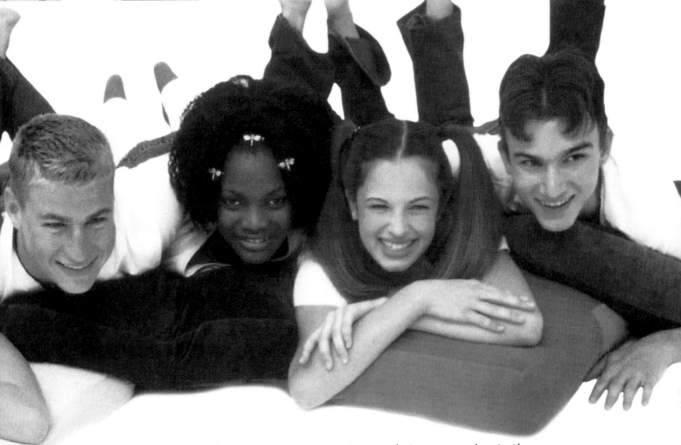

As if an unwanted pregnancy were not enough to worry about, there are also some nasty bugs out there, just waiting to take advantage of teenagers who engage in unsafe sex. What we are talking about, of course, are venereal diseases or sexually transmitted diseases – more commonly called STDs. Some STDs can be cleared up with antibiotics in a few days; others can go on for weeks. Then there are the real nasties that you have for life – or in the case of AIDS, that *take your life.* Not a pleasant picture, is it? Like pregnancy, your goal regarding STDs is to avoid them. The following are the most common STDs. At the first sign that you or your girlfriend may have any of these diseases, go see your school nurse or family doctor. Delays can be dangerous.

Bacterial Vaginosis
What is bacterial vaginosis?
Vaginosis or vaginitis is an inflammation which occurs in the vagina and includes several strains of germs that cause bacterial vaginosis yeast infections. Many women mistakenly believe that yeast infections are the most common type of vaginal infection, but bacterial vaginosis is

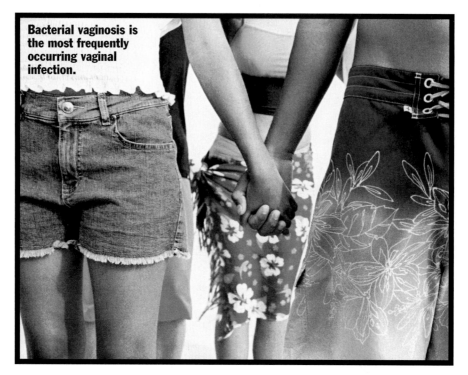

Bacterial vaginosis is the most frequently occurring vaginal infection.

the most frequently occurring vaginal infection, affecting from 10 percent to 64 percent of the population at any given time.

Although treatment is available and will quickly cure this infection, if left untreated bacterial vaginosis may increase a woman's risk of pelvic inflammatory disease (PID). Bacterial vaginosis occurs most during the reproductive years, although women of all ages are susceptible to this infection that affects the vagina, urethra, bladder and skin in the genital area.

What causes bacterial vaginosis?
Primary causes of bacterial vaginosis include an overgrowth of anaerobic bacteria and the Gardnerella organism. The healthy vagina includes a small amount of these bacteria and organisms. When the vaginal balance is disrupted by the *overgrowth* of these bacteria, another protective bacterium lactobacilli is unable to adequately perform its normal function. Lactobacilli normally provides a natural disinfectant (similar to hydrogen peroxide) which helps maintain the healthy and normal balance of microorganisms in the vagina.

E. coli (which is a normal inhabitant of the rectum) can cause bacterial vaginitis if it is spread to the vaginal area. Other factors which may contribute include hot weather, poor health, poor hygiene, use of an intrauterine device (IUD) for birth control, and routine douching.

What are the symptoms of bacterial vaginosis?

The most obvious sign of bacterial infection is an unpleasant, foul, sometimes fishy odor. Itching and/or burning sometimes accompany bacterial infections but are not a required symptom for a diagnosis of bacterial vaginosis.

Many times women are unaware they are infected until they are diagnosed during a routine pelvic exam and pap smear. It is important that the woman not douche during the few days before a visit to her gynecologist, as douching can hide signs of infection and may even make bacterial vaginosis worse.

What is the treatment for bacterial vaginosis?

The good news is that treatment is relatively simple and effective once proper diagnosis is made. Treatment usually consists of three to seven nights of Cleocin 2 percent vaginal cream. Oral antibiotic treatment is sometimes prescribed and may be available if it is requested from a physician. Although the symptoms may disappear before the medication is finished, it's important that the medication is completed exactly as directed by the physician.

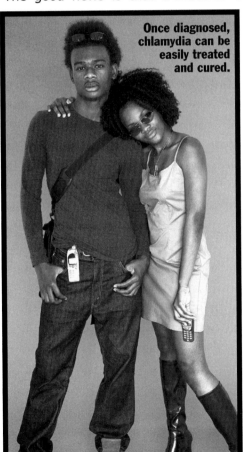

Once diagnosed, chlamydia can be easily treated and cured.

Chlamydial Infection

Chlamydial ("kla-mid-ee-uhl") infection is the leading sexually transmitted disease (STD) in the United States today, with an estimated 4 million new cases occurring each year. Once diagnosed, chlamydia can be easily treated and cured. Up to 40 percent of women with untreated chlamydia will develop pelvic inflammatory disease (PID), a serious complication of chlamydial infection. Undiagnosed PID caused by chlamydia is common. Of those with PID, 20 percent will become infertile, 18 percent will experience debilitating chronic pelvic pain, and 9 percent will have a life-threatening tubal pregnancy.

Chlamydial infection is caused by a bacterium, chlamydia trachomatis, and is transmitted during vaginal or anal sexual contact with an infected partner. A pregnant woman may pass the infection to her newborn during delivery, with subsequent neonatal eye infection or pneumonia. Chlamydia is also common among young men. Untreated chlamydia in men typically causes urethral infection, but may also result in complications such as swollen and tender testicles.

Symptoms of chlamydia – Men and women with chlamydial infections may experience abnormal genital discharge or pain during urination. These early symptoms of chlamydial infection may be absent or very mild. If symptoms occur, they usually appear within 1 to 3 weeks after exposure. One of every two infected women and one of every four infected men may have no symptoms whatsoever. As a result, the disease is often not diagnosed until complications develop.

In women chlamydial infections can result in PID; in men these infections may lead to pain or swelling in the scrotal area, which is a sign of epididymitis, an inflammation of a part of the male reproductive system located near the testicles. Left untreated, this condition (like PID in women) can result in infertility.

Chlamydial bacteria can cause proctitis (inflamed rectum) and conjunctivitis (inflammation of the lining of the eye). The bacteria have also been found in the throat as a result of oral sexual contact with an infected partner. A particular strain of chlamydia causes an uncommon

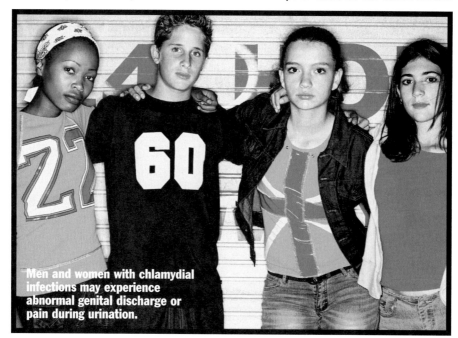

Men and women with chlamydial infections may experience abnormal genital discharge or pain during urination.

STD called lymphogranuloma venereum (LGV), which is characterized by prominent swelling and inflammation of the lymph nodes in the groin. Complications may follow if LGV is not treated.

Diagnosis – Chlamydial infection is easily confused with gonorrhea because the symptoms of both diseases are similar, and they often occur together. Until recently the only way to diagnose chlamydial infection was to take a sample of secretions from a patient's genital area and attempt to grow the organism in specialized tissue culture in the laboratory. Although still considered the most definitive test, this method is expensive and technically difficult, and test results are not available for up to 3 days.

Scientists have developed several rapid tests for diagnosing chlamydial infection that use sophisticated techniques and a dye to detect bacterial proteins. Although these tests are slightly less accurate, they are less expensive, more rapid, and can be performed during a routine checkup.

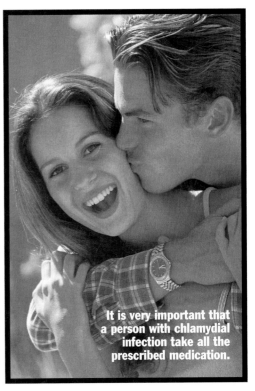

It is very important that a person with chlamydial infection take all the prescribed medication.

Treatment for chlamydia – A 7-day course of antibiotics such as tetracycline or doxycycline is the recommended treatment for chlamydial infection. Other antibiotics are effective, however, and can be used if tetracycline cannot be taken. For example, pregnant women should not take tetracycline, but rather can be treated with erythromycin. Penicillin, which is often used for treating some other STDs, is not effective against chlamydial infections. New medications are being developed that should greatly simplify treatment and help control the spread of chlamydia in the population.

It is very important that a person with chlamydial infection take all of the prescribed medication, even after symptoms disappear. To be sure that the infection is cured, a follow-up visit to the doctor or clinic 1 to 2 weeks after finishing the medication may be necessary. All sex partners of a person with chlamydial

At the first sign that you or your girlfriend may have an STD, go see your school nurse or family doctor.

infection should be evaluated and treated to prevent reinfection and further spread of the disease.

Pelvic Inflammatory Disease

Each year up to a million women in the United States develop PID, a serious infection of the reproductive organs. As many as half of all cases of PID may be due to chlamydial infection, and many of these occur without symptoms. PID can result in scarring of the fallopian tubes, which can block the tubes and prevent fertilization from taking place. An estimated 100,000 women each year become infertile as a result of PID.

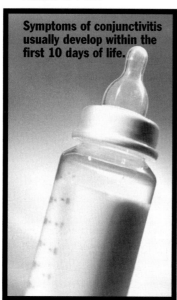

Symptoms of conjunctivitis usually develop within the first 10 days of life.

In other cases, scarring may interfere with the passage of the fertilized egg to the uterus during pregnancy. When this happens, the egg may implant itself in the fallopian tube. This is called ectopic or tubal pregnancy. This very serious condition results in the loss of the fetus and is a major cause of maternal death in the United States.

Effects of Chlamydial Infection in Newborns

A baby who is exposed to chlamydial bacteria in the birth canal during delivery may develop conjunctivitis (eye infection) or pneumonia. Symptoms of conjunctivitis, which include discharge and swollen eyelids, usually develop within the first 10 days of life. Symptoms of pneumonia, including a progressively worse cough and congestion, most often develop within 3 to 6 weeks after birth. Both conditions can be successfully treated with antibiotics. However, because of these risks to the newborn, many doctors now recommend routine testing of all pregnant women for chlamydial infection.

Prevention – Because chlamydial infection often occurs without symptoms, those who are infected may unknowingly pass the bacteria to their sex partners. Many doctors recommend that all persons who have more than one sex partner, especially women under 25 years of age, be tested for chlamydial infection regularly, even in the absence of symptoms. Using condoms (rubbers) or diaphragms during sexual intercourse may help reduce the transmission of chlamydial bacteria. In addition, recent research has shown that women infected with chlamydia have a three- to five-fold increased risk of acquiring HIV if exposed.

Genital Herpes

Forty-five million people in the United States are infected with the herpes simplex virus (HSV). According to estimates 500,000 new cases of herpes occur annually. A shocking 80 percent of those infected with HSV are never aware that they are infected because either they never develop symptoms or they fail to recognize the symptoms when they do occur.

There are two types of herpes and both can affect the genitals and the mouth. HSV 1 most commonly occurs on the lips in the form of fever blisters and cold sores. HSV 2 most commonly appears in the genitals. Once a person is infected with HSV it remains for life and people can experience periodic episodes of active herpes.

What are the symptoms of herpes?

Symptoms of herpes can vary widely from person to person. When symptoms do appear during a first episode they usually appear within 2 to 10 days after infection and last an average of 2 to 3 weeks. Some of the earliest symptoms can include an itching or burning sensation, pain in the legs, buttocks, or genital area, vaginal discharge, and/or a feeling of pressure or fullness in the abdominal area.

A few days following the initial symptoms, sores or lesions erupt at the site of the infection. These sores can occur inside the vagina or on the cervix in women, or in the urinary passage in both men and women. Herpes lesions may first appear as small red bumps that develop into blisters which become painful, open sores. After several

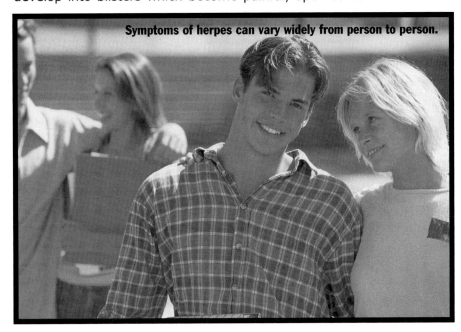

Symptoms of herpes can vary widely from person to person.

days these sores become crusted and then heal without scarring. The first episode of genital herpes can also include symptoms such as fever, headache, muscle aches, urinary pain or difficulty, and swollen glands in the groin area.

After genital herpes invades the skin or mucous membranes, the virus travels to the sensory nerves at the end of the spinal cord, where it remains inside the nerve cells in an inactive state. In most people the virus will become active again monthly. During a recurrent episode of genital herpes the virus travels along the nerves to the skin where it multiplies at or near the site of the original herpes lesions, causing new sores to appear.

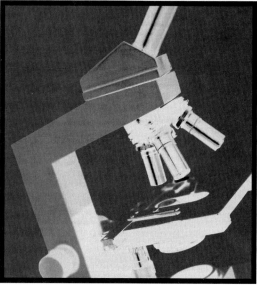

HSV can reactivate without any visible sores or lesions being present. During these periods of active virus, small amounts of the virus can "shed" at or near the site of the original lesions from genital secretions or from indiscernible lesions. Shedding occurs without any accompanying discomfort and may last only a day or two, but it is possible to infect a sexual partner during this time.

How is genital herpes diagnosed?
Although sores may be visible to the eye, several laboratory tests may be necessary to determine whether the sores are caused by HSV or another infection. The most reliable method of diagnosing genital herpes is by viral culture during which a new lesion is swabbed or scraped with the sample added to a laboratory culture that contains healthy cells. These cells are then examined, a day or two later, under a microscope that shows changes to the cells that indicate the growth of the herpes virus.

Other methods of diagnosing herpes are available to physicians, however, it's important to understand that the herpes virus is extremely hard to find and the fact that a physician fails to detect the virus in an active sore does not mean that a person does not have genital herpes. Because of the difficulty diagnosing herpes physicians may *misdiagnose* sores as something else such as ingrown hairs.

There is a blood test available that can detect antibodies to the virus, but this test cannot tell whether or not a person has an active genital herpes infection. The blood test can only determine if a person has been previously infected by HSV and has produced antibodies to the virus. Although antibodies are present they do not protect a person from subsequent outbreaks of herpes. This blood test also cannot distinguish between oral or genital herpes. New blood tests which have the ability to distinguish between HSV type 1 and type 2 are currently being developed; however, they are not available to the general medical population and are used mainly in research hospitals.

What are the treatments for genital herpes?
There are three drugs currently available to treat genital herpes – but these medications are not cures. Pharmaceutical treatment of genital herpes may shorten the length of first episodes and reduce the severity and frequency of recurrent episodes. Patients can help speed healing and avoid spreading the infection by following a few simple steps during periods of active herpes:
• Keep the infected area clean and dry.
• Don't touch the sores – if you do, wash your hands immediately.
• Refrain from sex from the time you first notice symptoms until sores/lesions are completely healed and covered by new skin.
Recurrent episodes of herpes can be triggered by minor trauma, by other infections including colds, and by menstruation and stress.

What risks or complications are associated with genital herpes?
In most cases genital herpes does not cause any long-term health consequences. Anyone with a weakened immune system can experience long-lasting and severe episodes of herpes. Pregnant women should be closely monitored for herpes activity. If the first episode of herpes occurs during pregnancy, she can pass the virus to her unborn baby, and may be at higher risk of premature delivery. Approximately 50 percent of babies born with neonatal herpes die or suffer neurological damage. Babies can develop encephalitis, severe rashes, and eye problems, however immediate treatment greatly improves the outcome for many infants.

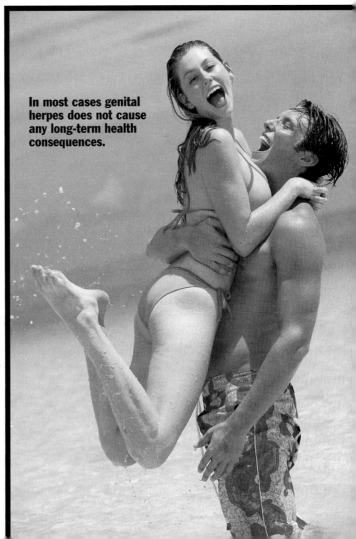

In most cases genital herpes does not cause any long-term health consequences.

The risk to babies depends greatly on whether the mother is experiencing a first episode or a recurrent episode of genital herpes. Because it takes days to weeks to get results from viral cultures that determine whether or not active herpes virus is present, many physicians will perform a Cesarean section on pregnant women diagnosed with genital herpes. However, if no *active* herpes is present at the time of birth there is little or no risk to the baby with vaginal delivery. If a woman is pregnant and has herpes, she should talk with her physician to determine the best delivery method for mother and baby.

In addition, because genital herpes creates open sores, people with herpes are at higher risk of contracting HIV and AIDS.

How can you protect yourself and your partner from HSV?
If you have herpes you can avoid transmitting it to your partner by not having sex during periods when you notice symptoms and not until any sores are completely healed and covered with new skin. Condoms offer some protection during the times when you are not experiencing symptoms, although it is possible that a condom will not cover all the affected areas. If you suspect you may have herpes, discuss your symptoms with your physician.

Gonorrhea

Gonorrhea is a bacterium that can cause sterility, arthritis and heart problems. In women, gonorrhea can cause pelvic inflammatory disease (PID), which can result in ectopic pregnancy or sterility. During preg-

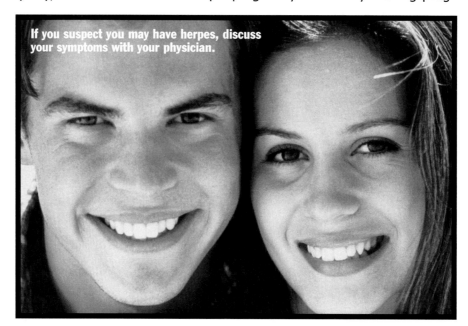

If you suspect you may have herpes, discuss your symptoms with your physician.

nancy, gonorrhea infections can cause premature labor and stillbirth. To prevent serious eye infections that can be caused by gonorrhea, drops of antibiotics are routinely put into the eyes of newborn babies immediately after delivery. More than 600,000 new cases of gonorrhea are reported every year in the US.

Common symptoms:
• For women: frequent, often burning urination, menstrual irregularities, pelvic or lower abdominal pain, pain during sex or pelvic examination, a yellowish or yellow-green discharge from the vagina, swelling or tenderness of the vulva, and even arthritic pain.
• For men: a pus-like discharge from the urethra or pain during urination. Eighty percent of the women and 10 percent of the men with gonorrhea show no symptoms. If they appear, they appear in women within 10 days. It takes from 1 to 14 days for symptoms to appear in men.

How gonorrhea is spread:
Vaginal, anal and oral intercourse.

Diagnosis – Microscopic examination of urethral or vaginal discharges. Cultures taken from the cervix, throat, urethra or rectum.

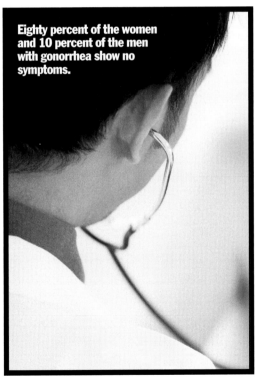

Eighty percent of the women and 10 percent of the men with gonorrhea show no symptoms.

Treatment – Both partners can be successfully treated with oral antibiotics. Often people with gonorrhea also have chlamydia. They must be treated for both infections at the same time.

Protection – Condoms offer very good protection against gonorrhea.

Hepatitis B Virus (HBV)
Although 90 to 95 percent of adults with HBV recover completely, this virus can cause severe liver disease and death. Unless they are treated within an hour of birth, 90 percent of the infants born to women with HBV will carry the virus. Pregnant women who may have been exposed to HBV should consider being

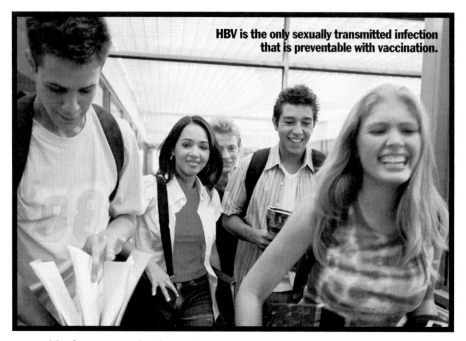

HBV is the only sexually transmitted infection that is preventable with vaccination.

tested before giving birth so that their babies can be vaccinated at birth or treated if they become ill. Like many other viruses, HBV remains in the body for life.

HBV is the only sexually transmitted infection that is preventable with vaccination. Yet approximately 77,000 Americans get HBV every year because they have not been vaccinated! There are now about 750,000 people with sexually acquired HBV in the US.

Common symptoms:
• extreme fatigue, headache, fever, hives
• lack of appetite, nausea, vomiting, tenderness in the lower abdomen.

Later symptoms include more abdominal pain, dark urine, clay-colored stool, yellowing of the skin and white of the eyes – jaundice. HBV may show no symptoms during its most contagious phases. If symptoms appear, they appear within 4 weeks.

How HBV is spread:
In semen, saliva, blood and urine by:
• intimate and sexual contact – everything from kissing to vaginal, anal and oral intercourse
• use of unclean needles to inject drugs
• accidental pricks with contaminated needles in the course of health care (hepatitis B is very contagious)

Diagnosis – Blood test is required.

Treatment – None. In most cases the infection clears within 4 to 8 weeks. Some people, however, remain contagious for the rest of their lives.

Protection – Condoms offer some protection against HBV during vaginal, anal, and oral intercourse, but the virus can be passed through kissing and other intimate touching. Children and adults who do not have HBV can get permanent protection with a series of HBV vaccinations.

Pelvic Inflammatory Disease

What is it?

Pelvic inflammatory disease affects millions of women each year in the United States and is an infection of one or more pelvic organs, including the uterus, cervix and fallopian tubes. PID occurs when a bacteria or organism enters the cervix and spreads upward. Symptoms of pelvic inflammatory disease include: lower abdominal pain, fever up to 103 degrees, rapid pulse, chills, back pain, pain during sex, and vaginal discharge.

PID is a serious condition and requires *immediate medical attention.* If a woman is experiencing pelvic pain or symptoms she should see her gynecologist right away. She should make a record of the pain and take it with her to her appointment to help the physician to understand exactly when the pain occurs, where the pain is located, and the severity of the pain. If pelvic inflammatory disease is left untreated it can become life-threatening!

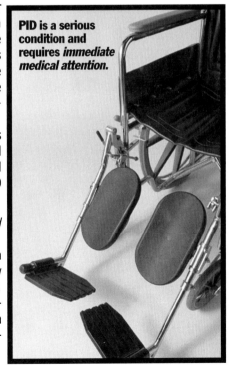

PID is a serious condition and requires *immediate medical attention.*

Pelvic inflammatory disease is usually contracted through sexual contact. Untreated gonorrhea and chlamydia cause an estimated 90 percent of all cases of PID.

What are current treatment and prevention recommendations?

Pelvic inflammatory disease can today be diagnosed through a new procedure called *falloposcopy.* Falloposcopy is a visual examination of the inside of the fallopian tubes; a simple procedure performed on an out-patient basis.

If PID is found and it hasn't progressed to a stage severe enough to require major reconstructive surgery to repair the fallopian tubes, antibiotic therapy may be tried. Floxin is now named by the FDA as the first oral medication approved for independent use to treat pelvic inflammatory disease. Previous recommendations included the use of intravenous antibiotics which required hospitalization.

The cervix dilates slightly just before, during and after a woman's period, increasing her risk of pelvic inflammatory disease by making it easier for an organism or bacteria to enter the cervix and cause infection. Douching significantly *increases* her risk of developing pelvic inflammatory disease and other pelvic infections and *is not* recommended. Douching removes the natural protective mucous from the cervix, giving bacteria a more receptive place to grow. Women should use caution if they must douche, and be aware of the risk.

The best protection against PID and other STDs is to always use a condom, unless you are in a long-term monogamous relationship and both of you have been tested for HIV and other STDs. A few inconvenient moments before sexual intercourse can prevent a lifetime of pain and even an untimely death.

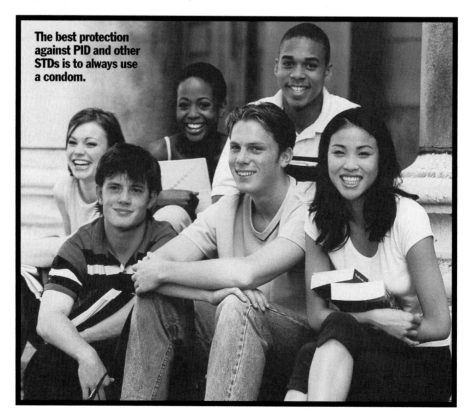

The best protection against PID and other STDs is to always use a condom.

Syphilis

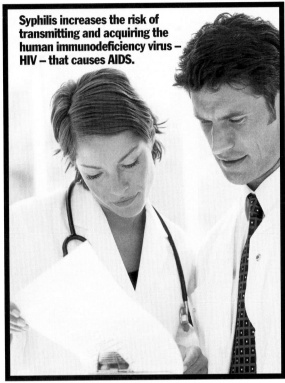

Syphilis increases the risk of transmitting and acquiring the human immunodeficiency virus – HIV – that causes AIDS.

At one time he was public enemy number one. He made millions of dollars a year selling prohibited alcohol, and was responsible for the deaths of hundreds of people. In the 1920s and 1930s Chicago's *Al Capone* was one of the most well known figures in the United States. Yet despite his almost absolute power, this terror of the Mafia gangs was brought down by a microscopic organism contracted in his teen years. Syphilis has respect for no one.

Syphilis is a sexually transmitted disease (STD) caused by a bacterium called Treponema pallidum. The initial infection causes an ulcer at the site of infection; however, the bacteria move throughout the body, damaging many organs over time. Medical experts describe the course of the disease by dividing it into four stages – primary, secondary, latent and tertiary (late). An infected person who has not been treated may infect others during the first two stages, which usually last one to two years. In its late stages, untreated syphilis, although not contagious, can cause serious heart abnormalities, mental disorders, blindness, other neurologic problems, and death. (In his later years Al Capone was reduced to spending his days trying to catch fish out of his swimming pool! Such was the extreme of his dementia.)

The bacterium spreads from the initial ulcer of an infected person to the skin or mucous membranes of the genital area, the mouth, or the anus of a sexual partner. It can also pass through broken skin on other parts of the body. The syphilis bacterium is very fragile, and the infection is almost always spread by sexual contact. In addition, a pregnant woman with syphilis can pass the bacterium to her unborn child, who may be born with serious mental and physical problems as a result of this infection. But the most common way to get syphilis is to have sex with someone who has an active infection.

Treatment – The good news is that syphilis, once a cause of devastating epidemics, can be effectively diagnosed and treated with antibiotic therapy. In 1996 a total of 11,387 cases of primary and secondary syphilis in the United States were reported to the US Centers for Disease Control and Prevention. Although treatment is available, the early symptoms of syphilis can be very mild, and many people do not seek treatment when they first become infected. Of increasing concern is the fact that syphilis increases the risk of transmitting and acquiring the human immunodeficiency virus – HIV – that causes AIDS.

Phthirus Pubis / Crab Louse / Pubic Lice

Description – Pediculosis pubis is the presence of the crab louse on a human host. This parasitic infestation is commonly referred to as "crabs" or "the cooties." Pubic lice are remarkably adapted for attachment to coarse body hairs and are grayish-white to pink in color. Crab louse can most often be found in the pubic and perianal areas, but some have been found on other areas of the body, including the eyebrows and eyelashes. The adult crab louse has (approximately) a 30-day life span, but can only survive up to 24 hours unattached to a human host. The louse mates frequently and adheres its eggs (known as nits) to the base of hairs. The nits require a week to hatch and will grow to adulthood in about 3 weeks.

Symptoms – The first signs of a crab louse infestation are persistent itching, irritation or annoyance in the infested area. Often, pustules form where lice bites have occurred and a severe skin reaction may develop as well. A definite sign of a pubic lice problem is the discovery of small white specks at the base of the hairs in the afflicted area.

Transmission – It is very unusual to find the crab louse anywhere but on the host, unless the louse is rubbed off or is carried off with a body hair. That's why pubic lice are typically transferred from person to person through sexual contact. Transfer may occur when two people sleep together or maintain other somewhat prolonged bodily contact. The louse can also be transmitted by coming into contact with contaminated bedding, clothing, toilet seats, etc., but this is highly unlikely in the case of crab lice.

Treatment – Nonprescription insecticides which can be used for human louse control include synergized pyrethrins A-200 Pyrinate, R&S, XXX, Liban, Pronto, Rid and YDP. Prescription insecticides include Topocide and various Kwell preparations. When used as directed, any of these compounds will be extremely effective in destroying both nits and lice. The dead nits can be removed from the hair by combing with a fine comb. Lice found on the eyelids or eyebrows can be removed with tweezers and, in addition, it might be advisable to add some vaseline to the edge of the eyelids to help kill the crabs. However, it is always best to consult a physician before using any sort of medication. Take note, itching will persist for several days after the application of an effective treatment. All clothing and bedding used throughout the infection should also be washed in hot water or dry cleaned.

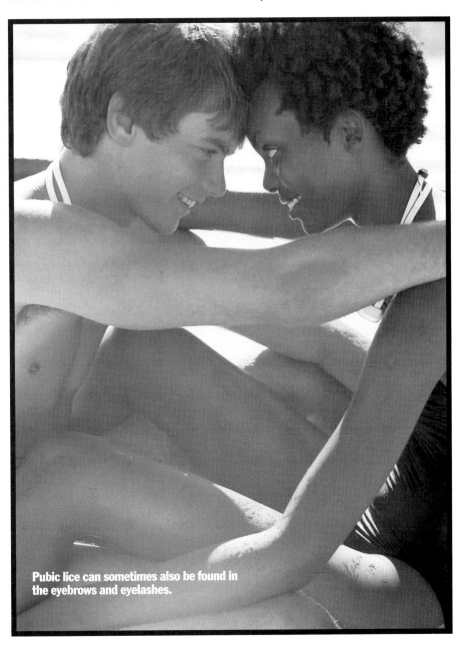

Pubic lice can sometimes also be found in the eyebrows and eyelashes.

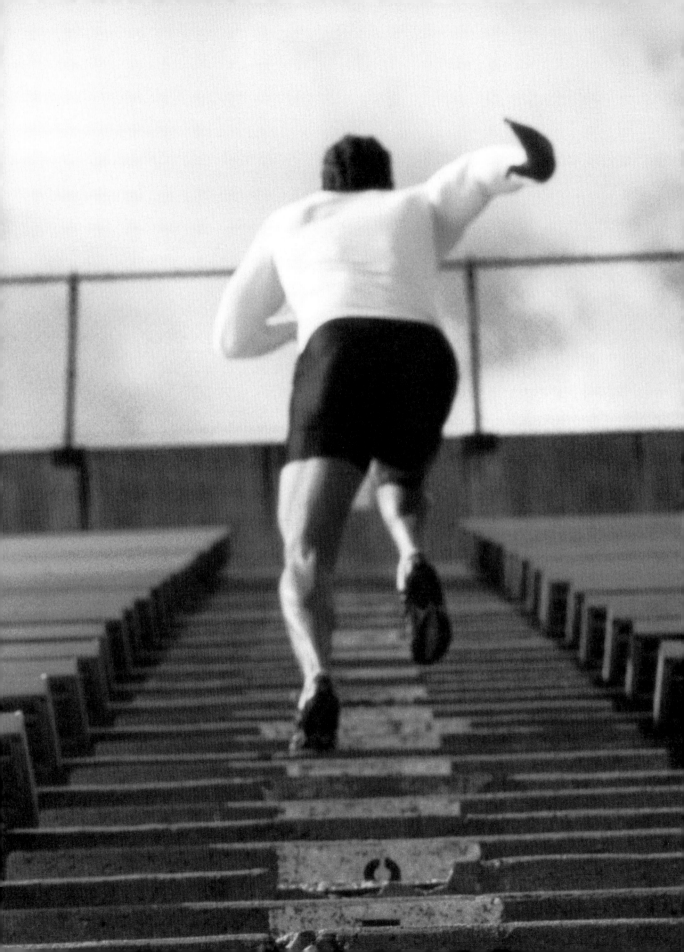

BOOK TWO

CHAPTER EIGHTEEN

Looking good may come easy at this stage of your life. Your skin and muscles are still firm and toned, even if you aren't exercising regularly. So why exercise as a teen? Well, because exercise will help you look and feel your best. Your body is still growing and changing throughout your teen years. Exercise will help you stay healthy and give you more energy to do the things you like to do. Regular exercise should become a habit. Start now, while you have the time. Then when you get to your 20s, 30s and 40s, exercise will already be a part of your life. Get a head start! Here's what exercise will give you, no matter what your age:

- improved weight control
- stronger heart and lungs
- greater physical endurance
- improved flexibility
- stronger and well toned muscles
- a means to burn off stress/better stress management
- improved self-esteem

Getting In Shape

Follow the F.I.T.T. Principle

F = Frequency of three types of exercise:
• Aerobic exercise: 3 to 5 times a week
  (swimming, vigorous walking or bicycling)
• Strength-building exercise: 2 or 3 times a week
  (weight training or calisthenics)
• Flexibility exercise: every day if possible
  (stretches or slow,
  concentrated movements)

I = Intensity

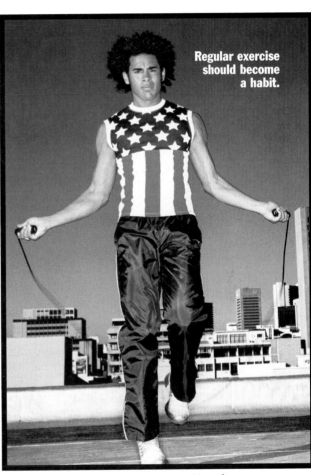

Regular exercise should become a habit.

• When you exercise, your body needs more oxygen and your heart starts pumping faster. That's why your pulse, or heart rate, is a good indicator of exercise intensity. Your target heart rate (THR) is the appropriate range of heartbeats per minute you should stay within during exercise (based on your age and physical condition). When you exercise within your THR, you are reaping the maximum benefit from that exercise. Aim for the low range when you begin the aerobic part of your fitness plan. Gradually work up to the higher range as you become physically fit.
• Target heart rate for healthy teens: Your range should be a maximum of 120 heartbeats per minute for beginners, and a maximum of 160 beats per minute for those who are already fit. Try to reach between 60 and 80 percent of your recommended maximum when you exercise. Here's how to find your target heart rate: At the wrist, use the first two fingers of one hand to feel along the thumb side of your other wrist, palm up. At the neck, place two fingers in the notch just to the right or left of your windpipe. Press lightly and practice counting for 10 seconds – this is how long you will take your pulse during exercise. Multiply by six to get your heartbeats per minute. Example: Counted 20 beats in 10 seconds, multiplied by 6 = 120 beats per minute.

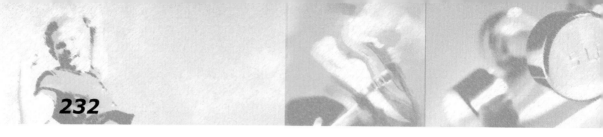
T = Time

A thorough exercise program can take as little as 45 minutes. Consider the following example:

• Take 5 minutes to warm up. Use low-intensity rhythmic exercises, such as walking, a full range of movement exercise, or a stationary bicycle.

• Continue with at least 20 minutes of aerobic conditioning. Select a continuous activity such as jogging, swimming, cycling or brisk walking. The activity you choose should put an increased demand on your heart and lungs by using large muscle groups (arms and legs).

• Then do 20 to 30 minutes of strength/endurance movements. Include strengthening exercises that focus on the major muscle groups. Try pushups, situps and weightlifting.

• Set aside 3 to 5 minutes for a cooldown. Cool off with low-intensity walking or exercises similar to the warmup portion. Try deep breathing and stretching.

• Finish with 5 to 7 minutes of flexibility movements. Use slow, controlled stretches and hold each for 30 to 60 seconds, targeting all major muscle groups.

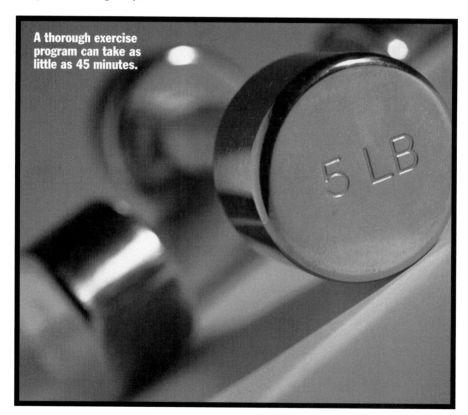

A thorough exercise program can take as little as 45 minutes.

T = Type
The type of exercise you do is completely up to you. The important thing is to find something you like and get started now!

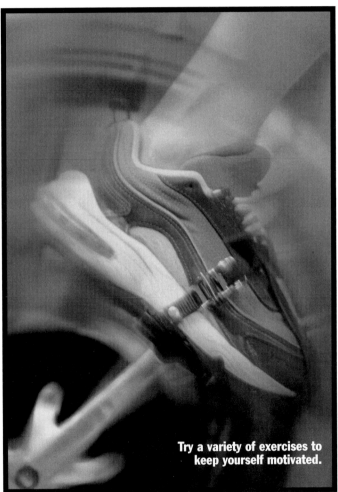
Try a variety of exercises to keep yourself motivated.

Overcoming Excuses
It's easy to find excuses for not exercising, so here are some tips to help overcome those big barriers to getting the exercise you need:

1. Find a training partner with a similar goal and exercise together. You'll be motivating each other.

2. Set realistic exercise goals. Don't be afraid to send out an SOS to friends, family, or a professional if you need help in sticking with your plan. If your mom likes to keep ice cream in the freezer, ask her if she will help by making it the low-fat, low-sugar variety instead.

3. Write a contract with yourself that includes what you are going to do, when you want to check your status in achieving your goal, and what you will reward yourself with when you achieve that goal.

4. Spend time with people who support your goal. There's nothing like hearing "You can do it!" and "Go for it!" to help make it all worthwhile.

5. Make your program portable, something you can do any time, any place.

6. Make your program fun. If you like to walk to a beat, take a radio or CD player and headset with you. If you like to talk with friends on the phone, suggest you go for a walk together instead.

7. Try a variety of exercises to keep yourself motivated. Swim one day, hike the next, weight train on the next.

CHAPTER NINETEEN

Back in the 1970s (when most of your parents were probably dating!), superstar Arnold Schwarzenegger starred in a moderately successful documentary called *Pumping Iron.* No, Arnold wasn't a superspy who went around blowing people up and saving the girl toward the end of the movie. Those roles would come later. *Pumping Iron* looked at the "whacky world of professional bodybuilding." You know, those beefy characters who get up onstage and show their muscles. Besides Arnold, the movie starred Lou Ferrigno, the same guy who later became famous as *The Incredible Hulk* (who turned green and got huge when he got angry). Besides the entertainment value, *Pumping Iron* showed that bodybuilders were no different than most athletes and trained just as hard and experienced the same emotions. This movie also introduced mainstream America to a fantastic new form of exercise – weightlifting.

A small percentage of people had been lifting weights for decades, but until *Pumping Iron* came along, weightlifting was seen as something that respectable people "didn't do." Gosh, who wants to get all sweaty and lift weights over their heads? That's just for egotistical jerks, right? Wrong!

Within a few short years following the release of *Pumping Iron,* researchers started taking a closer look at the benefits of weight training. What they found was that weight training had numerous

Pumping Iron: Not Just For Arnold!

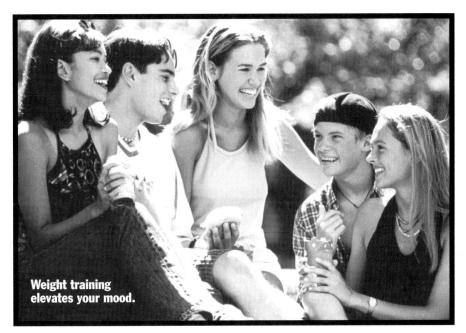

Weight training elevates your mood.

benefits to offer, and not just for jocks, either. People of all ages can benefit from a well-designed weight training program. If you don't believe us, just take a look:

Top 17 Benefits of Weight Training

1. Weight training tones your muscles, which looks great and raises your base rate of metabolism ... and that causes you to burn more calories 24 hours a day. You'll even burn more calories while you sleep.

2. Weight training can "reverse" the natural decline in your metabolism which begins around age 30. We know that's down the road, but hey ... it will happen.

3. Weight training energizes you.

4. Weight training has a positive effect on almost all of your 650-plus muscles.

5. Weight training strengthens your bones.

6. Weight training improves muscle tone and endurance.

7. Weight training makes you strong. Strength gives you confidence and makes daily activities easier.

8. Weight training makes you less prone to lower-back injuries.

9. Weight training decreases your resting blood pressure.

10. Weight training decreases your risk of developing adult-onset diabetes.

11. Weight training decreases your gastrointestinal transit time, reducing your risk for developing colon cancer.

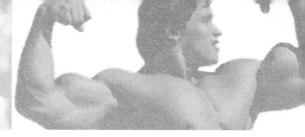

12. Weight training increases your blood level of HDL cholesterol (the good type).
13. Weight training improves your posture.
14. Weight training improves the functioning of your immune system.
15. Weight training lowers your resting heart rate, a sign of a more efficient heart.
16. Weight training improves your balance and coordination.
17. Weight training elevates your mood.

Despite everything we've just stated, amazingly most teenagers *still don't* work out with weights. Now, we realize there are practical reasons for not exercising, like cost and access to a gym, but one of the biggest reasons is the number of myths that have developed around weight training over the years.

Probably the most prevalent is the myth that weight training makes you muscle bound and uncoordinated. The fact that most sports teams have their own strength trainer should be enough proof to dispel that old myth. *Strength training will not make you muscle bound.* In fact it will do just the opposite – it will make you more athletic. Take a look at the

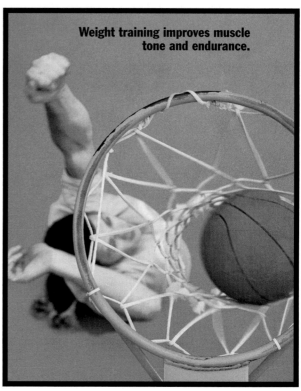

Weight training improves muscle tone and endurance.

average hockey, football or baseball player today vs. those of 20 years ago. Average bodyweight has gone up by 30 or 40 pounds – and it's not fat, either. Today's weight-trained athletes are for the most part bigger, stronger, *and better conditioned* than their counterparts of a few decades ago.

Another myth that just doesn't want to go away is the one that muscle turns to fat when you stop training. Sorry to deflate the anti-weight training gang, but muscle and fat are two distinct entities. You can't change one into the other or vice versa. What often happens is that athletes who retire don't adjust their eating habits accordingly. While competitive they could get away with eating 5000 to 6000 calories a day, but in retirement those excess calories simply get converted to fat. This, combined with the fact that unused muscle often takes on a saggy, untoned look, gives the appearance that the individual's muscle has "turned to fat." Trust us, it hasn't. The body follows a "use-it-or-lose-it" philosophy. Your muscle won't change into fat if you stop training. Instead it will gradually atrophy, a simple way of saying disappear.

A third myth about weight training is that it stunts growth in children. We have no idea where this myth came from. There is absolutely no physical evidence to suggest weight training causes the bones to stop growing. Granted, a boy who has not undergone puberty cannot build the same degree of muscle strength and size as someone who has, but that's because of hormone levels. It has nothing to do with his growth being stunted.

We hope by now you're getting the message that weight training has much to offer. Most of the negative comments you hear are from individuals who are stuck in a time warp. They are operating on a 1950s mindset. Let us reassure you – weight training is one of the most beneficial forms of exercise there is. It stimulates both your muscular and cardio systems. Few other forms of exercise can make this claim.

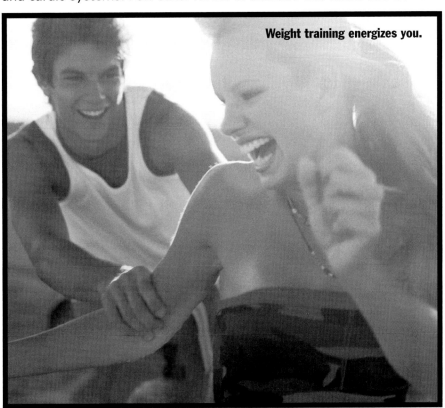

Weight training energizes you.

CHAPTER TWENTY

Know Your Body

Before we begin our introduction to the basic principles of strength training, we need to first review a few lessons you may have skipped or found boring in biology class. The human body is much the same as a car in that it's a collection of parts and systems that all work together to produce movement. Unlike a car, however, there's a lot going on in your body – even when you are not moving.

A number of years ago the National Geographic Society released a book called *The Incredible Machine.* The title of the book was very appropriate as nothing on earth comes close to the complexity of the human body. Let's take a closer look at this wondrous creation.

The Musculoskeletal System

Together, muscles and bones comprise what is called the musculoskeletal system of the body. The bones provide posture and structural support and the muscles provide the body with the ability to move (by contracting, and thus generating tension). The musculoskeletal system also provides protection for the body's internal organs. In order to serve their function, bones must be joined together by something. The point where bones connect to one another is called a joint, and this connection is made up mostly of ligaments (along with the help of muscles). Muscles are attached to the bone by tendons. Bones, tendons and ligaments do not possess the ability (as muscles do) to make your body move. Muscles are unique in this respect.

Muscles vary in shape and in size, and serve many different purposes. Most large muscles, like the hamstrings and quadriceps, control motion. Other muscles, like the heart and the muscles of the inner ear, perform different functions. At the microscopic level, however, all muscles share the same basic structure.

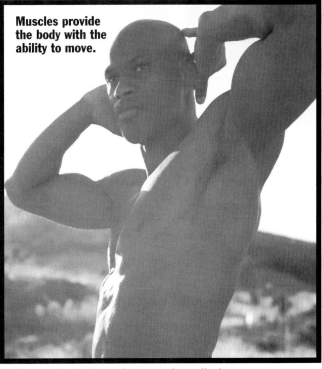

Muscles provide the body with the ability to move.

At the highest level, the (whole) muscle is composed of many strands of tissue called fascicles. These are the strands of muscle that we see when we cut red meat or poultry. Each fascicle is composed of fasciculi, which are bundles of muscle fibers. The muscle fibers are in turn composed of tens of thousands of thread-like myofibrils, which can contract, relax and elongate (lengthen). The myofibrils are (in turn) composed of up to millions of bands laid end to end, called sarcomeres. Each sarcomere is made of overlapping thick and thin filaments called myofilaments. The thick and thin myofilaments are composed of contractile proteins, primarily actin and myosin.

The way in which all these various levels of the muscle operate is as follows: Nerves connect the spinal column to the muscle. The place where the nerve and muscle meet is called the neuromuscular junction. When an electrical signal crosses the neuromuscular junction, it is transmitted deep inside the muscle fibers. Inside the muscle fibers the signal stimulates the flow of calcium, which causes the thick and thin myofilaments to slide across one another. When this occurs, it causes the sarcomere to shorten, which generates force. When billions of sarcomeres in the muscle shorten all at once, it results in a contraction of the entire muscle fiber.

When a muscle fiber contracts, it contracts *completely*. There is no such thing as a partially contracted muscle fiber. Muscle fibers are unable to vary the intensity of their contraction relative to the load against which they are acting. If this is so, then how does the force of a muscle contraction vary in strength from strong to weak? What happens is, more muscle fibers are recruited, as they are needed, to perform the job at hand. The more muscle fibers recruited by the central nervous system, the stronger the force generated by the muscle contraction.

The energy which produces the calcium flow in the muscle fibers comes from the mitochondria, the part of the muscle cell that converts glucose (blood sugar) into energy. Different types of muscle fibers have different amounts of mitochondria. The more mitochondria in a muscle fiber, the more energy it is capable of producing. Muscle fibers are categorized into two groups: slow-twitch fibers and fast-twitch fibers. Slow-twitch fibers (also called Type 1 muscle fibers) are slow to contract, but they are also very slow to fatigue. Fast-twitch fibers are very quick to contract and come in two varieties: Type 2A muscle fibers which fatigue at an intermediate rate, and Type 2B muscle fibers which fatigue very quickly.

> Muscles vary in shape and in size, and serve many different purposes.

The main reason the slow-twitch fibers are slow to fatigue is that they contain more mitochondria than fast-twitch fibers, and are therefore able to produce more energy. Slow-twitch fibers are also smaller in diameter than fast-twitch fibers, and have increased capillary blood flow around them. Because they have a smaller diameter and an increased blood flow, the slow-twitch fibers are able to deliver more oxygen and remove more waste products from the muscle fibers (which decreases "fatigability").

These three muscle fiber types (Types 1, 2A and 2B) are contained in all muscles in varying amounts. Muscles that need to be contracted much of the time (like the heart) have a greater number of Type 1 (slow) fibers. When a muscle first starts to contract, it is primarily Type 1 fibers that are initially activated, then Type 2A and Type 2B fibers are activated (if needed) in that order. Muscle fibers are recruited in this sequence – and that's what provides the ability to direct brain commands to execute such fine-tuned muscle responses. It also makes the Type 2B fibers difficult to train because they are not activated until most of the Type 1 and Type 2A fibers have been recruited.

One way to remember the difference between muscles with predominantly slow-twitch fibers and muscles with predominantly fast-twitch fibers is to think of "white meat" and "dark meat." Dark meat is dark because it has a greater number of slow-twitch muscle fibers and hence a greater number of mitochondria, which are dark. White meat consists mostly of muscle fibers which are at rest much of the time but are frequently called on to engage in brief bouts of intense activity. This muscle tissue can contract quickly, but is fast to fatigue and slow to recover. White meat is lighter in color than dark meat because it contains fewer mitochondria.

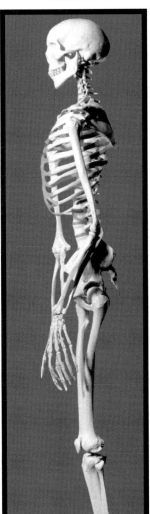

Located all around the muscle and its fibers are *connective tissues.* Connective tissue is composed of a base substance and two kinds of protein-based fiber. The two types of fiber are collagenous connective tissue and elastic connective tissue. Collagenous connective tissue consists mostly of collagen (hence its name) and provides tensile strength. Elastic connective tissue consists mostly of elastin and (as you might guess from its name) provides elasticity.

The base substance is called mucopolysaccharide and acts as both a lubricant (allowing the fibers to easily slide over one another), and as a glue (holding the fibers of the tissue together in bundles). The more elastic connective tissue there is around a joint, the greater the range of motion in that joint. Connective tissues are made up of tendons, ligaments, and the fascial sheaths that envelop, or bind down, muscles into separate groups. When muscles cause a limb to move through the range of motion of a joint, they usually act in the following cooperating groups:

Agonists – These muscles cause the movement to occur. They create the normal range of movement in a joint by contracting. Agonists are also referred to as prime movers since they are the muscles that are primarily responsible for generating the movement.

Antagonists – These muscles act in opposition to the movement generated by the agonists and are responsible for returning a limb to its initial position.

Synergists – These muscles perform, or assist in performing, the same set of joint motion as the agonists. Synergists are sometimes referred to as *neutralizers* because they help cancel out, or neutralize, extra motion from the agonists to make sure that the force generated works within the desired plane of motion.

Fixators – These muscles provide the necessary support to assist in holding the rest of the body in place while the movement occurs.

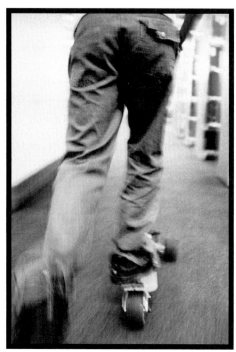

Fixators are also sometimes called stabilizers. As an example, when you flex your knee your hamstring contracts, and, to some extent, so does your gastrocnemius (calf) and lower buttock. Meanwhile, your quadriceps are inhibited (relaxed and lengthened somewhat) so as not to resist the flexion.

In this example the hamstring serves as the agonist, or prime mover; the quadriceps serve as the antagonist; and the calf and lower buttocks serve as the synergists. Agonists and antagonists are usually located on opposite sides of the affected joint (like your hamstrings and quadriceps, or your triceps and biceps), while synergists are usually located on the same side of the joint near the agonists. Larger muscles often call upon their smaller neighbors to function as synergists. The following is a list of commonly used agonist/antagonist muscle pairs:
• pectorals/latissimus dorsi (pecs and lats)
• anterior deltoids/posterior deltoids (front and back shoulders)
• trapezius/deltoids (traps and delts)
• abdominals/spinal erectors (abs and lower back)
• left and right external obliques (sides)
• quadriceps/hamstrings (quads and hams)
• shins/calves
• biceps/triceps
• forearm flexors/extensors

The contraction of a muscle does not necessarily imply that the muscle shortens; it only means that tension has been generated. Muscles can contract in the following ways:

Isometric contraction – This is a contraction in which no movement takes place, because the load on the muscle exceeds the tension generated by the contracting muscle. This occurs when a muscle attempts to push or pull an immovable object.

Isotonic contraction – a contraction in which movement does take place, because the tension generated by the contracting muscle exceeds the load on the muscle. Occurs when you use your muscles to successfully push or pull an object. Isotonic contractions are further divided into two types:

Concentric contraction – a contraction in which the muscle decreases in length (shortens) against an opposing load, such as lifting a weight.

Eccentric contraction – a contraction in which the muscle increases in length (lengthens) as it resists a load, such as lowering a weight in a slow, controlled fashion.

During a concentric contraction, the muscles that are shortening serve as the agonists – they do all the work. During an eccentric contraction the muscles that are lengthening serve as the agonists (and do all the work).

Naming Muscles

Before listing the various ways muscles are named, please keep this in mind: The human body didn't evolve to be conveniently categorized by scientists. It did so on its own terms. That's why some muscles need to be named in a few different ways. Scientists still debate as to whether a collection of fibers is *one muscle* or *multiple muscles.*

Characteristics for Naming Muscles

a. Size. The largest muscle within a group is usually distinguished from the rest of the muscles within the same group.
Example: The gluteus maximus is the largest muscle in the buttocks.
b. Shape. The shape that a particular muscle resembles may be a factor in naming it.
Example: The deltoid is shaped like a delta, or triangle.
c. Direction of fibers. The direction of muscular fibers within a muscle (longitudinal vs. lateral) may be considered when naming the muscle.
Example: The rectus abdominus is the longitudinal muscle within the abdomen (from the word *rectus,* meaning straight).
d. Location. The location of a muscle in relationship to another bodypart may also be reflected in the name.
Example: The frontalis overlies the frontal bone.
e. Number of attachments. Some muscles have more than one point of origin and/or attachment, which may factor in.
Example: The biceps brachii has two attachments or origins (from the word *bi,* meaning two).
f: Action. The manner in which the muscle moves the bodypart for which it is responsible may be considered when naming the muscle.
Example: The extensor digitorum extends digits (fingers).

CHAPTER TWENTY-ONE

Joining a gym for the first time? Sounds like a simple task, but selecting a gym or health club can be as mind-boggling as buying a new car. If you live in a medium-size community or larger, you're probably overwhelmed with choices. So how do you pick the right gym? Well, you wouldn't buy a car without shopping first and taking test drives, so be prepared to visit prospective clubs and "test drive" each one before signing on the dotted line. Here are some helpful guidelines to assist you in making an informed decision.

Selecting A Gym

Location – The more convenient your gym or health club is to get to, the more you'll use it. Decide at what time of day you are most likely to work out. Will you go to the gym on the way to or from school? How about on the weekend? How close is the gym to work or home, and how easily can you get there? If your gym is difficult to access, you'll be more likely to skip a workout. It's even possible your school has a weight room as most sports teams weight train nowadays. The nice thing about training at school is that it's very convenient and in most cases free. No monthly membership fees to worry about, no having to fight for a parking space. Here are a few factors to consider when shopping around for a place to train.

Facilities and amenities – What are the facilities like, and what type of equipment and classes are available? Are you looking for luxurious surroundings or simple and functional? Does the club have separate girls' and guys' locker rooms, changing rooms and showers? These amenities are very important if you work out on the way to school or during your lunch hour.

Focus – What is the focus of the club? Is it primarily aimed at weightlifters, or is it filled with exercise machines without a free weight in sight? Decide on the focus of your exercise program. If you mainly want to use aerobic exercise machines such as stair-steppers, bicycles and treadmills, don't join a hardcore, iron-pumping club that lacks this equipment.

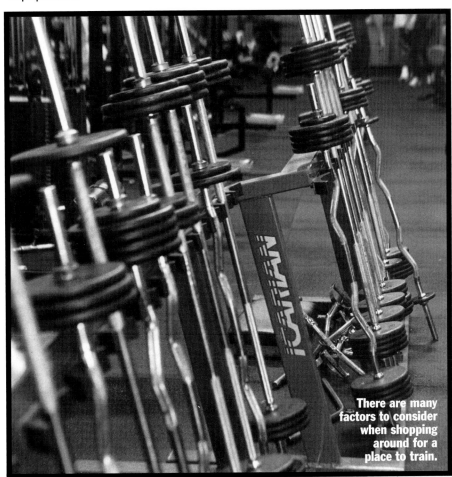

There are many factors to consider when shopping around for a place to train.

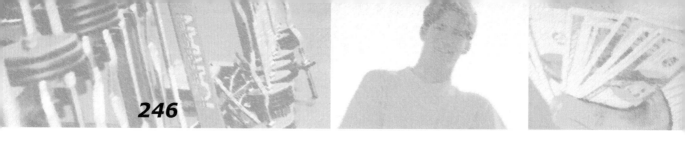

Conversely you probably don't want to join an uppity health spa either. These places mainly cater to well-to-do clientele and actually frown on serious training. Some won't even allow teens to access the facility, let alone become a member. And do you really want to be working out next to some stuffy librarian who's the same age as your mom? We think not.

Your best option is a middle-of-the-road fitness facility that has a good combination of aerobic and strength machines as well as free weights. Many of these facilities also have indoor tracks and swimming pools. You would have access to just about every form of indoor fitness activity there is.

Crowd control – How busy is the facility? How many members regularly use the club, and when are the busiest times? You won't want to go to a gym that is packed when you want to work out. On the other hand, if you have a flexible schedule and enjoy meeting people in the health club environment, pick a busy, popular gym.

Most gyms are moderately busy before work, lunch time and after school. Then at 4 p.m. the floodgates open and the place fills up. It usually stays busy until around 9 p.m.

As a teenager the best time for you to work out is just after school, which for most is about 3 p.m. This will give you a good hour or so before the bulk of the after work crowd starts to arrive. (You may want to check to see if the facility has membership restrictions. Some facilities require that teens be out the door by 5 p.m.)

Member profile – What are the members like? Is the gym filled with senior citizens listening to the Big Bands of the '40s? Or is it packed with Generation X-ers with grunge rock and gangster rap blaring over the sound system? If it's a typical fitness center you'll find the older folks tend to work out earlier in the day; the 20- and 30-somethings arriving at about 5 p.m.; and teens like yourself go in at around 3 or 3:30 p.m.

If you're not sure of the member profile of a particular gym, visit just after school. If you don't see many people in your age group, it probably means the place doesn't cater to teens.

Staff – Does the facility have experienced staff and instructors? Are they knowledgeable about the equipment, training and nutrition? Wearing a shirt with the facility's name on it doesn't guarantee any special ability, knowledge or training. Look for staff members who are friendly and competent. The better gyms have their instructors' certification diplomas posted around the main desk or in sales offices. Don't be shy in asking about qualifications. Anyone can call themselves a personal trainer.

Cost – Finally, how much does it cost? Does the club have a big initiation fee with large monthly payments? Must you sign a contract, or can you join on a month-to-month basis? Competition with other gyms can sometimes determine the cost. Be sure to look for advertised specials and coupons. Always ask if there are any special discounted membership packages available for teens.

Now that you know what to look for, jump in and start test driving those prospective gyms.

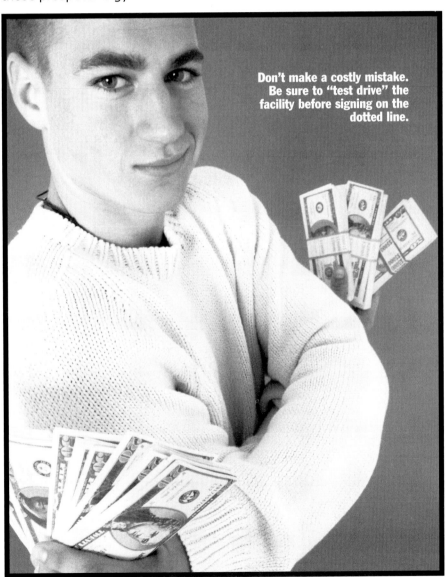

Don't make a costly mistake. Be sure to "test drive" the facility before signing on the dotted line.

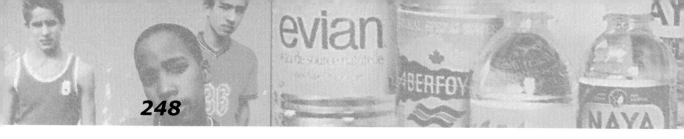

CHAPTER TWENTY-TWO

Gym Etiquette

Your first few weeks in the gym will probably be confusing, especially if you go there by yourself. Don't worry, it won't be long before you get the hang of things. To help you survive the first few workouts, we present to you a list of things we call "gym etiquette." Some items fall under the heading of *common sense,* while others are hard fast rules. Failing to abide by them will at the least create problems with other members. But really make a nuisance of yourself and you could be expelled.

Ask, ask, ask!

If you need help with anything – from how to work the treadmill to finding stretching mats, and from locating an exercise studio to learning how to use a machine – ask the fitness staff at the health club. It is not unusual for the staff to hear a variety of questions – and most likely, the question you will ask them is one they have already heard that day. There is no such thing as a stupid question.

Get to know the lingo.

If you are unfamiliar with words like *"rep"* and *"set,"* ask the fitness professionals at your club to give you an explanation of the terms. (We will be going into weightlifting principles in much greater detail later in the book.)

Go with the dress code.

Keep in mind, in some health clubs, it tends to be chilly when you first start for the day. Be

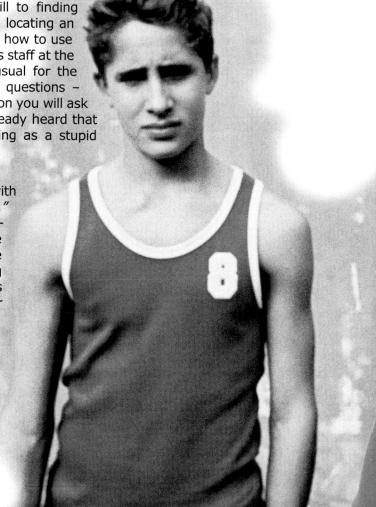

sure to dress comfortably. You might want to dress in layers. That way you can peel off as you get warmer. The standard gym outfit is a T-shirt and pair of shorts. If it's a bit cooler, change into a sweatshirt and pair of track pants. You can get really fancy with Spandex and what not, but the bottom line is to dress for maximum comfort.

Wipe down the equipment.

While health clubs maintain constant upkeep on the cleanliness of the facility and the equipment, gym etiquette dictates that you wipe down the equipment after you use it. No one wants to sit in another person's sweat. You don't want to grab the handles on the stepping machine and feel a layer of someone else's sweat. Likewise your sweat is not that appealing to another member. Most places have spray bottles and paper towel dispensers placed around the gym for cleaning the equipment. Please use them.

First come, first served.

If the cardio equipment you are interested in using is occupied, check for a sign-up sheet or board. Most clubs set a time limit for cardio equipment, so you can be sure your turn will come in a timely manner. If you can't access a piece of cardio equipment for half an hour or more, do some weightlifting first and then finish with the cardio. Although most people prefer to do cardio first, the rule is not etched in stone. And let's face it, it's no big deal for one workout.

Share.

If you are working on a piece of equipment and someone is waiting to use it, too – let him or her "work in." In other

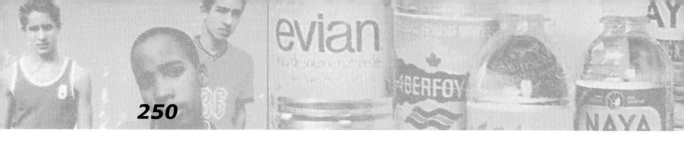

words, alternate sets. That way you can rest while the other person is lifting. This is especially true with weight training machines. Changing the weight is usually just a matter of moving a pin up or down the stack. About the only time you wouldn't ask to "jump in" is when someone has hundreds of plates loaded on a manually operated machine like the leg press. Simply ask the member to let you know when he or she is finished.

Don't forget a water bottle.

While health clubs have water fountains all over the place, it may be easier for you to stay hydrated if you carry a water bottle around with you. If you are on a cardio machine, having a water bottle handy is an easy way to keep drinking throughout the session.

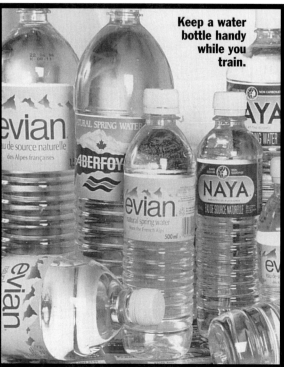

Keep a water bottle handy while you train.

Don't forget a towel.

If you plan on showering after your workout, check with the health club to see if they supply towels for you. If they do, grab one on your way into the locker room so you don't forget later. If the club does not supply towels, don't forget to pack your own.

Rerack your weights.

If you are using free weights, it is courteous to the other members to put your weights back on the rack when you are finished with them. One or two dumbells lying around on the floor is an accident waiting to happen; having to remove someone else's 500 pounds from the leg-press machine is downright annoying. Most gyms rigorously enforce this rule, so please follow it. Things will be a lot safer and more convenient for all members.

Be smell-conscious.

For the comfort of others, it's best to refrain from wearing any heavy aftershave or cologne. What smells good to you could be an allergy waiting to happen for the person next to you. (Many establishments have a "scent-free" policy, so check with your gym about this.) Also, please wash your workout clothes regularly. A sweat-soaked shirt lying around for a couple of days acquires an aroma that would drop an elephant at 50 paces!

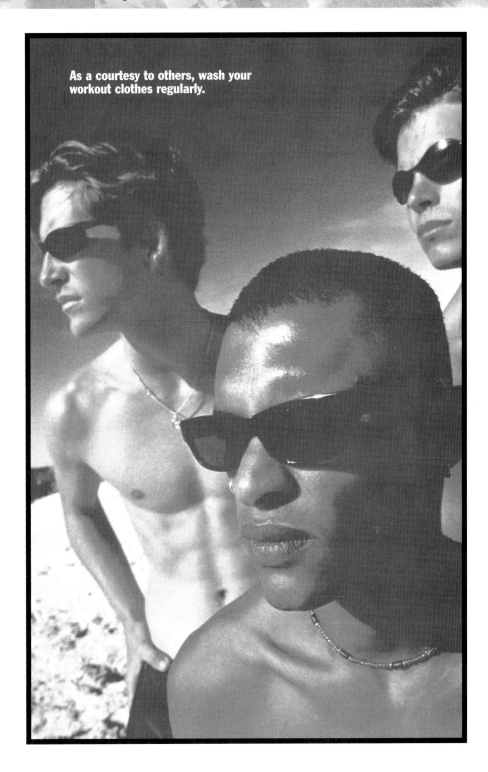

As a courtesy to others, wash your workout clothes regularly.

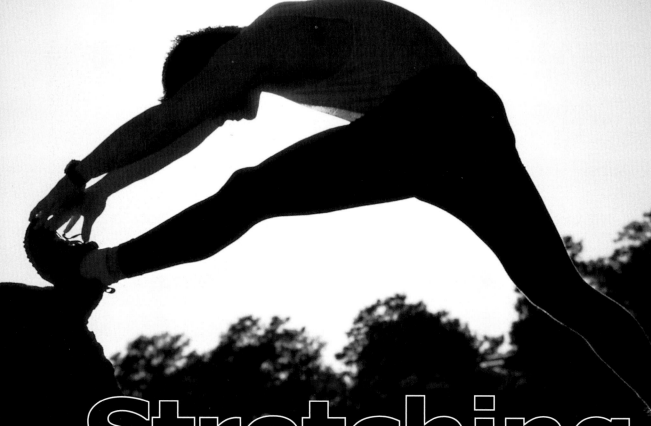

CHAPTER TWENTY-THREE

Stretching

Why stretch? Stretching is useful for both injury prevention and injury treatment. For the purposes of this discussion we will concentrate on *prevention*. If done properly, stretching increases flexibility and this directly translates into reduced risk of injury. That's because a muscle/tendon group with a greater range of motion passively, will be less likely to experience tears when used actively. Stretching is also thought to improve recovery and may enhance athletic performance. The latter has not been fully agreed upon in the medical literature, but improved biomechanical efficiency has been suggested as an explanation. Additionally, increased flexibility of the neck, shoulders and upper back may improve respiratory function.

How to Stretch

There are basically three methods of stretching: static, ballistic and PNF (proprioceptive neuromuscular facilitation). Static is the method recommended for the majority of athletes since it is the least likely to cause injury. Ballistic (bouncing) and PNF stretching are probably best reserved for a select few who are experienced with their use. To get the most benefit from your static stretching routine while minimizing injury, *stretching should be done after warmup exercises.* The increased blood flow to the muscles aids in the flexibility gains from stretching and is an important component for injury prevention.

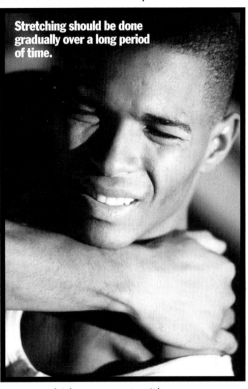

Stretching should be done gradually over a long period of time.

Static stretching is done by slowly moving a joint toward its end range of motion. A gentle "pulling" sensation should be felt in the desired muscle. This position is then held for 15 to 20 seconds. Do not stretch to the point of pain and do not bounce – this may cause injury to the muscle. Within a session, each subsequent stretch of a particular muscle group seems to give progressively more flexibility. A set of 3 to 5 stretches is probably sufficient to get the maximum benefit from the routine.

Alternate between agonist and antagonist muscle groups (eg. quadriceps and hamstrings) and alternate sides. It is also a good idea to start with the neck and progress down to the feet. This progression enables you to take advantage of gains in flexibility from the previously stretched muscle groups. *Stretching should also be done after the workout.* The postworkout stretch is thought to aid in recovery. Cold packs can be applied to sore areas in those of you who are recovering from injuries.

Why am I so tight?

There is considerable variation in baseline flexibility between individuals. There may also be variation within a given individual (e.g., flexible shoulders but inflexible hips, or flexible right hamstring, but tight, inflexible left hamstring). Genetics, injuries and abnormal biomechanics all play a role in these differences. One shouldn't try to make big gains in flexibility in a short period of time. Stretching should be done gradually over a long period of time and then maintained to prevent you from slipping back toward inflexibility. Some people will enthusiastically embark on a stretching program, but then quit two weeks later because they haven't seen any benefit. Be patient and consistent. It takes a long time.

Relax

You *must* relax during the stretching routine. It should not be a rushed event. Don't think about school or your job and don't look at others working out. The "I've got to hurry up and do this so I can go" attitude is counterproductive. This is a time to slow your breathing and to *free your mind.* Some athletes will employ mental imagery while stretching. In this relaxed state, the athlete visualizes proper form in preparation for training or competition.

Concentrate on Technique

If you have any back, neck, bone or joint problems consult your doctor before beginning a stretching program. No stretching routine should be painful. Pain indicates either incorrect technique or a medical problem. If in doubt, ask a qualified health professional. These two stretches are good:

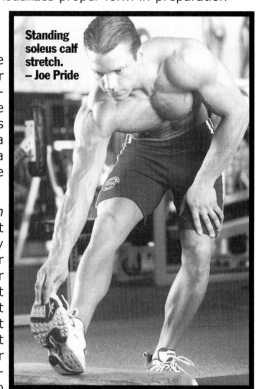

Standing soleus calf stretch. – Joe Pride

1. *Standing soleus calf stretch (using a step)* – Place your right heel on a step with the knee slightly bent. Lean forward and grasp your right toe with your right hand. Your left knee should be slightly bent and your back should be straight (not rounded). Support your weight on the left leg and place your left hand on the left thigh. Pull your right toes toward the knee, keeping the knee slightly bent. Get to the point of a mild stretch and hold for 30 seconds.

2. *Standing gastrocnemius calf stretch (using a step)* – Place your right heel on a step with the knee extended. Lean forward and grasp your right toe with your right hand. Your left knee should be slightly bent and your back should be straight (not rounded). Support your weight on the left leg and place your left hand on the left thigh. Pull your right toes toward the knee keeping the knee slightly bent. Get to the point of a mild stretch and hold for 30 seconds.

Hamstring Stretches

The hamstrings (hams) consist of the biceps femoris, semitendinosis and semimembranosis. They are located on the back of the upper leg. Their function is to extend the hip and flex the knee.

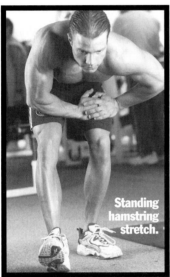

Standing hamstring stretch.

1. Standing ham stretch (can be performed using a step or with the leg on the floor) – Place your right heel on a step (or in front of you on the floor) with the knee slightly bent. Lean forward placing your hands on the left leg. Your left leg knee will be slightly bent (this is the leg that is supporting your bodyweight). As you lean forward, your lower back should curve slightly inward. Try to press the buttocks and back up, pushing the hips away from the front knee. Get to the point of a mild stretch and hold for 30 seconds.

2. Sitting ham stretch – Sit on the floor with the right leg extended and the left leg bent (the left knee will be next to your chest). Slide the bent leg down to stretch the right hamstring keeping the chest pressed against the thigh of the left leg. Your lower back should be slightly curved. Make sure you don't round the upper back (if you keep your chest pressed against your knee, the upper back will be okay). Get to the point of a mild stretch and hold for 30 seconds.

Sitting hamstring stretch.

3. Supine ham stretch – Lie on your back with the left leg extended. Raise the right leg with the knee slightly bent. Grasp the right calf or thigh and gently pull the right leg toward your body. (As the muscle relaxes, you may be able to pull the leg a little closer.) Get to the point of a mild stretch and hold for 30 seconds.

Quadriceps Stretches

The quadriceps (quads) consist of four muscles located on the front of your thigh. The muscles are the vastus lateralis, vastus intermedius, vastus medialis and rectus femoris. These four muscles act together to extend the knee. The rectus femoris also helps flex the hip.

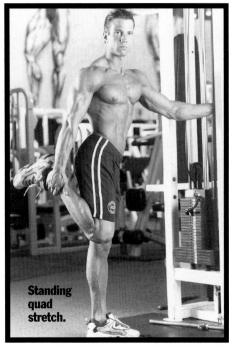

Standing quad stretch.

1. Standing quad stretch – Contract the abdominals to hold the pelvis in a neutral position *(do not arch your back* – you may need to tilt the pelvis back if you feel your back begin to arch). Lift the right ankle toward the glutes. Reach back with the right or left hand and gently hold the ankle (the right knee should be pointing toward the floor). Press the front hip bone forward and slightly extend the hip. Keep the torso lifted with your head up. Get to the point of a mild stretch and hold for 30 seconds.

2. Side-lying quad stretch – Lie on your left side with the left arm extended and head resting on it. Contract the abdominals to hold the pelvis in a neutral position. Bring the right ankle back toward the glutes. Reach back with the right hand and gently hold the ankle (the right knee should be parallel to the floor). Press the front hip bone forward and slightly extend the hip. Get to the point of a mild stretch and hold for 30 seconds.

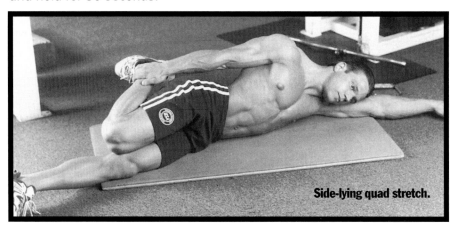

Side-lying quad stretch.

Shoulder Circles
• Stand tall, feet placed slightly wider than shoulder width apart, knees slightly bent.
• Raise your right shoulder toward your right ear, take it backwards, down and then up again to the ear in a smooth action.
• Repeat with the other shoulder.

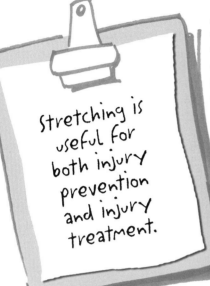

Stretching is useful for both injury prevention and injury treatment.

Arm Circles
• Stand tall, feet slightly wider than shoulder width apart, knees slightly bent.
• Lift one arm, reach forward, then lift it up and backwards in a continuous circling motion.
• Keep the back straight at all times.
• Repeat with the other arm.

Chest Stretch
• Stand tall and place your feet slightly wider than shoulder width apart, knees slightly bent.
• Hold your arms out to the sides parallel with the floor, palms of the hands facing forward.
• Stretch the arms back as far as possible.
• You should feel the stretch across your chest.

Biceps Stretch
• Stand tall, feet slightly wider than shoulder width apart, knees slightly bent.
• Hold your arms out to the sides parallel with the floor, palms facing forward.
• Rotate the hands so the palms face to the rear.
• Stretch the arms back as far as possible.
• You should feel the stretch across your chest and in the biceps.

Upper-Back Stretch
• Stand tall, feet a little bit wider than shoulder width, knees slightly bent.
• Interlock your fingers and push your hands as far away from your chest as possible, allowing your upper back to relax.
• You should feel the stretch between your shoulder blades.

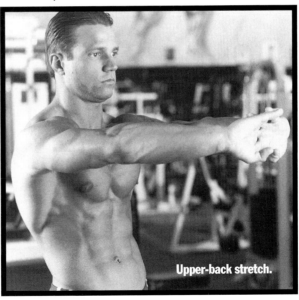

Upper-back stretch.

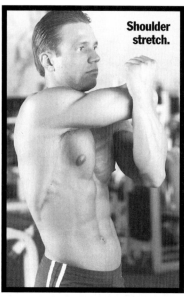

Shoulder stretch.

Shoulder Stretch
- Stand tall, feet slightly wider than shoulder width apart, knees slightly bent.
- Place your right arm across the front of your chest parallel with the floor.
- Bend the left arm up and use the left forearm to ease the right arm closer to your chest.
- You will feel the stretch in the shoulder.
- Repeat with the other arm.

Shoulder and Triceps Stretch
- Stand tall, feet slightly wider than shoulder width apart, knees slightly bent.
- Place both hands above your head and then slide both of your hands down the middle of your spine. Return to the starting position, then repeat.
- You'll feel it in the shoulders and triceps.

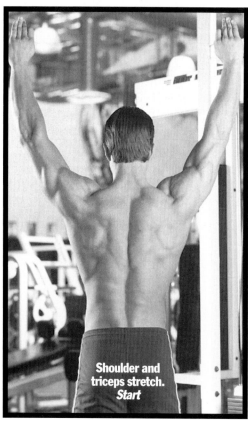

Shoulder and triceps stretch.
Start

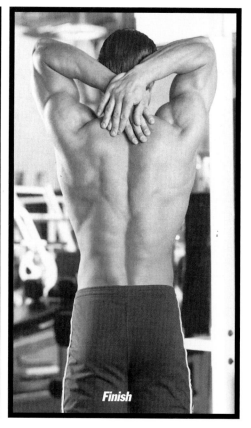

Finish

Trunk Twists
• Stand tall with your feet slightly wider than hip width apart, knees slightly bent, hands resting on hips.
• Rotate the upper body slowly and smoothly to bring right shoulder to the front.
• Rotate the upper body slowly and smoothly to bring left shoulder to the front, keeping your back straight and your hips facing forward.

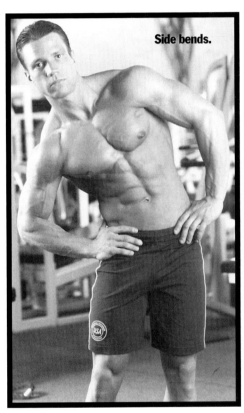
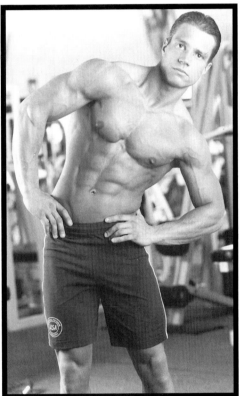

Side bends.

Side Bends
• Stand tall, feet slightly wider than shoulder width apart, knees slightly bent, hands resting on the hips.
• Bend slowly to one side, come back to the vertical position, then bend to the other side.
• Do not lean forward or backward.

Abdominal and Lower Back
• Lie face down on the floor in a prone position
• Lift your body off the floor so that you are supported only by your forearms and toes. The elbows should be on the floor and should be

almost directly behind your shoulders. Your forearms and hands should be resting down, pointed straight ahead. Toes and feet should be shoulder width apart with your head in line with your spine.

• Contract your gluteus (butt) muscles gently. Hold for ten seconds.
• Lift your right arm off the floor, straighten it and point it straight ahead, holding it in the air for 10 seconds.
• Return to the starting position.
• Repeat with the left arm.
• Return to starting position.
• Lift your right leg off the floor and hold it there for ten seconds (keep back straight).
• Return to starting position.
• Repeat with left leg.
• Return to starting position.
• Lift your right arm and left leg simultaneously and hold that position for ten seconds.
• Return to starting position.
• Lift your left arm and right leg simultaneously and hold them in position for ten seconds.
• Return to the starting position.

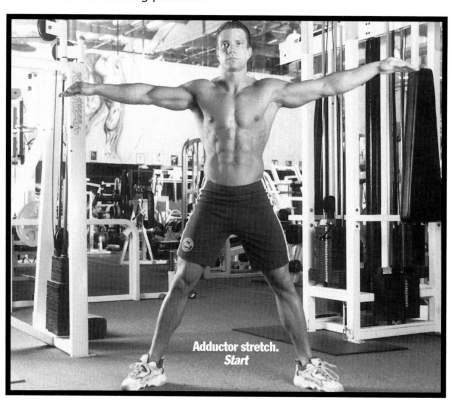

Adductor stretch.
Start

Adductor Stretch
• Stand tall with your feet approximately twice shoulder width apart.
• Bend the right leg and lower the body.
• Keep your back straight and use the arms to balance.
• You will feel the stretch in the left leg adductor.
• Repeat with the left leg.

Groin Stretch
• Sit with tall posture.
• Ease both of your feet up toward your body and place the soles of your feet together, allowing your knees to come up and out to the sides.
• Resting your hands on your lower legs or ankles, ease both knees toward the floor.
• You will feel the stretch along the insides of your thighs and groin.

Front of Trunk Stretch
• Lie face down on the floor, fully outstretched.
• Bring your hands to the sides of your shoulders and ease your chest off the floor, keeping your hips firmly pressed into the floor.
• You will feel the stretch in the front of the trunk.

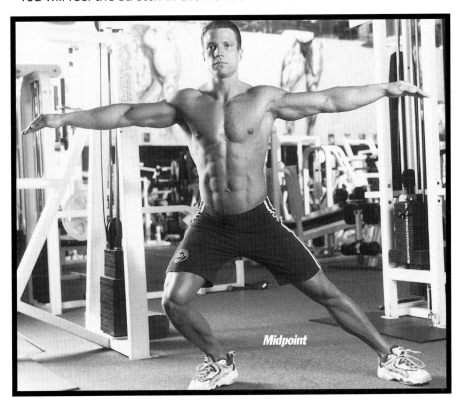

Midpoint

CHAPTER TWENTY-FOUR

Basic
Strength-Training
Principles

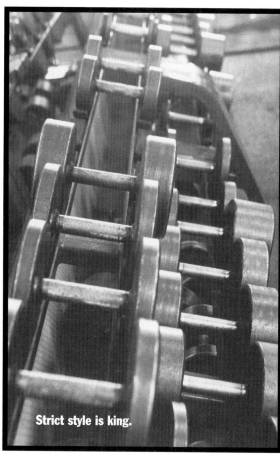

Strict style is king.

Strength training is no different than most forms of fitness in that there are basic concepts and principles to guide you. Unfortunately, in their desire to get in shape in the quickest time possible, many teens fail to abide by these guidelines. Without sounding like your mom or teacher, these basic principles are for your own good, so to speak. Follow them wisely and you'll reap the rewards for years to come. Skip them in favor of the teachings of some "gym rat" know-it-all and you could be setting yourself up for a major injury. At the very least you could be wasting your time in the gym. In this chapter we present the very important principles and guidelines for a safe and effective strength-training program.

The Overload Principle

Development is based on adaptation to demands: This general principle refers to the fact that stress (in this case the amount of weight you use) should be progressively increased in order to cause adaptation or change. Factors that can be used to overload your muscles include: load (intensity), volume (repetitions and sets), rest and frequency.

Load refers to the intensity (poundage) of the exercise. Strength development occurs when the muscle works against increased loads (weight resistance). Load is usually stated as a percent of the maximum weight the individual can lift in that position. Strength training uses loads of 70 to 100 percent of a person's one-rep max (1RM).

Repetition refers to how many times the load is moved, or in simple terms how many times you lift the weight up and down. "Rep" is probably the most basic term used in weight training. Reps are grouped together into the second most basic term in weightlifting – "sets." To develop muscle endurance a program incorporates a high number of reps (12 to 25) and low load (less than 70 percent). Greater load (more than 70 percent) and lower reps (fewer than 12) will develop muscular strength.

Rest is the time interval between groups of repetitions. The amount of rest depends on your fitness goals. If you are trying to develop a combination of strength and endurance, rest 1 to 2 minutes between sets. The goal of strength training is to work against maximum resistance during each set.

Frequency is the number of training sessions per week. As intensity and volume increase, the muscle and nervous systems need time to restructure in order to handle the greater workloads placed upon them. Lifting programs for specific muscles are usually scheduled twice or three times per week. *Split routines* are used when an exercise program has too many exercises or too much intensity for a single workout session. An example of a split routine would be to divide exercises into upper body and lower body days. Your program

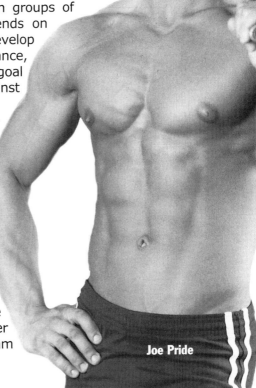

Joe Pride

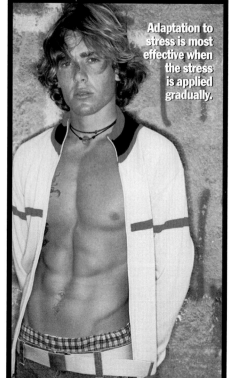

Adaptation to stress is most effective when the stress is applied gradually.

might have lower-body exercises on Mondays and Wednesdays, and upper-body exercises on Tuesdays and Thursdays. Muscles increase in strength and size *following* the workout – therefore adequate rest and recovery time is absolutely necessary. Sometimes rest is as important as the level of overload. If you are getting injured, having trouble recovering, or are exceedingly sore, the overload is *excessive* and you must make adjustments to your routine.

Progression

Take gradual steps. Adaptation to stress is most effective when the stress is applied gradually. High levels of change take time to develop. You will not develop a high level of physical fitness overnight – that's impossible. Development is the result of many small gains. It is generally accepted that training should concentrate on volume (reps and sets) first, and then on intensity (increased poundages).

Training Specifically

Train the way you want to develop. Strength-training experts call this the "S.A.I.D. Principle" – specific adaptation to imposed demands: The body develops specifically according to stresses that are placed upon it. Any training program should reflect the desired adaptation you wish to bring about. For example, the adaptation to endurance exercise such as biking or running differs from that of strength training. As the level of training progresses, even the training for biking and running will become specialized. In some cases training for one activity might actually *hamper* the development in another.

Individual Differences: Genetics

We are not all created equal. Genetics limits our capacity to develop fitness and skill. People have different body types and develop at different rates. It is important, however, to realize that anyone can improve if he or she is consistent and hardworking. Lifestyle is far more important than genetics in determining health and well-being.

Reversibility: Use it or lose it!

This principle is the reverse of the overload principle. The body develops according to the stress placed upon it. As progressive stress is increased you gain strength; when it is removed, you lose it.

Proper Technique and Correct Form

The most common training error or mistake is the tendency to use poor form or to "cheat" on the exercise. One cause of poor form is trying to use too much weight (resistance) too quickly, and using body momentum to aid in completing the movement. Development is based on how the body adapts to the stress, so cheating does not yield significant gains. Another cause is the use of poor posture or limb alignment – *improper form can cause injury!* If you take nothing else from this chapter take this: *Strict style is king.*

Order of Exercises

If strength is your goal, start with multijoint large muscles first and then proceed to single-joint small muscles. Doing small muscle exercises first might fatigue them too quickly, thereby limiting the performance of the large muscles. For example the biceps are used on most back exercises. Because they are smaller they tend to tire quicker, limiting the effectiveness of your back exercises. If you train biceps before back, you won't be able to lift enough weight to adequately stimulate your larger back muscles. The same holds true for triceps, which come into play on chest and shoulder exercises. Here's a general rule of thumb: *Train largest to smallest.*

Breathing

Most books and experts give the following advice on breathing: "Holding your breath and straining can cause the Valsalva effect, which increases blood pressure and can cause unconsciousness. Exhale

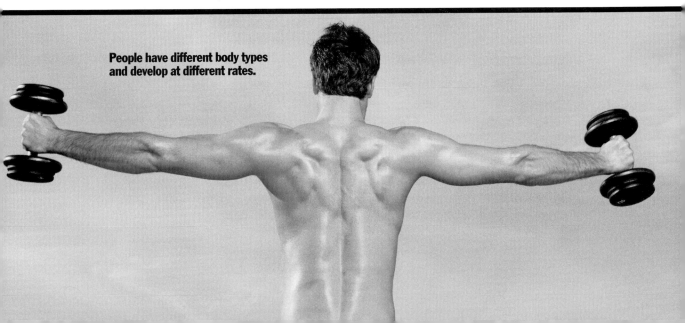

People have different body types and develop at different rates.

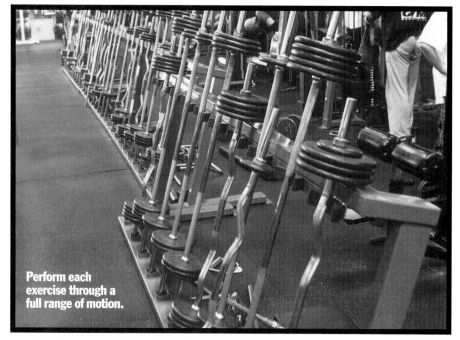

Perform each exercise through a full range of motion.

during the concentric (muscle-shortening) part of the contraction and inhale during the eccentric (muscle lengthening) part of the lift. For example during the bench press: exhale while you press the weight up, inhale as you lower the weight down."

Now we should add that the previous method is called "going by the book." Some writers and strength-training experts make a big deal out of breathing, but in our opinion it shouldn't be. In over 20 years of training, the authors have yet to see someone faint because they forgot to breath. The body will do a marvelous job of breathing for you without any conscious effort on your part. The only exception to this would be in cases if someone has a habit of holding his or her breath for more than a couple of reps. In this case the individual should concentrate on breathing on every rep. But to say you *absolutely must* breath on every rep is making a mountain out of a molehill. Let the body take care of breathing; you concentrate on proper technique.

Always be sure to warm up!
Although we went into this in more detail earlier in the book, it's worth repeating. Warmups increase the temperature of the muscles and increase synovial fluid in the joints. This helps the muscles work better and protects against injury. Good warmup practice is to do a light aerobic workout and then do a couple of low intensity sets of exercises before performing the actual work sets.

Exercise Speed

Lifting fast creates momentum and doesn't promote blood flow to the muscle. Slow movement creates less momentum and less internal muscle friction. The control needed for the slow lifting requires more application of muscle power throughout the range of the movement, and promotes rapid blood flow to the muscle. It is even more important to slow down the eccentric (negative) part of the lift, because this action promotes increased blood flow to the muscle. This causes microtrauma (beneficial temporary muscle breakdown) that then yields muscle development. It is recommended that the concentric (shortening) phase lasts one to two seconds and the eccentric (lengthening) phase lasts three to four.

Exercise through the full range of motion.

Perform each exercise through a full range of motion, with emphasis on the end of the positive phase. Full-range exercise movements are advantageous for strengthening the prime mover muscles, or agonists – these are the muscles directly trained in the exercise, such as the biceps in the biceps curl. Lifting in the full range of motion is also good

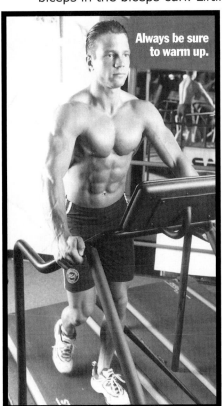

Always be sure to warm up.

for stretching the antagonist muscles, the muscles that act in opposition to the agonist. In the biceps curl, the triceps muscle group is the antagonist. Training through the full range of motion enhances both muscle strength and joint flexibility.

Selection of Exercises

Very important. You must select at least one exercise for each major muscle group to promote well-balanced overall muscle development. Training only a few muscle groups or training one muscle group more increases the risk of hurting yourself. This is one of the primary reasons for many sports-related injuries. Many athletes have some muscle groups that are much stronger than others – usually those they use the most in their sport – and that results in muscle imbalances that often lead to injury. Even though you may not currently participate in competitive sports, you should still strive for overall muscle balance.

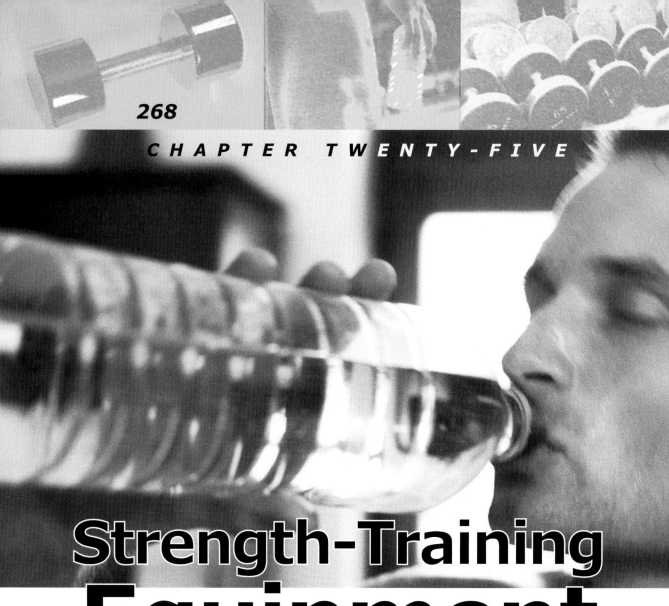

CHAPTER TWENTY-FIVE

Strength-Training
Equipment

We'll be the first to admit it – the modern strength-training gym can be an intimidating place, especially for beginners. You got all these crazy-looking contraptions that do *who knows what*. Some look downright dangerous (they are!), while others can be found in most basements or attics. What we are going to try to accomplish over the next few pages is help you sort through the maze that makes up the gym. More specifically, we are going to describe the various pieces of equipment you will use in your workouts. Some cost thousands of dollars and are owned by the gym. The others cost a few dollars and can be purchased by you. Don't let the cost fool you, either. A few of these pieces of personal equipment are just as important as that $5000 treadmill.

Equipment: Yours and Yours Alone

Water bottle – Even though our ancestors left the oceans hundreds of millions of years ago, humans are still very dependent on this life-giving liquid. In fact your body is over 90 percent water, which is why you have all those conservation mechanisms to retain water. Still there are situations when water loss outpaces water conservation; and you guessed, exercise is one of those times.

Most gyms have water fountains and you can easily take a few sips between exercises, but the same cannot be said when you are on the cross-trainer or treadmill for half an hour. You must also consider the matter of hygiene. How many people use those water fountains over the course of a day? Hundreds if not thousands in a busy gym, and some of those individuals are carrying around some very nasty germs.

The easy solution is to carry a water bottle. You can buy one for $3 or $4 at most gyms or sporting-goods stores. Many gyms will even give them away as a marketing gimmick. Cheaper still, reuse a mineral water bottle. You don't need to spend big bucks to keep yourself well hydrated during your workouts. Every few minutes take a few mouthfuls. On hot and humid days you may need to sip continually to keep your water levels high.

Headbands – Much of the water you consumed in the previous paragraph will be leaving the body in the form of sweat. Now while sweating is great for cooling the body, it does have its undesirable side. For those of you who wear glasses, sweat makes exercise a tad difficult. Every few minutes you have to reposition your glasses. And we probably don't need to describe what sweat feels like when trapped under a contact lens. As with water bottles, preventing sweat from getting into your eyes is relatively easy and inexpensive. For a few dollars you can buy a headband. They come in different colors and styles, but they all do the same thing. They soak up sweat and stop it from getting into your eyes. If purchasing one does not appeal to you, why not make your own! All you need is a bit of cloth and some basic sewing skills.

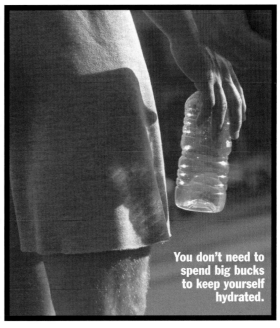

You don't need to spend big bucks to keep yourself hydrated.

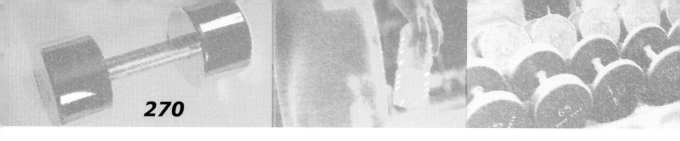

***Gloves* –** For some people it's a rite of passage. For others it's downright disgusting. What we are talking about are *calluses* – those thicker areas of the hands caused by a buildup of dead skin from repeated usage. A callus is a defense mechanism to prevent breakage of the skin – the body's first line of defense against invading organisms. After a couple of workouts you'll notice your hands starting to blister at the base of the fingers. This is caused by a chafing of the outer skin layer over the lower layers. Repeated chafing causes a buildup of fluid, which in turn leads to blisters. If the chafing keeps up, the body basically says "I don't need this anymore" and starts laying down a layer of dead skin to thicken the area and prevent more blisters. For some people this is no big deal, but to be honest many don't like the look or feel.

The way to avoid getting calluses is to wear gloves. Protective gloves are not unique to weightlifting. Many sports require the use of gloves – from golf and hockey to baseball and racquetball. Gloves provide a barrier between the hands and whichever piece of weight training equipment you are holding on to. If you wear gloves from day one, your hands will never blister or form calluses.

If using gloves has a downside, it's *dependence.* Once you start using them you are committed. If you forget them one day and proceed with your workout you'll develop a set of blisters that may take a week to heal properly. With time you'll be using more weight and thus placing more pressure on the hands. Another factor is *feel.* Many people find that gloves prevent them from getting a good grip on the bar or machine handle.

The choice to wear gloves is ultimately yours. Our advice is to skip gloves unless you need soft hands for delicate activities (playing a musical instrument, for example). A few calluses are not that bad and once you develop calluses you'll never have to worry about getting blisters.

***Wraps* –** For those readers who regularly engage in sports, there's nothing new about wraps. Even with proper technique, sooner or later one or more of your joints may start to act up. Let's face it, repetitious movement places stress on the soft tissue that surround the body's joints. Eventually inflammation may occur to the point that performing exercises involving that joint is very painful. Even though we'll be talking about injuries in more detail later in the book, suffice to say this: As soon as a joint begins to hurt, take a few days off from training. If the problem still doesn't clear up, go see your doctor.

There may come a point, however, when even with the usual amount of rest and medical intervention, certain joints continue to cause slight pain. We say *slight* because if there is severe pain you have to listen to your doctor. But if it's only minor, one solution is to use wraps. Wraps are nothing more than long, narrow pieces of cloth – usually bandage material – that you wrap around the offending joint. Wraps add security to the area as well as heat. The heat keeps the area soft and supple, which not only reduces the chance of injury but also reduces the pain from previous injuries.

Contrary to popular belief, belts don't make you physically stronger.

For obvious reasons avoiding injuries is your primary goal. But when minor injuries come along that just don't want to go away, wraps offer a means to keep training in relative comfort.

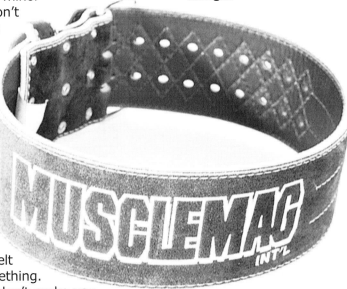

Belts – Name almost any sport and you'll find a piece of equipment that is unique to that sport. Baseball has its bat, hockey its puck, and tennis its racket. For weightlifting no piece of equipment has become more associated than the weightlifting belt. You've probably seen cartoons where some character squeezes his waist to half its size with a belt and then lifts a car or something. Contrary to popular belief, belts don't make you physically stronger. Instead they give extra protection and security to the lower back. For some this may provide a psychological boost, but there's nothing about the belt that is making the muscles stronger. On some exercises like squats, rows and overhead presses, there is extra pressure placed on the lower back. A belt acts almost like a splint you'd put on a broken leg – it adds support. Weightlifting belts come in three basic styles: velcro, heavy-duty powerlifting, and middle-of-the-road. Let's look at all three.

Velcro belts – Velcro belts are usually made of a type of cloth or webbing material, and fasten at the front with velcro. From an appearance and fit perspective, velcro belts are great. But from a practical point of view they are almost useless. Sure their tight fit adds a little extra warmth to the area, but their flimsy construction gives little or no lower back support – the primary function of belts. If you are wearing a belt just for looks, then so be it, but if you want good lower-back support, read on.

Powerlifting belts – Powerlifting belts are the largest and thickest of the various belt styles. Some of them are up to six inches wide and half an inch thick. Powerlifters use them to provide support on superheavy lifts like squats and deadlifts. If such belts have a drawback it's the way they fit. For someone with a small or medium-size waist, the belt won't hug as tight as you'd want. For a 300-pound powerlifter with a 40-inch waist, this is not an issue, but for most readers a powerlifting belt is too large and ungainly. Your best option is the middle-of-the-road belt.

Middle-of-the-road belts – As the name implies, middle-of-the-road belts are designed for the average person. They'll fit just about everyone, while at the same time provide good lower-back support. They offer more support than the velcro belts, but being slightly thinner than the powerlifting belts, the middle-of-the-road belts fit much better. They are usually made of leather, but other materials may also be used. They range in price from $20 to $50 or more.

Should I wear a belt?

There's a school of thought that wearing a belt is *dangerous* in the long run. The theory is that if you continually wear a belt, the lower

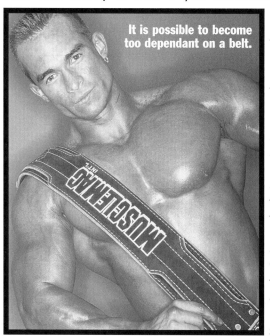

It is possible to become too dependant on a belt.

back muscles become so dependent on the belt that they never strengthen as well as they should. The belt is sort of a crutch that they rely on. In some respects this is true, it is possible to become too dependent on a belt. Some guys put the belt on in the locker room like a gladiator going into battle and don't take it off until they leave the gym. The authors routinely see guys running on the treadmill while wearing a belt! How the treadmill compares to a set of squats, we don't know, but for some a belt is like a security blanket. Our advice

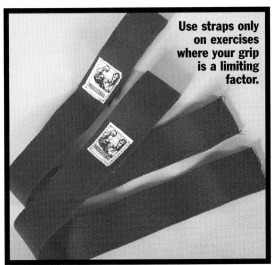

Use straps only on exercises where your grip is a limiting factor.

is to wear a belt on those exercises that add a bit of extra pressure to the lower back region, but take it off for everything else.

Straps **–** After a couple of weeks of working out you'll realize that there are a few exercises where the forearm muscles give out before the bigger muscle being worked – especially true when training the back. Most back exercises require you to hold on tight with your forearms while you pull the bar or handle toward you. You may reach the point where the back muscles are capable of pulling more weight than the forearms are capable of gripping. One solution is to do more direct forearm-training to strengthen your grip, but even this may not be enough. Bodybuilders and other weightlifters get around this "weak link in the chain" effect by using straps.

Straps are narrow pieces of woven cloth or leather that you wrap around your wrists and the bar or handles you are gripping. Some have a loop on one end that you can feed the other end through, other straps are straight and you simply position your wrist in the middle and wrap both ends around the object you are gripping. When wrapping around the bar or handle you wrap under and over, not over and under. Sounds trivial but wrapping under and then over means the strap will get *tighter* as you pull on it. This means the bar or handle won't slip out of your hand as you perform the exercise.

You can buy straps for $15 to $20 or make your own. For a couple of bucks you can buy a few yards of leather, dense cloth, or woven material. Simply cut the strip into 24 to 30-inch lengths. Fold back about 4 inches of one end and stitch it to the main section. Feed the other end through the loop and away you go.

Straps are like belts in that you can get too dependent on them. Use them only on exercises where your grip is the limiting factor.

Chalk **–** We are sure many of you readers either engage in or have engaged in gymnastics. Therefore a detailed accounting of chalk is not needed. Chalk is one of those training aids that costs mere pennies but can make a huge difference to your workouts. One of the byproducts of exercise is *sweat* and it has this nasty habit of getting on everything, including your hands and the equipment. It won't be long before a buildup of sweat causes you to lose your grip. Gymnasts get around this by using fine powdered chalk. Chalk soaks up water and allows you to maintain a firm grip on whatever you are holding on to.

Chalk comes in small blocks of 3 to 4 inches and costs a couple of bucks. As a word of caution, check to see your gym's policy before purchasing. Some gyms don't like the mess chalk leaves behind. Most hardcore and middle-of-the-road gyms don't usually mind, but forget it if you train at an upscale fitness spa-type facility. The last thing they want is chalk on their nice clean carpet!

The Training Journal

One of the best ways to know where you are going is to know where you have been. In other words, you can reach your goals faster if you keep a detailed record of your training progress. For a few bucks you can pick up a neat little *log book* to record all sorts of important information about your workouts. Almost all the advantages of keeping a training journal come from regular comparisons that you are able to make by

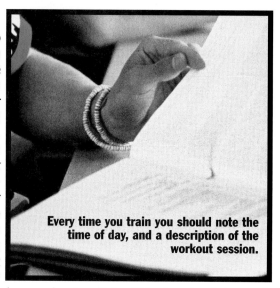

Every time you train you should note the time of day, and a description of the workout session.

logging and tracking day-to-day workouts, diet, attitude, etc. A journal lets you chart the peaks and valleys of your performances. You may think you will never forget a particular event or practice, but could you remember the exact workout the day or weeks before, that prepared you for that peak performance?

A training journal is also a great place to record the results of competitive events. By jotting down the name of the event, the people you competed against, and the outcome, you can compare your accomplishments from event to event, from year to year.

Your Personal Record

Because each person's training needs are different, the type of information recorded is completely up to the individual. Your training journal should be just that – yours. Sports physiologists, athletic trainers and coaches, as well as former Olympic medalists agree that there are several areas *every athlete* involved in a serious program should include in his or her journal.

Daily Workouts

Every time you train you should note the time of day, and a description of the workout session. Specify the type of exercise and how you felt before, during and after training. Also note the *intensity* level of each session and the number of workouts that day. Record the number and length of rest intervals during the session. Write it down if you are recovering from illness or injury. In noting the time of day of your training, you can compare early morning workouts to afternoon sessions, for example, to see if the time of day influences how well you train or how you feel.

Sleep Patterns

Note in your journal the ease at which you fell asleep the night before, and how well and how long you slept. Jot down any changes or disturbances in sleep patterns as well as the total hours slept each night.

Injuries

How you recover from an injury can be documented in your journal, and can be used as a reference for future injuries. Regular record keeping will show what type of treatment was used for a particular injury. How long did it take for a complete recovery? Was complete rest or moderate exercise the way you rehabilitated? A journal will help you

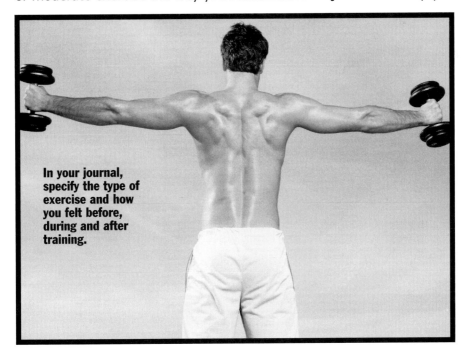

In your journal, specify the type of exercise and how you felt before, during and after training.

track the cause of injuries more easily, too. For example, if a knee problem develops for no apparent reason, a journal will allow you to look back over your activities of the previous days for clues. Recovering from any illness such as a cold or the flu also should be noted in your journal. Frequent illnesses may indicate a low resistance to germs and infections as a result of stress or overtraining.

Supplementary Training

All supplementary training should be recorded and monitored. If you are weight training for greater muscular strength, note the poundages and repetitions, or weight resistance machines used in your training. When running or cycling is part of your program, record the distance and time (speed) for each workout.

Common Journal Pitfalls

The most common pitfall of keeping a regular journal is to record too much information. Keep only information that is important to you and your training program. Don't become bogged down with recording trivial details or more data than you need. Jot down only the main details. Otherwise, you may tire altogether of keeping any notes.

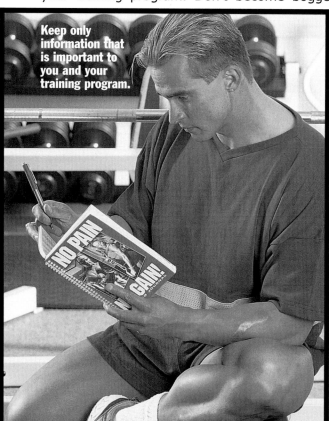

Keep only information that is important to you and your training program.

Looking Back ...

The greatest benefit you will get from keeping a training journal is the ability to look back over past weeks, months and years. You might not have to recall the difficulty, once you are through a particularly tough training period, but flipping back through the pages in your journal will remind you of just how hard you have worked.

Equipment: The Gyms

Generally speaking gym equipment falls into two categories – machines and free weights. Even though we'll be describing the operation of each later in the book, we'll give you a brief overview of both types here.

Machines

Strength-training machines come in many shapes and sizes, and even though there are dozens of different manufacturers, they all operate on similar principles. Most have a weight stack made up of flat plates weighing 5, 10 or 20 pounds each. The weight is selected by a pin that is inserted into a hole in the plate. Most machines have a set of upright columns that let the plates travel up and down.

Some of the first machines developed were multistations that had an exercise for each muscle arranged around a central core. Your high school probably has a Universal multistation located close to the gym. Many commercial gyms still use this popular piece of equipment (hey, it takes up less space), but the trend nowadays is to have the exercises performed on separate machines. Machines have been developed to work just about every muscle group, but some are far more effective than others.

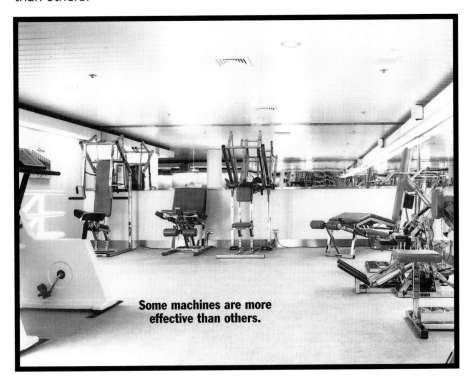

Some machines are more effective than others.

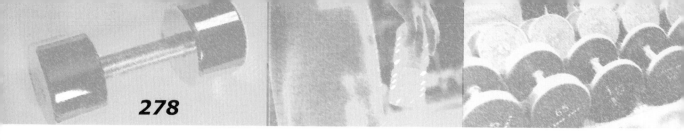

Free Weights

Free weight is the term given to barbells and dumbells. Barbells are the long bars you see Olympic lifters trying to lift over their heads. A standard Olympic barbell is about seven feet long and weighs 45 pounds. The bar consists of a narrower inner section, and a thicker section on each end called *sleeves.* The sleeves are about two feet long and are designed to accept round weight plates. Speaking of plates, they come in seven sizes – 2.5, 5, 10, 25, 35, 45 and 100 pounds. You put one or more on each end of the barbell and secure it in position with a collar. Collars may be large heavy-duty contraptions that have multiple bolts to be tightened, or simple one-piece springs that you squeeze and slide on outside the plates to keep them in place.

Besides Olympic bars, barbells come in other shapes and sizes. Many gyms have shorter, straight bars (four to five feet long) that are one piece and have two collars on each end that act like a vise and trap the plates in between.

EZ-curl bars are about three and a half feet long and have a series of bends in the middle. The bends in the bar allow the hands to be angled slightly while gripping the bar. For some this places less stress on the wrists and forearms.

Dumbells are the baby brothers of the weightlifting world. They consist of a short bar about a foot long and (like barbells) have plates on each end. Dumbells are designed to be held one in each hand, although a few exercises can be done using just one dumbell.

Despite their simplicity, you can use barbells and dumbells to work every muscle group. In fact, despite the advances made in machine technology, most experts agree that barbells and dumbells are still the most effective way to work muscles.

Free Weights vs. Machines

Should you do your strength workouts using free weights or machines or both? This is probably one of the most popular questions asked in the world of fitness. Many articles have been written about the topic and it continues to be a controversial issue among fitness enthusiasts and experts alike. Some believe that free weights are superior to machines, while others will bet their bottom dollar that training on a machine is the only way to go!

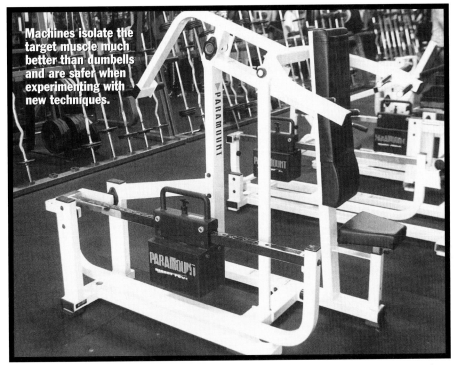

Machines isolate the target muscle much better than dumbells and are safer when experimenting with new techniques.

Actually, we don't see what all the fuss is about. The fact is that both free weights and machines have a lot to offer, but each also has its *disadvantages.* We believe any strength-training workout should include exercises using both machines and free weights.

Machines isolate the target muscles much better and are safer to use when you want to experiment with new or different techniques. Furthermore a machine provides you with much better control and stability and requires less coordination and skill. It also saves a lot of time, because you don't have to go around stacking plates and carrying dumbells all the time.

The disadvantage of using machines is that they do not offer you much variety and can become boring after a while. Another problem is that machines are often designed for the average person, and may be uncomfortable to use for a very tall or very short person.

Free weights, on the other hand, allow you to use your body in a more "natural" way, simulating real-life movements more accurately. It encourages you to employ your stabilizer muscles properly and to use correct body alignment. Free weights also offer much more variety and can be used in many different ways to target different muscle groups.

Free weight exercises are normally suitable for most people who train, but often beginners need a lot of guidance to ensure they are using proper form and technique. Those who do not have the necessary

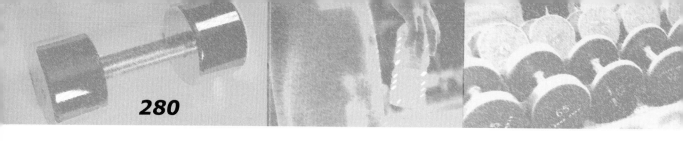
skills may develop serious injuries by training incorrectly. Training with free weights is also a very time-consuming process.

As you can see there is no reason to exclude free weight or machines. Both have a place in any strength workout, depending on your goals, fitness level, skill and time constraints. To put it simply, a chef does not debate whether pots are better than pans. He uses both in cooking. The most important thing is that the end result is a success. Maybe the fitness industry should start thinking the same way.

Note that free weights and machines are not the only option you have when you train for strength. Using your own natural bodyweight can be just as effective in resistance exercise. In fact, those traditional, "old-fashioned" pushups, pullups, dips and situps are still some of the best strength exercises one can do. You don't need expensive, state-of-the-art gym equipment to get results!

The Advantages of Machines

1. They are great for beginners because they are safe and easy to use.
2. Machines guide your body through a certain range of motion.
3. You don't have to worry about balancing the weight as much as with free weights.
4. Machines don't require as much coordination.
5. Machines isolate each muscle group.
6. Machines let you get in a fast workout. You go through a circuit of machines and then you are finished.
7. Machines are usually arranged so that you work large muscle groups and then smaller muscle groups.

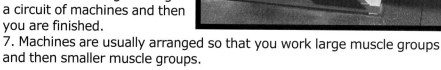

Machines don't require as much coordination.

The Disadvantages of Machines

1. Machines don't fit every body. They can be hard to adjust.
2. Machines don't build as much balance or coordination.
3. Machines can put your body into a bad range of motion. If you feel uncomfortable move to another machine.
4. Machines are not portable. They can't be moved around very easily.
5. Many bodybuilders believe that working out with machines alone doesn't build a very good body.

The Advantages of Free Weights

1. Free weights are versatile. One set of dumbells can be used for many different exercises.
2. Using free weights builds better balance and coordination.
3. Free weights work your muscles in a way that matches real life.
4. Bodybuilders primarily use free weights to gain their massive size.
5. Free weights allow you to strengthen muscles and tendons that wouldn't get much work when using machines.

The Disadvantages of Free Weights

1. Free weights can be difficult because of the balance and coordination required.
2. A free weight workout will take longer than a machine workout.
3. You can get injured easier using free weights.

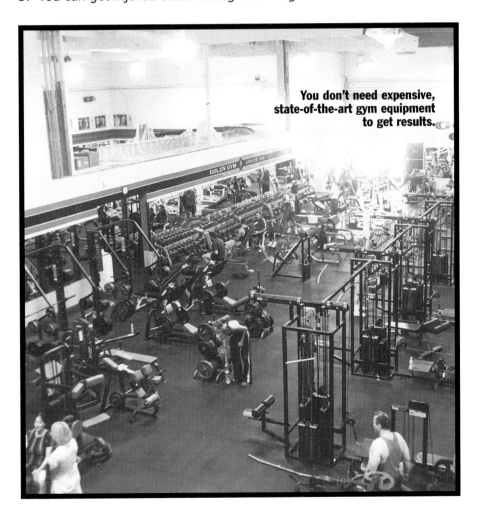

You don't need expensive, state-of-the-art gym equipment to get results.

CHAPTER TWENTY-SIX

If you take note of the following statement, and accept it now, it will help you throughout your training. Remember this: *About 30 percent of your results depends on your actual workouts; the other 70 percent depends on your diet and sleep.* Of course, this depends on your goals. If a nice shapely physique hidden beneath an inch and a half of fat is desirable to you, then you can pretty much ignore this rule; otherwise, you should live by it.

Getting in shape requires much dedication. It's far from over when you zip up the gym bag and head home. In fact, *postworkout* is one of the most crucial time periods in your training regimen. That's the time to replenish and fuel your body for maximum recovery. There, we got that out of the way. Now let's start with the physical workout, and we can concentrate on the diet later in the book.

I'm Here, So Now What Do I Do?

As a beginner (less than 6 months of steady training) we recommend you start doing something like a total-body workout three times a week. The reasoning here is, it won't take much to get your muscles completely worked at this point, so it's best to hit them all with a couple basic movements. If you use the same workout as "Joe Pro Bodybuilder" in the latest issue of *MuscleMag International* or *Flex* at this point, you'll probably be out of the gym for days because of soreness. Better to take it slow at first so you don't burn out.

Try something like this, three times a week.
Stationary bike – 30 minutes on lowest setting
Leg presses – 2 sets x 15 reps
Leg curls – 2 sets x 10-12 reps
Calves: Seated calf raises – 2 sets x 15-20 reps
Chest: Flat dumbell presses – 2 sets x 8-12 reps
Back: Lat pulldowns – 2 sets x 12-15 reps
Biceps: Incline dumbell curls – 2 sets x 10-12 reps
Triceps: Triceps pushdowns – 2 sets x 12-15 reps
Abs: Crunches on incline bench – 3 sets x 30 reps
Cardio is optional: Treadmill, stepping machine or jumping rope

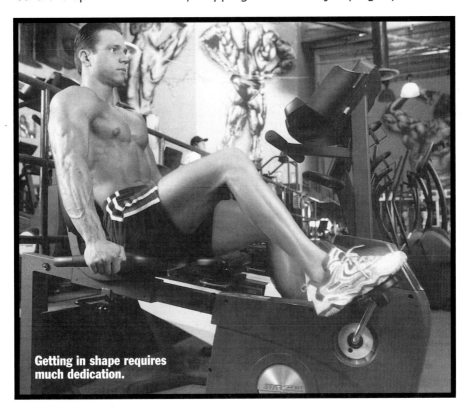

Getting in shape requires much dedication.

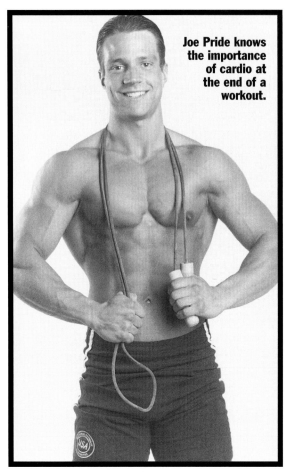

Joe Pride knows the importance of cardio at the end of a workout.

The optional cardio at the end of the workout is always good, even more so if you have some fat to lose (which most of us do). It's usually pretty relaxing once you get used to it, and we'd recommend spending some money on a Walkman and some good music. It helps a lot! The heart is one of the most neglected muscles, and we don't want you to fall into the habit of cardiovascular neglect right from the beginning!

The above workout routine is pretty vigorous for a beginner, but you'll learn a lot of the basic movements – and you'll build the foundation of your fitness lifestyle! If you don't know what some of these exercises are, you'd be best to ask a trainer on staff at your gym. He or she will usually show you, and make sure you're performing the movements properly.

Now what?

We would recommend you follow this workout for about 3 to 4 months, with proper sleep and a solid healthy diet full of whole foods, and then move on to a four-day split. (We'll explain this in an upcoming chapter.) Stay motivated, and try to lift with a training partner. We know it's tough to find someone really motivated, but if you do, you'll be surprised how much you'll push each other. Stay educated on nutrition and the latest findings in the fitness world by reading everything you can – on-line, in magazines, books, talking to bodybuilders, fitness competitors, and other athletes who strength train on a regular basis. Don't just romp around in the gym for an hour a day and expect to have Arnold Schwarzenegger's body in a couple of months. It won't happen. Don't spend a thousand dollars a month looking for that "magic supplement" that will melt fat off either. What *will* get you looking good is persistence, time, determination and education. Stick to your diet, don't miss any workouts, and get plenty of sleep and rest between workouts. Set some smaller goals for yourself – and achieve them!

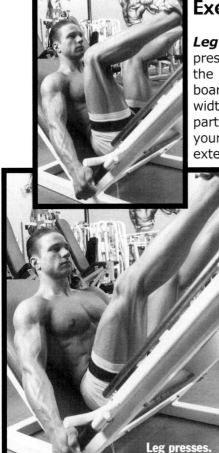

Exercise Descriptions

Leg presses – You will need to use the leg-press machine to perform this exercise. Sit in the seat and place your feet on the pressing board. Your stance should be about shoulder width, but this can be varied to work different parts of the thigh. Lower your legs slowly until your knees touch your chest, then press and extend your legs to the locked out position, pause, then repeat. Perform the movement in a slow, controlled manner.

Comments – Although the leg press doesn't give the degree of thigh development as squats, it is a close second. And if you have knee or back problems, the leg press will adequately work the thighs without aggravating these areas. As with squats, the wider the stance, the more glute involvement. By making a V with the feet (heels together, toes apart) you can do wonders with the inner thigh region (vastus medialis).

Perhaps the greatest advantage of the leg press is the amount of weight you can use. Unlike squats, where the lower back is a limiting factor, the leg press allows you to pile on hundreds of pounds of plates. It won't be long before you have six, eight, or more 45-pound plates on

Leg presses.

each side. Provided you do the exercise in good style, you can really let the ego go wild on this exercise. The lower back is virtually eliminated, and even the knees don't have the same stress placed on them.

If there is as word of caution it concerns *hyperextending* the legs. Place the feet too low on the pressing board, and you risk locking out your legs and actually forcing them into a hyperextended position at the knee joint. When performing the exercise, *do not* forcefully lock out the legs. Doing so may damage the supporting connective tissues (ligaments, tendons and cartilage) of the knees.

Muscles worked – The design of the leg-press machine is intended to place most of the stress on the thighs. There is very little glute involvement, and the spinal erectors are all but eliminated from the exercise. The calves and hamstrings only play a small role in stabilizing the legs during the exercise.

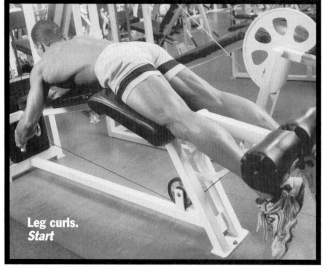

Leg curls.
Start

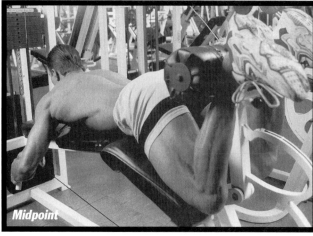

Midpoint

Leg curls – Lie down on the leg-curl machine, with your feet placed under the round foot supports (often called rollers). Pretend you are doing biceps curls (which in fact is what the hamstrings are – leg biceps), and curl the legs toward your buns. Pause at the top, and slowly lower the legs back to the starting position.

Comments – Some gyms have three variations of leg-curl machine. Two of them require that you lie face down on a bench. The bench may be either straight or partly angled. The angled bench forces you to do the exercise more strictly. It keeps you from *swinging* the legs up. Many gyms have a third type of leg-curl machine that allows you to stand up and work one leg at a time. It's similar to one-arm concentration curls for the biceps.

Just as you wouldn't do biceps curls in an awkward manner, so too must leg curls be performed in a slow, rhythmic style. No jerking or bouncing the weight, and try to avoid lifting your butt off the bench. If you have to raise your glutes, you're probably using too much weight.

Muscles worked – Leg curls primarily work the leg hamstrings, although there is some calf involvement. The glutes and thighs only come into play to stabilize the legs during the exercise.

Seated calf raises – You will need a special machine to do this exercise. Sit down on the seat of the machine and place the padded knee rests on your legs. With your toes on the block of wood, stretch up and down as far as you can.

Comments – Because it works the lower calf, you will need to use less weight. Go for at least 20 reps and try to feel every one of them. No

bouncing the weight on your legs. Even though the supports are padded, improper style can injure your knees.
Muscles worked – Since the legs are bent, most of the stress is placed on the lower calf (soleus), but there is some secondary, upper calf involvement.

Triceps pushdowns – You will need to use the lat pulldown machine for this exercise. Grab the bar with a narrow grip, anywhere from 2 to 8 inches. With your elbows tight to your sides, press the bar down to a locked-out position. Pause and flex the triceps at the bottom, and then return the bar to about chest high.

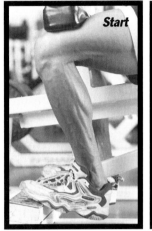
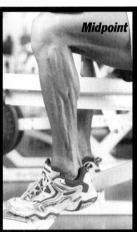

Seated calf raises.

Comments – Take a false grip (thumbs above the bar) for triceps pushdowns, and resist the urge to flare the elbows out to the sides. If you have to swing to push the bar down, you probably have too much weight on the bar.
Muscles worked – Triceps pushdowns work the entire triceps region, especially the outer head.

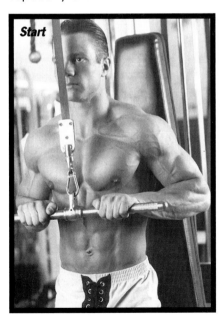

Triceps pushdowns.

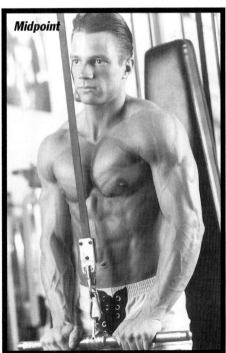

Flat dumbell presses – This exercise is similar to the barbell version, but you use two dumbells instead. Start by sitting on a flat bench, and cleaning (lifting) a pair of dumbells to your knees. Lie back on the bench, and with the dumbells pointing end to end (i.e. they form a straight line across your chest like a barbell), lower them down to your sides. Pause at the bottom, and then press to arms' length.

Comments – The advantage of using dumbells is the greater range of movement at the bottom. A barbell can only be lowered to the rib cage, whereas the dumbells can be lowered below the rib cage, which gives the chest muscles a greater stretch. But be careful! The lower part of the movement is the most dangerous, and if you drop the dumbells in an uncontrolled manner, you run the risk of tearing the pec-delt tie-ins. Although there is much personal preference, most bodybuilders find a dumbell spacing of about 6 to 8 inches wider than the shoulders to be the most effective.

About 30 percent of your results depend on your actual workouts; the other 10 percent depends on your diet and sleep.

Muscles worked – Dumbell presses are great for developing the pec-delt tie-ins. If you squeeze together at the top, the inner pecs are also worked. And no matter how much you try to eliminate them, the triceps and shoulders will be involved. That's fine. At the beginning stage you *want to* work as many muscles in conjunction as possible.

Lat pulldowns – Although not quite as effective as chinups, pulldowns enable you to adjust the amount of weight. Chins force you to use your body weight, whereas the lat machine allows the user to select the desired poundage. Instead of pulling yourself up to an overhead bar, the bar is brought down to you. Take a wide grip (about twice shoulder width) and sit on the attached seat, or kneel down on the floor. Now pull the bar down, either behind your head, or to the front and touch your chest. Pause at the bottom and squeeze your shoulder blades together. Return to the outstretched arms position.

Comments – Pull to the front or pull to the back, it's a personal decision. There is little difference between the two. Either version will add tremendously to back width, giving that much coveted V-shape. Generally speaking, when you pull to the front, you hit more of the lower upper back (i.e. the lower insertions of your lats). Pulling behind the neck works the upper regions of the lats and the rear delts. There is so much overlap between the two movements, however, that at the beginning level, either is sufficient. You might want to rotate both movements, either on the same day or alternate back days.

Keep your grip fairly wide as narrow-grip pulldowns place much of the stress on the biceps. In fact many bodybuilders often perform narrow-grip chins and pulldowns as *biceps* exercises! And finally, because you have to grip the bar, the muscles of the forearms get a good workout. In fact they may be the weakest link in the chain.

Muscles worked – Lat pulldowns work the whole back region, from the large latissimus muscles to the smaller teres, rhomboids and rear deltoids. They also stress the biceps and forearms.

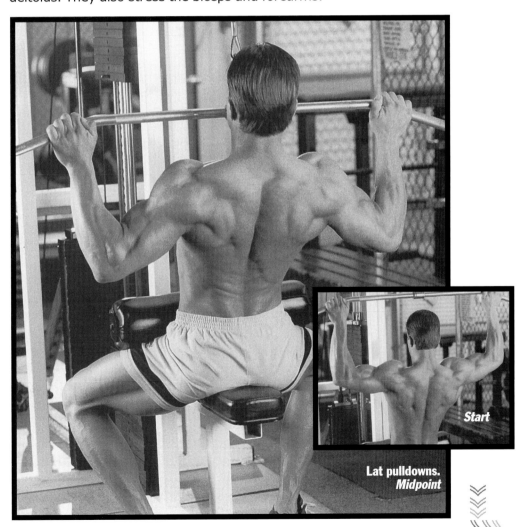

Start

Lat pulldowns.
Midpoint

Incline curls – You will need an incline bench to perform this one. Unlike incline presses for your chest, use a bench with an angle of at least 45 degrees. Anything less will place too much strain on your front delts. Lie back on the bench and grab two dumbells. Curl the bells up until the biceps are fully flexed. All the tips suggested here would apply for standing dumbell curls as well. Rotate the hands from a facing in, to a facing up position. Don't swing the weight up.

Comments – You have the option of curling both dumbells simultaneously or alternately. When you lower the dumbells, be careful not to hit the side of the incline bench. In fact, this is another reason for starting the dumbells in a forward pointed position. If they were in the standard end to end position, they would have less clearance with the bench. The advantage of using the incline bench is that it limits the amount of cheating you can do. Let's face it, you can't swing very much with your back braced against a rigid board.

Muscles worked – Incline curls work the whole biceps region. Many bodybuilders find them great for bringing out the biceps peak. Of course this attribute is more genetic than anything else. The exercise does provide some forearm stimulation, but not to the same extent as the various barbell curls.

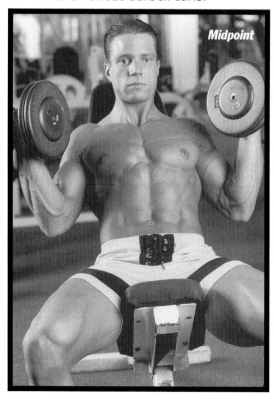

Midpoint

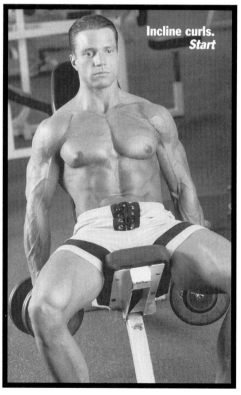

Incline curls.
Start

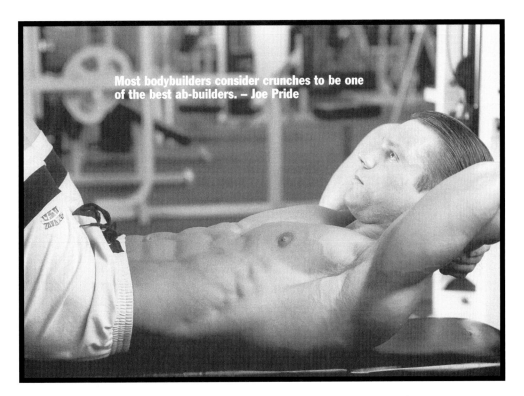

Most bodybuilders consider crunches to be one of the best ab-builders. – Joe Pride

Crunches – You will need a flat bench or chair to perform this exercise. Lie down on the floor and rest your calves on the bench. Adjust your distance from the bench so that your thighs are perpendicular to the floor. Now bend forward and try to touch your thighs with your upper body.

Comments – Most bodybuilders consider crunches to be one of the best ab-builders. At first you may want to perform the movement with your hands by your sides. As you get stronger, place your hands at the sides of your head. Doing so adds the weight of the arms to your upper body, thus making the exercise more difficult.

Muscles involved – Crunches primarily work the upper abs, but there is some lower ab stimulation as well. The exercise also brings the hip abductors into play, although to a much lesser extent than situps.

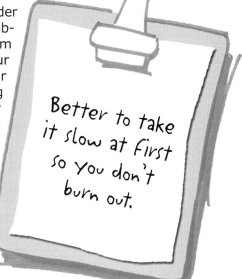

Better to take it slow at first so you don't burn out.

CHAPTER TWENTY-SEVEN

With three to six months of introductory training behind you it's time to progress to the intermediate ranks. At this point, the waters get a bit cloudy regarding what is "right," "best" or whatever. We are not going to try to tell you that after three months you must start following intermediate routines. Most teens progress at different speeds. What's best for you may be useless for someone else. Hopefully, however, the suggestions in the next few pages will enable you to keep progressing and perhaps more important, help keep your motivation levels high.

It's time to split!

Perhaps the biggest change you'll make in your training during the intermediate phase is to divide or split your training into sections. Up until now you've been training the whole body on non-consecutive days, performing only one exercise per bodypart.

The Intermediate Level

Although such training is productive, and certainly has advantages, most serious strength trainers eventually switch to a split routine.

By *split routine* we mean training certain muscles on one day and others the next. One of the disadvantages to full body workouts is the diminished intensity factor that creeps in toward the end of the routine. Often you are only going through the motions on the last couple of muscle groups. Splitting, however, allows you to do more for the muscles, as you don't have to budget your energy reserves to hit the entire body. In fact this is the primary advantage to split routines; the reduced number of muscles trained allows you to do more for them during each workout. Instead of one exercise for 3 sets, you can do two, three, even four exercises for the same muscle. There are several ways you can split up your routine.

Push-pull – This routine consists of training your *pulling muscles* (back and biceps muscles) on one day and your *pushing muscles* on the next (chest and triceps muscles). You can then divide your legs, shoulders and abdominals between the other two workout days.

Upper body/lower body – This split routine consists of training your upper body one day, and your lower body the next. Even though the legs are only one muscle group, they constitute 50 percent of the body's muscle mass.

Random – Random muscle combinations are perhaps the most common split routines. There's really no right way to combine muscle groups. It probably doesn't make sense to combine legs, chest and back on one day, as these are the three largest muscle groups. Instead put legs with a smaller muscle like arms or shoulders. The bottom line is, try to divide the body evenly so that you are training about the same amount of muscle mass on each day.

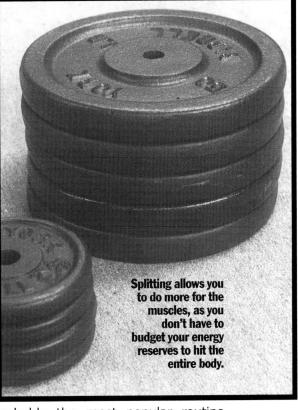

Splitting allows you to do more for the muscles, as you don't have to budget your energy reserves to hit the entire body.

How often should I train?
Besides deciding which muscle groups to combine, you also need to decide how often to train. As there are many options from which to choose, let's look at the pros and cons of each.

Four Days per Week
Training four days a week is probably the most popular routine followed. You divide the body into two halves and then train two days in a row followed by a day off. You can go two on/one off indefinitely, or follow the traditional week as follows:

> Monday – Day 1
> Tuesday – Day 2
> Wednesday – Off
> Thursday – Day 1
> Friday – Day 2
> Weekends – Off

The four-day split has many advantages; chief of which is that you are only in the gym two days in a row. The day off in between gives the body ample time to recover. For some, even two days in a row is too taxing on the recovery system and a modified version of the four-day split is followed. In this case you train one day, take a day off, and then train the other half of the body on the third day. The one-on/one-off routine gives the body 48 hours of rest between workouts.

A third variation of the four day split is great for those who want to divide the body in two but can only get to the gym three times per week. In this case the two-week split can be followed:

Week 1	Day 1
	Day 2
	Day 1
Week 2	Day 2
	Day 1
	Day 2

Notice how in the first week the Day 1 routine is followed twice, while Day 2 exercises are followed only once, but during the second week you switch things around. This means that during a two-week period you hit the same muscles three times each. Such a split is great as it allows time for school and work. With an average workout lasting an hour, it takes a total time investment of only three hours per week. Even the busiest teens can usually scrounge three hours of time to train.

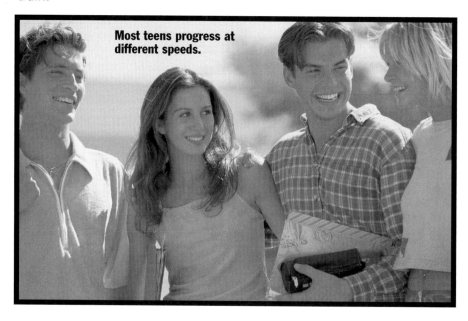

Most teens progress at different speeds.

SAMPLE ROUTINE "A"

Day 1

Thighs:	Squats	3 sets x 8-12 reps
	Leg extensions	3 sets x 8-12 reps
Hamstrings:	Lying leg curls	3 sets x 8-12 reps
	Stiff-leg deadlifts	3 sets x 8-12 reps
Calves:	Standing calf raises	3 sets x 6-8 (15-20)
	Seated calf raises	3 sets x 6-8 (15-20)
Biceps:	Cable curls	3 sets x 8-12 reps
	Incline curls	3 sets x 8-12 reps
Triceps:	Lying dumbell extensions	3 sets x 8-12 reps
	Cable pushdowns	3 sets x 8-12 reps
Abdominals:	Lying leg raises	3 sets x 15-20 reps
	Crunches	3 sets x 15-20 reps

Note: Alternate low reps (6-8) and high reps (15-20) for the calves.

Day 2

Chest:	Flat dumbell presses	3 sets x 8-12 reps
	Incline dumbell flyes	3 sets x 8-12 reps
Back:	Front lat pulldowns	3 sets x 8-12 reps
	One-arm rows	3 sets x 8-12 reps
Shoulders:	Machine presses	3 sets x 8-12 reps
	Side lateral raises	3 sets x 8-12 reps
	Bent-over laterals	3 sets x 8-12 reps

SAMPLE ROUTINE "B"

Day 1

Chest:	Flat barbell presses	3 sets x 8-12 reps
	Incline dumbell presses	3 sets x 8-12 reps
Back:	Chinups	3 sets x 8-12 reps
	T-bar rows	3 sets x 8-12 reps
Biceps:	Preacher curls	3 sets x 8-12 reps
	Concentration curls	3 sets x 8-12 reps
Abdominals:	Crunches	3 sets x 15-20 reps
	Reverse crunches	3 sets x 15-20 reps

Day 2

Thighs:	Leg presses	3 sets x 8-12 reps
	Leg extensions	3 sets x 8-12 reps
Hamstrings:	Seated leg curls	3 sets x 8-12 reps
	Lying leg curls	3 sets x 8-12 reps
Calves:	Toe presses	3 sets x 6-8 (15-20)
	Seated calf raises	3 sets x 6-8 (15-20)
Shoulders:	Dumbell presses	3 sets x 8-12 reps
	Cable lateral raises	3 sets x 8-12 reps
	Reverse pec-dek flyes	3 sets x 8-12 reps
Triceps:	Dumbell extensions	3 sets x 8-12 reps
	Bench dips	3 sets x 8-12 reps

SAMPLE ROUTINE "C"

Day 1

Thighs:	Lunges	3 sets x 8-12 reps
	Leg presses	3 sets x 8-12 reps
Chest:	Incline dumbell presses	3 sets x 8-12 reps
	Flat dumbell flyes	3 sets x 8-12 reps
Shoulders:	Front barbell presses	3 sets x 8-12 reps
	Upright rows	3 sets x 8-12 reps
	Bent-over laterals	3 sets x 8-12 reps
Triceps:	Lying barbell extensions	3 sets x 8-12 reps
	Kickbacks	3 sets x 8-12 reps
Calves:	Standing calf raises	3 sets x 6-8 (15-20)
	Seated calf raises	3 sets x 6-8 (15-20)

Day 2

Back:	Front pulldowns	3 sets x 8-12 reps
	Seated cable rows	3 sets x 8-12 reps
Hamstrings:	Lying leg curls	3 sets x 8-12 reps
	Stiff-leg deadlifts	3 sets x 8-12 reps
Biceps:	Standing dumbell curls	3 sets x 8-12 reps
	One-arm cable curls	3 sets x 8-12 reps
Abdominals:	Hanging leg raises	3 sets x 15-20 reps
	Crunches	3 sets x 15-20 reps

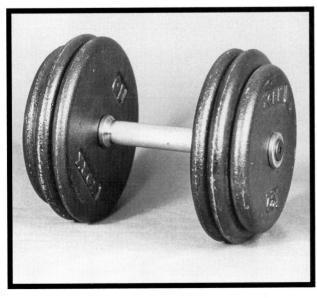

Six-Day Splits

If four-day splits have one disadvantage it is that they require you to train three muscle groups during one workout. Even by only doing two exercises per muscle group, there's still a lot of ground to cover. By the time you get to the third muscle group you may be just going through the motions. One solution to this is to follow the three-day split, where you divide the body into three distinct areas. This means you only have to hit two muscles per workout.

Besides the time factor, the six-day split allows you to do three or more exercises for each muscle group. Even though increasing the weight is often enough to keep the muscles responding, sometimes an increase in volume is needed. By having to train only one or two muscle groups you have the extra time to add a few extra exercises.

There are two primary ways to implement a six-day split routine. The most popular is to train three on, and then take a day off. A few individuals prefer training six on and then resting on the seventh. Of the two we recommend the former. Training six days straight can leave the body in a state of overtraining. Even three on, one off may be too taxing as you are essentially working out six days out of eight. Or put another way, in a two-week period you are in the gym 12 days. The top strength trainers in the world usually limit six-splits to a few months of the year – just enough time to shock the body without draining it entirely. Of course you are going to be the best judge of when you need to reduce your training volume. As soon as you start to recognize the symptoms of overtraining either reduce your workload or take a few days (perhaps weeks) off.

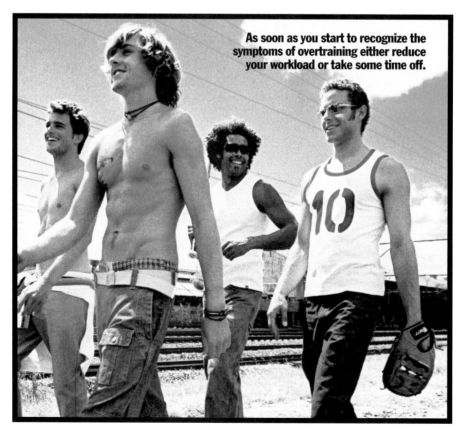

As soon as you start to recognize the symptoms of overtraining either reduce your workload or take some time off.

SAMPLE ROUTINE "A"

Day 1: Chest and Arms

Chest:	Flat barbell presses	3 sets x 8-12 reps
	Incline dumbell presses	3 sets x 8-12 reps
	Pec-dek flyes	3 sets x 8-12 reps
Biceps:	Standing barbell curls	3 sets x 8-12 reps
	Concentration curls	3 sets x 8-12 reps
Triceps:	Pushdowns	3 sets x 8-12 reps
	Dumbell extensions	3 sets x 8-12 reps

Day 2: Legs and Abs

Legs:	Squats	3 sets x 8-12 reps
	Leg extensions	3 sets x 8-12 reps
	Lunges	3 sets x 8-12 reps
	Lying leg curls	3 sets x 8-12 reps
	Stiff-leg deadlifts	3 sets x 8-12 reps
	Standing calf raises	3 sets x 6-8 (15-20)
	Seated calf raises	3 sets x 6-8 (15-20)
Abdominals:	Reverse crunches	3 sets x 15-20 reps
	Crunches	3 sets x 15-20 reps
	Rope crunches	3 sets x 15-20 reps

Day 3: Back and Shoulders

Back:	Front pulldowns	3 sets x 8-12 reps
	Seated cable rows	3 sets x 8-12 reps
	One-arm rows	3 sets x 8-12 reps
	Back extensions	3 sets x 15-20 reps
Shoulders:	Dumbell presses	3 sets x 8-12 reps
	Lateral raises	3 sets x 8-12 reps
	Reverse pec-dek flyes	3 sets x 8-12 reps
	Dumbell shrugs	3 sets x 8-12 reps

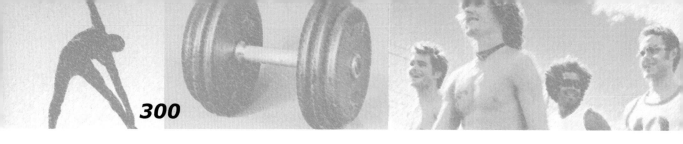

SAMPLE ROUTINE "B"

Day 1: Chest and Back

Chest:	Incline dumbell presses	3 sets x 8-12 reps
	Flat barbell presses	3 sets x 8-12 reps
	Flat dumbell flyes	3 sets x 8-12 reps
Back:	Chinups	3 sets x 8-12 reps
	T-bar rows	3 sets x 8-12 reps
	One-arm rows	3 sets x 8-12 reps

Day 2: Legs and Abs

Legs:	Leg presses	3 sets x 8-12 reps
	Hack squats	3 sets x 8-12 reps
	Seated leg curls	3 sets x 8-12 reps
	Stiff-leg deadlifts	3 sets x 8-12 reps
	Donkey calf raises	3 sets x 6-8 (15-20)
	Seated calf raises	3 sets x 6-8 (15-20)
Abdominals:	Hanging leg raises	3 sets x 15-20 reps
	Crunches	3 sets x 15-20 reps
	Rope crunches	3 sets x 15-20 reps

Day 3: Shoulders and Arms

Shoulders:	Machine presses	3 sets x 8-12 reps
	Cable lateral raises	3 sets x 8-12 reps
	Reverse pec-dek flyes	3 sets x 8-12 reps
	Upright rows	3 sets x 8-12 reps
Biceps:	Barbell curls	3 sets x 8-12 reps
	One-arm preacher curls	3 sets x 8-12 reps
Triceps:	Rope extensions	3 sets x 8-12 reps
	Bench dips	3 sets x 8-12 reps

ROUTINE "C" (MACHINES ONLY)

Day 1: Legs and Abs

Thighs:	Leg presses	3 sets x 8-12 reps
	Leg extensions	3 sets x 8-12 reps
Hamstrings:	Lying leg curls	3 sets x 8-12 reps
	Seated leg curls	3 sets x 8-12 reps
Calves:	Standing calf raises	3 sets x 6-8 (15-20)
	Seated calf raises	3 sets x 6-8 (15-20)
Abdominals:	Machine crunches	3 sets x 15-20 reps

Day 2: Chest and Back

Chest:	Flat machine presses	3 sets x 8-12 reps
	Incline machine presses	3 sets x 8-12 reps
	Pec-dek flyes	3 sets x 8-12 reps
Back:	Front pulldowns	3 sets x 8-12 reps
	Seated cable rows	3 sets x 8-12 reps
	Pullover machine	3 sets x 8-12 reps

Day 3: Shoulders and Arms

Shoulders:	Machine presses	3 sets x 8-12 reps
	Lateral raise machine	3 sets x 8-12 reps
	Reverse pec-dek flyes	3 sets x 8-12 reps
Biceps:	Machine preacher curls	3 sets x 8-12 reps
	Cable curls	3 sets x 8-12 reps
Triceps:	Pushdowns	3 sets x 8-12 reps
	Rope extensions	3 sets x 8-12 reps

ROUTINE "D" (FREE WEIGHTS ONLY)

Day 1: Legs and Abs

Thighs:	Squats	3 sets x 8-12 reps
	Lunges	3 sets x 8-12 reps
Hamstrings:	Stiff-leg deadlifts	3 sets x 8-12 reps
	Back extensions	3 sets x 8-12 reps
Calves:	Donkey calf raises	3 sets to failure
	One-leg calf raises	3 sets to failure
Abs:	Lying leg raises	3 sets x 15-20 reps
	Crunches	3 sets x 15-20 reps
	Reverse crunches	3 sets x 15-20 reps

Day 2: Chest and Arms

Chest:	Flat dumbell presses	3 sets x 8-12 reps
	Incline dumbell presses	3 sets x 8-12 reps
	Dumbell pullovers	3 sets x 8-12 reps
Biceps:	Barbell curls	3 sets x 8-12 reps
	Incline dumbell curls	3 sets x 8-12 reps
Triceps:	Dumbell extensions	3 sets x 8-12 reps
	Bench dips	3 sets to failure

Day 3: Back and Shoulders

Back:	Chinups	3 sets x 8-12 reps
	Barbell rows	3 sets x 8-12 reps
	One-arm rows	3 sets x 8-12 reps
Shoulders:	Dumbell presses	3 sets x 8-12 reps
	Lateral raises	3 sets x 8-12 reps
	Bent-over laterals	3 sets x 8-12 reps

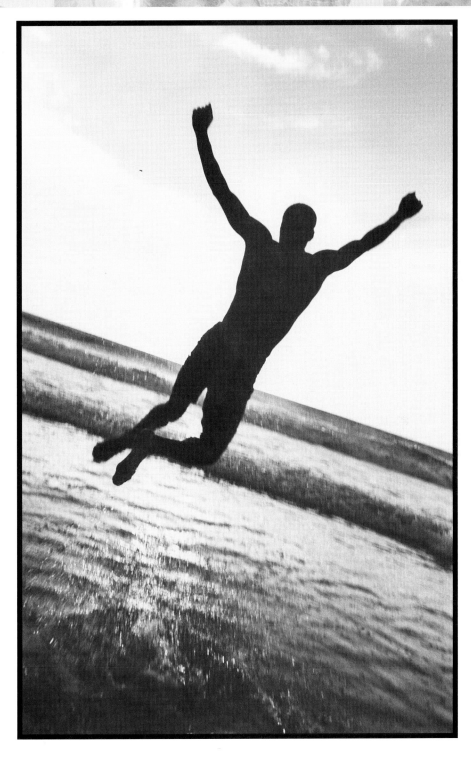

CHAPTER TWENTY-EIGHT

Like most aspects of life, boredom occasionally rears its ugly head in the gym. For the first month or so you'll probably be a little bit sore after every workout – that's normal, and in fact good. The soreness indicates the muscles are still responding to the exercises.

Eventually, however, you will reach a point when the exercises we initially put you on fail to adequately stimulate the muscles. Further, even if they did, you may be getting tired and bored with doing them. As much as the authors love working out, we'll be the first to admit that the activity can easily get to be boring. The easiest solution to this problem is, of course, to change exercises on a regular basis and follow a split routine of some kind. But even

Techniques to Jazz Up Your Workouts

this can lead to boredom and stagnation after a period of time. What you need to do is employ a series of advanced training techniques to stimulate and challenge the muscles in different ways. Not only will your muscles start responding again but perhaps more important – it will be fun!

In no particular order we suggest the following techniques be incorporated into your routines to jazz things up so to speak. As a word of caution, please don't perform these techniques on all your exercises during every workout. The end result would be an overstressed and overtrained body. Instead use them sparingly.

Supersets

For our purposes here, a *superset* is the completion of two consecutive sets without a rest. Supersets can be consecutive exercises for the same muscle, opposing muscles, or two completely unrelated muscle groups. When performing supersets for opposing or unrelated muscle groups, there is an opportunity for one muscle to recover while another is worked, therefore you are able to use a heavy weight for both exercises. Because minimal rest is prescribed, try to arrange for exercises that can be performed within a close proximity of one another (i.e. a flat dumbell press and a single-arm dumbell row). Training

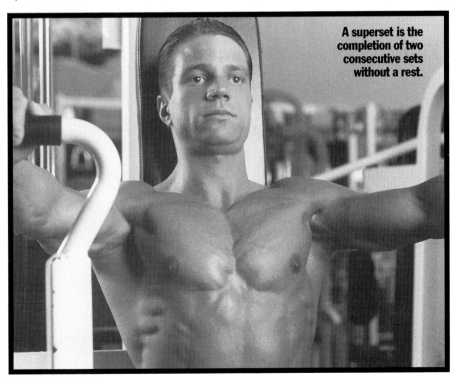

A superset is the completion of two consecutive sets without a rest.

opposing muscle groups in this manner ensures the development of balanced muscular strength. You can design an entire workout using multiple supersets, *or* you can add a superset at any point in the workout (such as the transition from chest to back).

An example of two opposing muscle groups are the chest and back. Pick a back exercise that pulls the arms into the torso (a row) and balance that with an exercise that pushes away from the torso (flat dumbell press). You can also use supersets for the anterior and posterior heads of the deltoids (shoulders) which somewhat oppose one another. An example exercise combination would be a front dumbell raise followed by a bent-over dumbell raise. Muscles of shoulder extension (lats) can be paired up with the antagonistic shoulder flexors (deltoids) using a pulldown/shoulder press combination. And finally, for the ultimate arm superset, choose one triceps exercise and follow it with an exercise for your biceps.

Supersets can also be performed using two successive exercises for the same bodypart. This technique is sometimes referred to as "pre-exhaustion," where an isolation exercise is performed for a muscle group (i.e. dumbell flye for the chest) followed by a compound exercise for the same muscle group (i.e. bench press). The second exercise will be performed using a lighter weight than is normally needed because the muscle group will have been previously fatigued.

A second superset method for the same muscle group is referred to as "drop-setting." In this technique, a set of an exercise is performed to failure, at which time you would reduce the weight and perform subsequent repetitions with the lighter weight.

Advanced training techniques will stimulate and challenge your muscles in different ways.

Trisets

A triset is three exercises performed consecutively with no break in between. For example, for the first triset in this chest routine you would start with a 15-rep set of bench presses, follow immediately with 15 reps of incline flyes, then 15 reps of decline flyes. You'd rest 15 to 30 seconds, then repeat, doing a second triset of 12 reps each exercise.

Giant Sets

The next step up the ladder of intensity, giant sets are quite similar to supersets except you perform four or more exercises back to back. This method of training is excellent for the larger muscle groups like the thighs, chest and back. The progressive workload and variation of movements will cause a maximum amount of muscle fiber utilization, a great stimulus for muscle growth.

Pre-Exhaustion

The pre-exhaust technique is one form of resistance weight training that brings large amounts of muscle fibers immediately into play by effectively isolating the area being worked. This principle was introduced by Bob Kennedy, founder and publisher of *MuscleMag International,* and documented in *IronMan* magazine in 1968. Using this principle you can work almost any muscular structure much harder than would normally be possible.

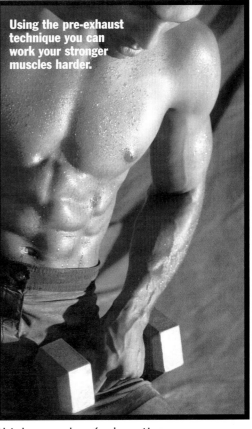

Using the pre-exhaust technique you can work your stronger muscles harder.

The theory is this: In any exercise that involves two or more muscle groups, failure is reached when the weakest muscle group can no longer function. In a case like this, very little growth stimulation is provided for the stronger muscles involved in the same exercise because they were not worked to their fullest potential.

Let's use the barbell squat as an example. The point of failure is normally reached when the lower back muscles fail. This usually happens before the larger and stronger thigh muscles have been worked to their potential. By *pre-exhausting* the thigh muscles (exhausting them without the use of the lower back) the problem can be solved. The easiest way to do this would be to perform a set of leg extensions and then do a set of squats or leg presses. You'll hit your quads like never before.

The back is another area that can be targeted with pre-exhaustion. On most back exercises the smaller biceps fail first. To get around this do a set of straight-arm pushdowns and then perform a set of regular pulldowns or some rowing movement.

Let's not forget the chest either. The weak links in chest-training are the triceps and front shoulders. Perform a set of flat dumbell flyes to tire out the chest and then switch to dumbell or barbell presses. That way the large muscle fibers are brought into play and growth is stimulated.

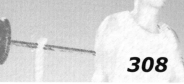
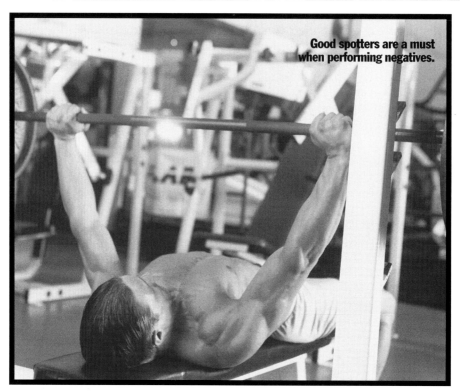

Good spotters are a must when performing negatives.

Negatives

To perform a negative-style exercise you must first warm up in the standard fashion. Next, load the bar with 40 percent more weight than you would normally use for 8 repetitions (specific number of reps may vary for you, but 8 is a good number to start with). Let us use the bench press for our example. Get into the standard position to perform bench presses (body positioning, grip, etc.). You will need two training partners, one to stand on either end of the bar.

When you are ready, ask your partners to unrack the weight and hand it to you, with your arms in the locked-out position. Begin movement by slowly lowering the weight to your chest. Take 8 to 10 seconds to perform the eccentric (lowering) portion of the movement. Once you have touched your chest with the bar your partners will lift the weight off you and then let go in the locked-out position. Continue this until you can no longer control the descent of the weight (obviously good spotters are a must). Try to get 8 repetitions in this manner. If you cannot, then continue to use the same resistance in your training sessions until you can. Once you get 8 repetitions increase the weight by 5 percent during your next training session.

You can *lower* more weight than you can *lift* – and that's because of friction. Intramuscular friction impedes your strength when you lift a weight, but aids it when you lower a weight. Most trainees can lower 40 percent more weight than they can lift in proper form. The same average trainee can hold (statically) 20 percent more than they can lift and 20 percent less than they can lower. So for example, if you can curl 100 pounds, you can lower 140 pounds, and you can hold statically 120 pounds. Standard training can reduce your positive strength greatly, but hardly affects your negative strength. That is why negative training is so much more demanding on the muscles. You can far more greatly fatigue the muscle than with standard training.

Negatives can be performed with any weightlifting exercise. For each bodypart you should pick one exercise and perform one set of negatives to failure. This type of training is very intense and can fatigue the muscle to a greater degree than you can possibly imagine. If you train in a negative fashion, you can train each bodypart once per week at the most, and possibly once every 2 or even 3 weeks.

Cheat Reps

Obviously, cheating should be discouraged. Try to keep perfect form on all exercises to minimize risk of injury and maximize isolation effort on the muscle. However, if you have reached failure with perfect form, cheat reps performed carefully can help you squeeze an extra few reps out and go beyond failure. The best example we can use is the standard barbell curl. Pick a weight with which you can get 8 or 9 reps in good style. Once you reach the last rep, use just enough body swing to keep the bar moving upward, then lower it in a slow and controlled manner.

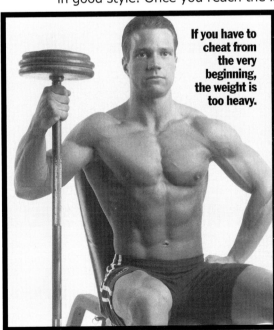

If you have to cheat from the very beginning, the weight is too heavy.

We should point out that cheating is one of the first advanced techniques people learn in the gym. Unfortunately it is also the most abused. Next time you're at the gym watch how many guys are cheating the weight up from the very first rep. Stimulating the biceps is the last thing on their minds. Their only goal is lifting the weight for a given number of reps. For them proper style and technique has gone out the window. You should only use cheat reps on the last couple of reps of a set. If you have to cheat from the very beginning, the weight is too heavy.

Drop Sets

When you come to the end of a set, and you cannot do another rep, it doesn't mean that all the fibers in that muscle are fatigued. It just means that enough fibers are tired enough to prevent you from lifting the poundage you are trying for. If you were to reduce the weight, you would be able to lift it for more reps, thus placing a more thorough overload on the target muscles. This concept is the basis for *drop sets.*

Drop sets are a little different than supersets, but they still reap the same awesome benefits. For drop sets, here's what you do. At the end of a set, when you are unable to do any more reps, set the weight down, strip some plates off, pick the weight back up, and get as many more reps as you can. Depending on how you construct your workout, you could even arrange to do a series of drop sets, so perform even more of these, dropping the poundage a third or even a fourth time.

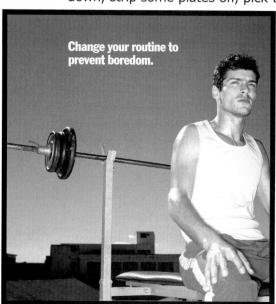

Change your routine to prevent boredom.

Usually you do drop sets on your last set of an exercise. However, one thing that we must mention is that when you do these, you have to be very quick in stripping the weight off the bar. You must minimize the time that you are not actually lifting the weight. That's why a training partner is very helpful when performing these. Of course, cables and machines are particularly good for drop sets because all you have to do to change the poundage is slide a pin out, or push a button. But that's not to say these machines are actually better for building muscle, just easier to do drop sets with.

Running the Rack

The method of "running the rack" stems from the technique of drops sets as well. The case of lateral raises provides the perfect demonstration. When doing lateral raises, pick up a pair of dumbells and start doing your reps. Then, when you can't do another rep, rerack the dumbells, immediately pick up the next lightest weight, and squeeze out as many more as you can. Simply work your way down the rack until you reach the lightest dumbells on the rack or the ones you choose to go down to. You can use this technique for any exercise that requires moderately weighted dumbells.

10 x 10: German Volume Training

In strength-coaching circles, this method is often called the "10 sets of 10" method. Because this technique has its roots in German-speaking countries, it often gets called "German volume training."

The program works because it targets a group of motor units, exposing them to an extensive volume of repeated efforts – specifically, 10 sets of a single exercise. The body adapts to the extraordinary stress by hypertrophying the targeted fibers.

The goal of the German volume training method is to complete 10 sets of 10 reps with the same weight for each exercise. You want to begin with a fairly light weight, one you could lift for 20 reps to failure if you had to. For most people, on most exercises, that would represent 60 percent of their 1RM load. Therefore, if you can bench press 100 pounds for 1 rep, you would use 60 pounds for this exercise.

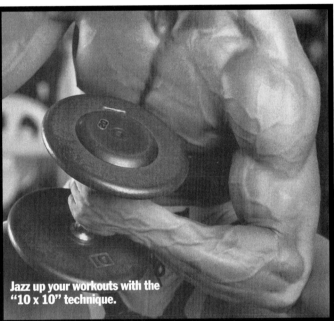

Jazz up your workouts with the "10 x 10" technique.

Rest intervals – When bodybuilders try this technique, they often question its value for the first several sets because the weight doesn't feel heavy enough. However, there is minimal rest between sets (about 60 seconds when performed in sequence and 90 to 120 seconds when performed as a superset), which incurs cumulative fatigue. (Interestingly enough, you might find you get stronger again during the eighth and ninth sets, because of a short-term neural adaptation.) It's important to take rest intervals, so you should definitely use a stopwatch to keep track. This recommendation is very important, as you will become tempted to lengthen the rest time as you fatigue.

Number of exercises – One, and only one, exercise per bodypart should be performed in the 10 x 10 routine. Therefore, choose an exercise that will recruit a lot of muscle mass. Triceps kickbacks and leg extensions are definitely out – squats and bench presses are definitely in. For supplementary work for individual bodyparts (like triceps and biceps), you can do 3 sets of 10 to 20 reps.

Staggered Sets

Staggered sets are usually used to help develop an underdeveloped area. For instance if your calves were a little smaller than you like, you might incorporate an extra session of calf exercises on a day when they aren't scheduled. So when chest day comes around you would work in a set of calf raises between each exercise you do that day. By the end of the day you may have done 20-30 sets! The same holds true for forearms. While resting between sets of a leg exercise, perform a set of forearm curls.

The best muscle groups to hit with staggered sets are calves, forearms, and front or rear shoulders. That's because, while hurting like the dickens when trained, these muscles don't require much energy to fatigue them. As a word of caution, perform staggered sets for calves on upper body days, and staggered sets for forearms and front or rear deltoids on leg days. Once again we must consider the weakest link in the chain. Fatiguing calves may interfere with thigh and hamstring training, while the forearms and deltoids are involved in chest- and back-training.

"I Go You Go"

This technique is great with a training partner. As soon as you finish a set, your partner performs his or her set, then the pattern repeats. As soon as your partner completes his or her set, you jump in and perform your set. This pace of training can be very intense. When using the "I Go You Go" system, there are unlimited variations for interest. This method can be used for a particular exercise or it can be used throughout the entire workout. This type of training allows very little time for the muscle to recuperate.

If you are used to resting 2 to 3 minutes between sets, this technique will seem very difficult at first, but the muscles will adapt. Don't be surprised to see a loss of strength in the particular exercise you are performing in comparison to your normal poundages. This is caused by inadequate time for 100 percent muscle recovery. There is a direct correlation between rest and strength. Shorter rest periods usually result in less strength. Do not worry about this. You are exhausting numerous muscle fibers with this system – and that's the name of the game.

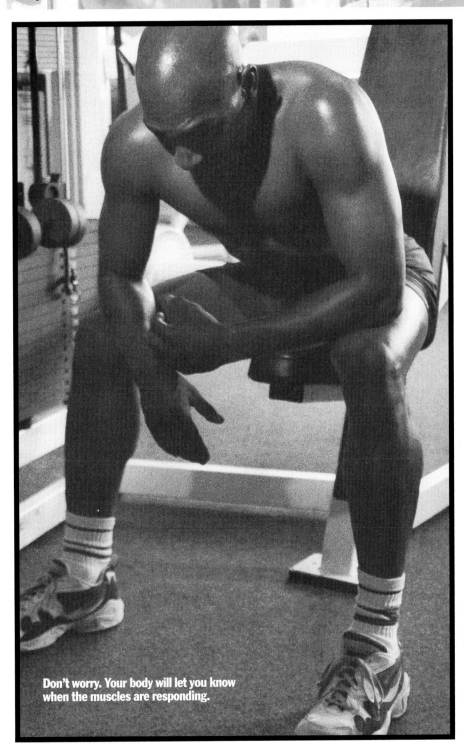

Don't worry. Your body will let you know when the muscles are responding.

CHAPTER TWENTY-NINE

For those you who don't like the gym scene, or don't have access to one, all hope is not lost. Some of the fittest people around do it all at home. No parking hassles, no membership fees, no fighting for equipment, *no sweat!*

Home Sweat Home

Getting in shape can be cheap!

For mere pennies you can set up a nice little gym in your basement or spare room. All you need is a couple of pairs of dumbells (or one adjustable set), a barbell, and an adjustable bench that can go from flat to 90 degrees with a couple of angles in between. Now, you could buy everything we just mentioned at Wal-Mart or any other department store, but there's a cheaper way. Just about every teenage guy buys himself a barbell set and dumbells or receives them for Christmas, as do some girls. And you know what? Most people never use them! Probably 99 percent of barbells and dumbells end up in the attic or basement. If you don't already have a set of your own, check with someone in your class or at work to see what's available. You may get the whole set for $20 or less. In fact we're sure many people will happily give them to you. If the classmate route falls through, try hitting a few flea markets and garage sales. Barbells and dumbells are usually one of the first things to go during spring cleaning.

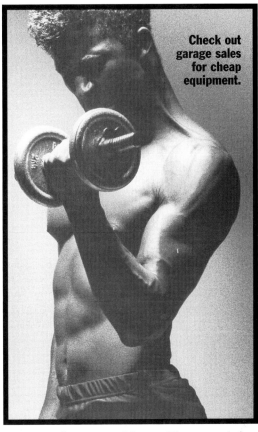

Check out garage sales for cheap equipment.

The Dust-Collector

If you have a few extra dollars, you can buy a *multigym.* These weird-looking contraptions range in price from a couple of hundred to a couple of thousand dollars. (The big ones in commercial gyms may cost $20,000 or more – that's a lot of days working at McDonald's!) Multigyms are great in that you can work just about the entire body in a small area of floor space. Most multigyms have attachments for both upper and lower body.

You know what's the nice thing about multigyms? They make great dust collectors and towel racks! Seriously, multigyms are like barbells and dumbells in that they get used for one or two weeks and then they're stored away somewhere. You can use this to your advantage. Check around with relatives or friends (don't be afraid to check with your friends' parents either). You may be able to pick up a complete multigym for a fraction of what you'd have to pay at a department store.

A final piece of equipment you may want to add is a *squat rack.* You can pick up a home-model squat rack for less than a hundred dollars, but a cheaper solution is to have someone who's handy with a

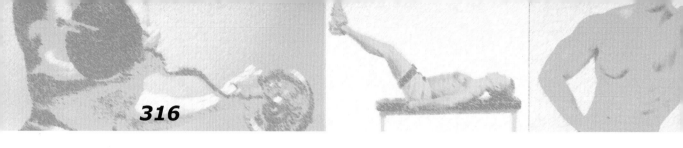

316

blowtorch weld one together for you out of a few scraps of iron. All you need are two long iron beams joined with a couple of cross beams. Have the long beams placed at about a 75-degree angle to the floor, and a series of pegs (short pieces of iron) welded to the bars every foot or so. These pegs are what you rest the barbell on between sets.

The Routines

With your home gym set up, it's time to begin. The following programs can be followed three, four or six days a week. As a word of caution, don't skip the three-day routines in favor of the six-day splits, thinking you will get in shape faster. Jumping to an advanced routine before the body is ready is a great way to get injured. You also run the risk of burnout.

Three-Day Routines
Three day splits are the simplest but most effective routines for beginners to follow. They adequately stimulate the muscles without overtaxing your recovery system. In a three-day routine you train the entire body every second day. Even though most people follow the traditional Monday/Wednesday/Friday split, in reality your body doesn't know the difference. If Tuesday/Thursday/Saturday works best for your weekly schedule, so be it. The bottom line is that you are training!

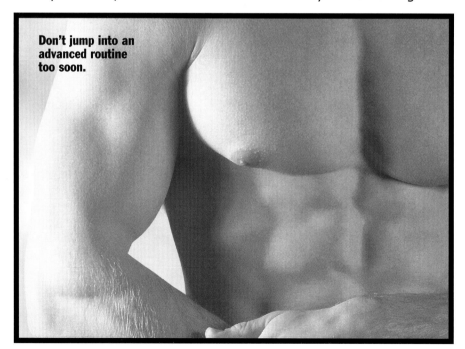

Don't jump into an advanced routine too soon.

Routine #1

Legs:	Squats	3 sets x 12-15 reps
	Stiff-leg deadlifts	3 sets x 12-15 reps
	Dumbell calf raises	3 sets x 12-15 reps
Chest:	Flat dumbell presses	3 sets x 12-15 reps
	Incline dumbell flyes	3 sets x 12-15 reps
Back:	One-arm rows	3 sets x 12-15 reps
	Dumbell pullovers	3 sets x 12-15 reps
Shoulders:	Dumbell presses	3 sets x 12-15 reps
	Side lateral raises	3 sets x 12-15 reps
Biceps:	Incline dumbell curls	3 sets x 12-15 reps
Triceps:	Dumbell extensions	3 sets x 12-15 reps
Abdominals:	Crunches	3 sets x 20-30 reps

Routine #2

Legs:	Lunges	3 sets x 12-15 reps
	Stiff-leg deadlifts	3 sets x 12-15 reps
	Dumbell calf raises	3 sets x 12-15 reps
Chest:	Incline barbell presses	3 sets x 12-15 reps
	Flat dumbell flyes	3 sets x 12-15 reps
Back:	Two-arm dumbell rows	3 sets x 12-15 reps
	Barbell pullovers	3 sets x 12-15 reps
Shoulders:	Front dumbell raises	3 sets x 12-15 reps
	Upright rows	3 sets x 12-15 reps
Biceps:	Barbell curls	3 sets x 12-15 reps
Triceps:	Dumbell kickbacks	3 sets x 12-15 reps
Abdominals:	Reverse crunches	3 sets x 20-30 reps

Four-Day Splits

If three-day splits have a disadvantage it's that you may be getting tired by the time you reach the last couple of muscle groups. To avoid overtraining you can split the body in half and train four times a week. Four-day splits are probably the most common routines people follow.

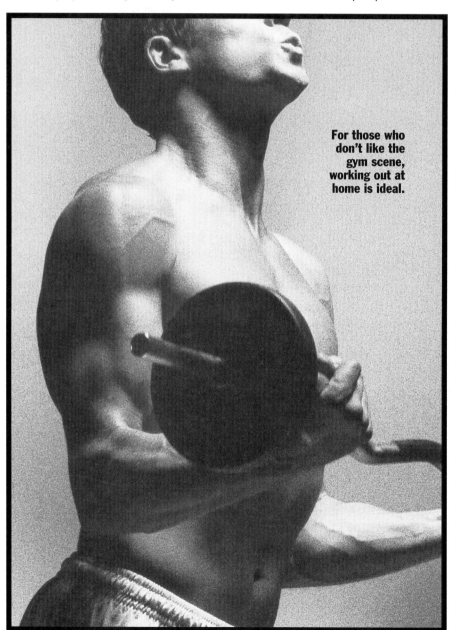

For those who don't like the gym scene, working out at home is ideal.

Routine #1
Day 1

Legs:	Squats	3 sets x 12-15 reps
	Lunges	3 sets x 12-15 reps
	Stiff-leg deadlifts	3 sets x 12-15 reps
	One-leg dumbell calf raises	3 sets x 12-15 reps
Biceps:	Standing barbell curls	3 sets x 12-15 reps
	Incline dumbell curls	3 sets x 12-15 reps
Triceps:	One-arm dumbell extensions	3 sets x 12-15 reps
	Dumbell kickbacks	3 sets x 12-15 reps

Day 2

Chest:	Incline dumbell presses	3 sets x 12-15 reps
	Flat dumbell flyes	3 sets x 12-15 reps
Back:	Dumbell rows	3 sets x 12-15 reps
	Barbell rows	3 sets x 12-15 reps
Shoulders:	Dumbell presses	3 sets x 12-15 reps
	Lateral raises	3 sets x 12-15 reps
	Bent-over laterals	3 sets x 12-15 reps
Abdominals:	Crunches	3 sets x 20-30 reps
	Reverse crunches	3 sets x 20-30 reps

Routine #2
Day 1

Chest:	Flat barbell presses	3 sets x 12-15 reps
	Incline dumbell flyes	3 sets x 12-15 reps
Back:	T-bar rows	3 sets x 12-15 reps
	Dumbell pullovers	3 sets x 12-15 reps
Biceps:	Standing dumbell curls	3 sets x 12-15 reps
	Concentration curls	3 sets x 12-15 reps

Day 2

Legs:	Lunges	3 sets x 12-15 reps
	Stiff-leg deadlifts	3 sets x 12-15 reps
	Dumbell calf raises	3 sets x 12-15 reps
Shoulders:	Front dumbell raises	3 sets x 12-15 reps
	Upright rows	3 sets x 12-15 reps
Triceps:	Lying dumbell extensions	3 sets x 12-15 reps
	Kickbacks	3 sets x 12-15 reps
Abdominals:	Crunches	3 sets x 20-30 reps
	Reverse crunches	3 sets x 20-30 reps

Six-Day-Splits

Six-day splits are one of the most advanced forms of training. They place a great demand on the recovery system over the long term, and should only be followed for short periods of time, i.e. four to six weeks.

There are generally two ways you can perform the six-day split. You can train three days in a row and take the fourth day off, and then repeat, or train six days in a row and take the seventh day off. Our advice is to follow the first method. Few people can subject their bodies to six straight days of training without burning out. And we don't mean in a couple of months either. Most people will be physically exhausted after just one or two weeks of such training.

The advantage of training the body over three days is that you only have to hit one or two muscle groups per session. Not only does this give you more time to focus on weak areas, but it allows you to complete your workout in 30 to 45 minutes. We're sure with school, work, and in many cases sports activities, you don't have the time to be spending hours in the gym. But we bet you can find 30 or 40 minutes on most days to get in a short workout.

As one final piece of advice, at the first sign of overtraining take a week or two off to reevaluate your training. You may have to cut back on the number of workouts you are performing each week.

Day 1

Legs:	Squats	3 sets x 12-15 reps
	Lunges	3 sets x 12-15 reps
	Stiff-leg deadlifts	3 sets x 12-15 reps
	One-leg calf raises	3 sets x 12-15 reps

Day 2

Chest:	Incline barbell presses	3 sets x 12-15 reps
	Flat dumbell presses	3 sets x 12-15 reps
Back:	Barbell rows	3 sets x 12-15 reps
	One-arm rows	3 sets x 12-15 reps

Day 3

Shoulders:	Dumbell presses	3 sets x 12-15 reps
	Side lateral raises	3 sets x 12-15 reps
Biceps:	Barbell curls	3 sets x 12-15 reps
	Incline dumbell curls	3 sets x 12-15 reps
Triceps:	Kickbacks	3 sets x 12-15 reps
	Lying dumbell extensions	3 sets x 12-15 reps

Leg Exercises

Squats – Place the barbell on the squat rack at about shoulder height. Step under the bar and rest it across your traps and shoulders. Step back, away from the rack, and place your feet slightly closer than shoulder width apart. Now in a slow and controlled manner bend your knees and descend toward the floor until your thighs are approximately parallel with the floor. Pause for a second and then return to the upright starting position.

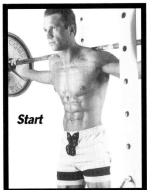

Start

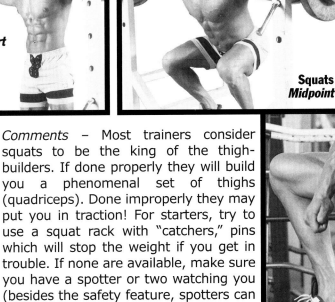

**Squats
Midpoint**

Comments – Most trainers consider squats to be the king of the thigh-builders. If done properly they will build you a phenomenal set of thighs (quadriceps). Done improperly they may put you in traction! For starters, try to use a squat rack with "catchers," pins which will stop the weight if you get in trouble. If none are available, make sure you have a spotter or two watching you (besides the safety feature, spotters can tell if you are performing the exercise properly).

Always wear a belt when performing squats, even though you seldom see them used in exercise photos and demonstration. Also don't bounce at the top or bottom of the exercise. Remember, you have a loaded barbell on your shoulders – and that's putting a lot of stress on your spine. Keep control of the weight throughout the movement.

Make sure you rest the bar across your shoulders and traps, not on the bony protrusion at the base of your skull. Do so and you will need regular chiropractic visits!

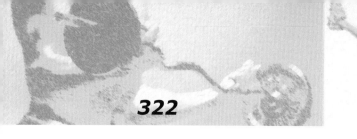
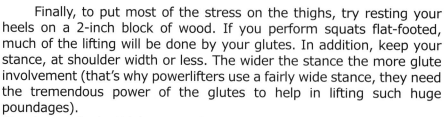
Finally, to put most of the stress on the thighs, try resting your heels on a 2-inch block of wood. If you perform squats flat-footed, much of the lifting will be done by your glutes. In addition, keep your stance, at shoulder width or less. The wider the stance the more glute involvement (that's why powerlifters use a fairly wide stance, they need the tremendous power of the glutes to help in lifting such huge poundages).

Muscles worked – While primarily a thigh-builder, squats will stimulate the whole leg region. Even with a narrow stance, the glutes will come into play. Also, the calves and hamstrings are used in stabilizing the legs as you move up and down. Finally, and much less obvious, the spinal erectors (lower back muscles) are needed to keep the body upright. In fact they are often the weak link in the chain. Most injuries obtained while doing squats center around the lower back region. That's why you must concentrate when performing this exercise.

Lunges – Hold a dumbell in each hand and position the legs in sort of a runner's stance, i.e. one leg in front of the other. Bend at the hips and knees until the front thigh is parallel with the floor. Return to the starting position by straightening the legs.

Comments – You can perform this exercise with dumbells or a barbell. In either case make sure your knee *does not* move out past the toes on the front foot. Some people literally "lunge" forward. This may give the thigh and glute muscles a slightly better stretch, but it places much more stress on the knees. You may have to experiment with your stance to ensure that this doesn't happen.

Muscles worked – Like squats, lunges hit most of the lower body region. The thighs and glutes do the main work, but the hamstrings also come into play.

Stiff-leg deadlifts – Place an Olympic bar on the floor in front of a block of wood, or on the end of a flat bench. Stand on the block or bench. With knees slightly bent, grab the bar with a shoulder-width grip. Raise the torso up to the top position, pause for a second and then bend forward until the plates are just short of touching the floor.

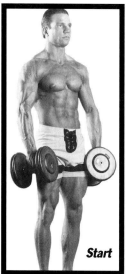
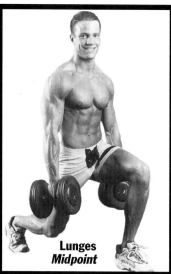

Start

**Lunges
Midpoint**

Comments – Although the name says *stiff-leg,* keeping the legs completely locked can put excessive stress on the lower back. Always keep a slight bend at the knee. Also, for the same reason, never bounce. The lower back ligaments receive enough abuse in life without you giving them another reason to act up.

Muscles worked – Although the lower legs do not bend as in a traditional leg curl, the hamstring muscles do cross the hip joint and are thus stimulated by extension at the hip. The lower spinal erectors and glutes also come into play on this exercise.

Dumbell calf raises – Hold a dumbell in one hand and stand on one foot on the lower step of a set of stairs or the edge of a piece of wood that is at least 2 inches thick. With the opposite leg curled up (you should now look like a flamingo!), flex up and down on your toes. Go for maximum stretch at both the top and bottom.

Comments – To keep your balance you may need to hold onto some sort of upright support (edge of a wall, sturdy piece of furniture, etc).

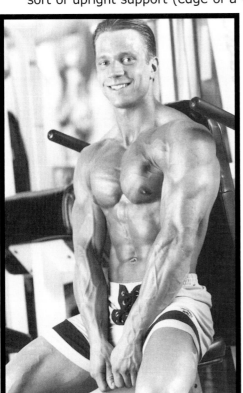

Rather than doing all 3 sets with one leg and then switching, alternate back and forth between sides.

Muscle worked – Dumbell calf raises primarily work the upper part of the calf (gastrocnemius), but the lower calf (soleus) also comes into play.

Chest Exercises

Flat barbell bench presses – Lie on your back and take the barbell from the supports, using a grip that is 6 to 8 inches wider than shoulder width. Lower the bar slowly to the nipple region, and then press it back up to lockout.

Comments – Considered the king of chest exercises, bench presses are performed by virtually every top bodybuilder. A few points to consider, though. Don't drop the bar and bounce it off the chest. Yes, you can lift more weight that way, but you are robbing the exercise of its effectiveness. You also run the risk of breaking ribs or splitting your sternum. Then there is the pec-delt tie-in to worry about. Dropping the

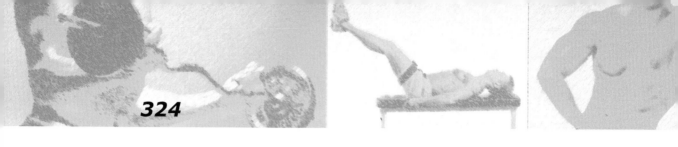

bar in a loose fashion increases the risk of tearing the area where your chest muscles connect to your shoulder muscles. To avoid the previous nasties, lower the weight in a slow, controlled manner, and then push it back to arms' length.

Whether you lock the arms out or not is your personal choice. Some bodybuilders prefer to stop just short of a lockout. That keeps the tension on the muscles throughout the movement. Others find locking out feels more comfortable. As the split is about 50-50 on the issue, try both methods and choose for yourself (this choice applies to virtually all the exercises).

Another point to mention, don't arch your back off the bench. Once again by cheating you may increase your lift by a few pounds, but at what cost? Arching decreases the amount of pectoral stimulation, and it certainly is no benefit to your lower back.

Incline barbell presses.
Start

Midpoint

If you have trouble keeping your back on the bench, perform the movement with your knees bent and legs up in the air. You will not be able to use as much weight, but there is no way you can arch your back when in this position.

Muscles worked – Flat bench presses primarily work the lower chest region, but the whole pectoral-deltoid area is stimulated. You will also find your triceps receive a great deal of stimulation. Finally, the muscles of the back and forearm are indirectly involved in stabilizing the upper body during the exercise.

Incline barbell presses – If using an adjustable bench, set it to an angle of about 25 to 30 degrees. Incline bench presses are performed in the same manner as flat benches, the only difference being instead of lowering the bar to the nipple region, bring it down to the center of the chest, just under the chin.

Comments – Most people find angles above 30 degrees place too much stress on the front delts, and not the upper pectorals. Of course your bone structure may dictate the opposite. You may have to play around with the angle to see what works best for you. If you don't have access to an adjustable bench, make do with the fixed version. In many cases these fixed benches are closer to 45 degrees, which is too steep for working the upper pecs. You may find that slightly arching the back, can shift most of the stress from the shoulders to the chest. But be careful, as the lower back was not designed to be arched to any degree. Here's a better solution – raise one end of a flat bench. You can use a couple of pieces of wood, another bench, or a specially constructed wooden block (most gyms have these for performing bent-over rows) to prop up the flat bench.

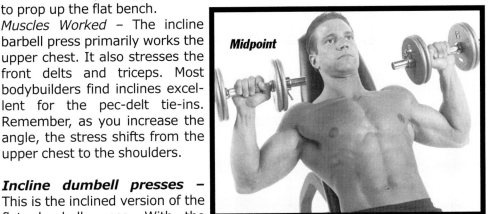

Midpoint

Muscles Worked – The incline barbell press primarily works the upper chest. It also stresses the front delts and triceps. Most bodybuilders find inclines excellent for the pec-delt tie-ins. Remember, as you increase the angle, the stress shifts from the upper chest to the shoulders.

Incline dumbell presses – This is the inclined version of the flat dumbell press. With the exception of the angle, the exercise is performed in the same manner.

Comments – Because you have to hoist the dumbells up higher, to get them into starting position, it might be a good idea to obtain the help of a spotter. Most bodybuilders lift one of the dumbells up, and have a partner pass them the other one. If possible have both passed to you. Without sounding too repetitious, we must warn you to *lower the dumbells slowly,* and go for a full but controlled stretch at the bottom.

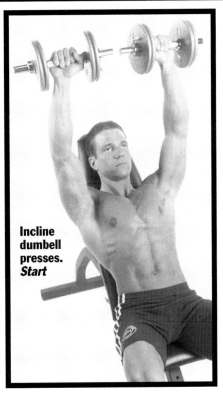

Incline dumbell presses. Start

Muscles worked – Incline dumbell presses are an excellent exercise for developing the upper chest. Because of the increased angle, they also hit the front deltoids. And like most chest exercises, there is some secondary triceps involvement. If your shoulders are taking too much of the weight, drop the angle of the bench a few degrees.

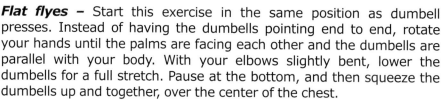

Flat flyes – Start this exercise in the same position as dumbell presses. Instead of having the dumbells pointing end to end, rotate your hands until the palms are facing each other and the dumbells are parallel with your body. With your elbows slightly bent, lower the dumbells for a full stretch. Pause at the bottom, and then squeeze the dumbells up and together, over the center of the chest.

Comments – Flyes are more of a stretching exercise than a mass-building movement. Still, with practice, you'll eventually be using considerable weight. Always lower the dumbells in a controlled manner, no matter what the poundage. Let them drop and you'll rip the pec-delt tie-in. Treatment for such an injury is surgery and many months of rehabilitation.

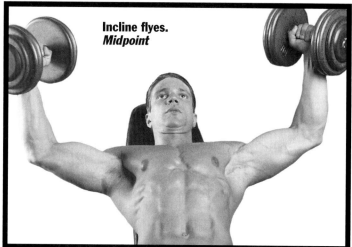

Incline flyes.
Midpoint

Muscles worked – Flyes work the whole chest region. Fully stretching at the bottom works the outer chest region and squeezing together at the top develops the inner chest. This gives your chest that clean line up the middle. As there will be some pec-delt tie-in strain, be careful at the bottom of the movement.

Incline flyes – This is the same exercise as the previous, but you use an incline bench. Once again go for a slow, full stretch at the bottom, and take care.

Comments – As with incline dumbell presses, the angle dictates lifting the dumbells up higher. You may need a partner to hoist the dumbells into position. In fact it's probably a good idea to have them passed to you, whether you can lift them or not. Jerking heavy dumbells from the floor puts a great deal of stress on the biceps and lower back. Better to be safe than macho.

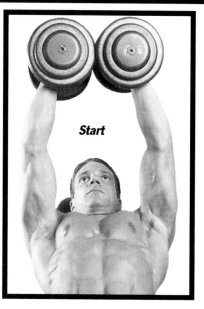

Start

Muscles worked – Incline flyes put most of the stress on the upper pectorals. They also strongly affect your chest-shoulder tie-ins. Once again, by squeezing the bells together at the top, the inner chest can be worked.

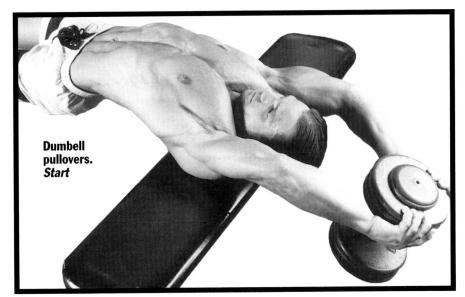

Dumbell pullovers. Start

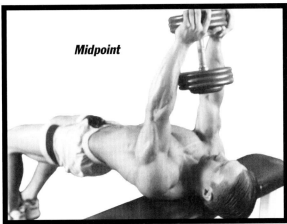

Midpoint

Dumbell or barbell pullovers – Grab a dumbell (or barbell) and lie face up *across* a flat bench. With the hips dropped below bench height, and the arms kept nearly straight, lower the dumbell behind your head to a comfortable stretch. Pull the weight up until the dumbell is positioned at arms' length above the chest. Contract your pecs and return slowly to a full stretch at the bottom.

Comments – Some people prefer doing this exercise while lying lengthways on the bench; others prefer doing the movement with an EZ-curl bar. Try all three and see which works best for you.

Muscles worked – Pullovers are one of those exercises that incorporate a large number of muscles. For some it's a great lat exercise, while others get a great chest stretch. Serratus and shoulders also play a role.

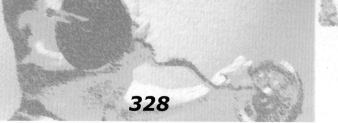
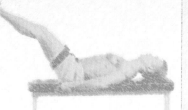
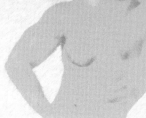
Back Exercises

***Bent-over barbell rows* –** Bend over at the waist so that your upper body is just short of parallel with the floor. Grab a standard barbell, and using a wide grip, drag it up the abdomen. Lower slowly and then repeat. Concentrate on using the upper back muscles (lats) and not your spinal erectors.

Comments – You must be especially careful on this exercise. Any sudden bouncing or jerking will put great stress on your lower back. If you have to "throw your lower back into it" you are using far too much weight. Take off a few plates and do it more strictly. The only part of the body that should move is your arms. Your upper body and legs should remain stationary. To get a full stretch, stand on some sort of low platform. Most gyms have specially constructed boxes for you to stand on while performing bent-over rows. The extra 10 to 12 inches of stretch will add greatly to the effectiveness of this exercise. As a final point, bend your knees slightly. This will help reduce the stress on your lower back.

Muscles worked – This exercise is considered by most to be one of the best back strengtheners. It's particularly effective in working the center area. Besides the back muscles, bent-over rows stress the biceps and forearms. Finally, because of the bent over position, the exercise stretches the hamstrings and spinal erectors.

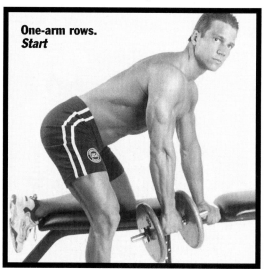

One-arm rows.
Start

***One-arm and two-arm rows* –** Instead of using a barbell or cable, you can do your rows using a dumbell. Bend over and grab a bench for support. Place one leg behind the other, in a running type stance, or on the bench. Grab a dumbell with the arm that is furthest from the bench (i.e. the bracing arm is closest to the bench) and stretch it down and slightly forward. From that position at the bottom, pull the dumbell up until the elbow is fully bent, contract, then lower slowly. The movement is comparable to that of sawing wood.

For the two-arm version set your adjustable bench at about 30 degrees and lie face down. Grab the dumbells and pull them toward the upper body as if sawing wood. Return to the starting position with arms just short of a lockout.

Comments – One- and two-arm rows are great because they allow you to brace your upper body. This is essential if you have a lower back injury. Even though your biceps will be involved in the movement, try to concentrate on using just your back muscles. Once again, no bouncing or jerking the weight. If you have to contort the body to lift the it, the dumbell is too heavy.

Muscles worked – One- and two-arm rows are great *overall* back exercises. They are particularly effective at hitting the outer edges of the lats. The smaller back muscles like the teres, rear shoulders, and rhomboids also come into play.

T-bar rows – Although many gyms have a long bar that has one end bolted to the floor you can make do with a regular barbell. Simply place one end in a corner and place one or two weight plates on top to keep the end down. Place the weights on the other end and keep them from sliding inward by a collar. Either grab the bar with both hands just behind the plates, or hold a small bar positioned underneath (this is where the name T-bar comes from as the long and short bars form a letter T. With legs bent and your torso held slightly above parallel, pull the bar up to your lower rib cage. Squeeze at the top, then lower back

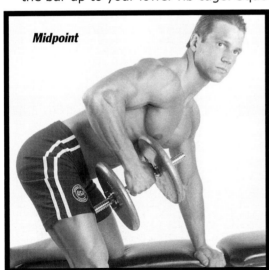

Midpoint

to the floor. Don't touch the plates to the floor, but stop a few inches from it.

Comments – Once again don't bounce or jerk the weight up. Like barbell rows, T-bar rows place a great deal of stress on the lower back. Keep your upper body stationary, and lift the plates with your back muscles and arms only. Always keep the lower back slightly arched by keeping your butt stuck out and back (sounds crude but trust us, this stance is a lot less stressful on your lower back).

Muscles worked – T-Bar rows work the same muscles as the regular barbell row. The lats, teres, rhomboids, rear delts, biceps, forearms and lower back all come into play. Because of the assortment of muscles worked, both types of rows are excellent mass builders.

Note: If you have lower back problems, you might want to avoid these exercises. If you must do them, start off by using light weight. Gradually build up the poundage over time. Don't make the mistake of

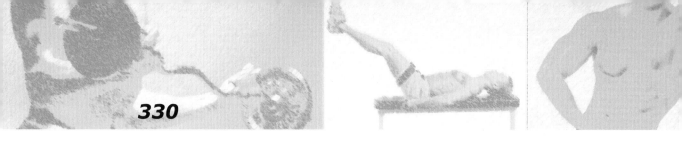

slapping on 45-pound plates from day one. Take your time. Keep in mind that lower back injuries often don't heal. You're likely to have them for life. Therefore the emphasis should be on preventing them. In a manner of speaking, rows can be a double-edged sword. Done properly they will help strengthen the lower back, thus reducing the chances of future injuries. Done improperly they may be the cause of the injury! So pay strict attention to your exercise style. Don't get carried away with the weight, and don't lift with the lower back.

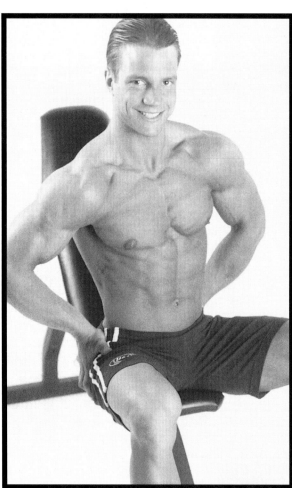

Shoulder Exercises

Dumbell presses – Instead of performing your pressing movements with a barbell, grab a pair of dumbells and hoist them to shoulder level. You can stand or sit when pressing the dumbells, but if standing, be careful not to excessively arch the lower back.

Comments – You can press both dumbells at the same time or in an alternating fashion. As with the barbell version, be careful of the lower back. Try not to arch excessively, and don't drop the dumbells back to the starting position.

Muscles worked – This exercise stresses the whole deltoid region. Particular emphasis is placed on the front and side deltoids. There is some secondary trap and rear deltoid involvement, too.

Upright rows – Start the exercise by holding a barbell at arms' length. Using a narrow grip (about 3 to 5 inches) lift the bar up the front of the body, keeping the elbows flared to the sides. Squeeze the traps together at the top, and then lower into the starting position.

Comments – Which muscles are worked depends on the grip used.

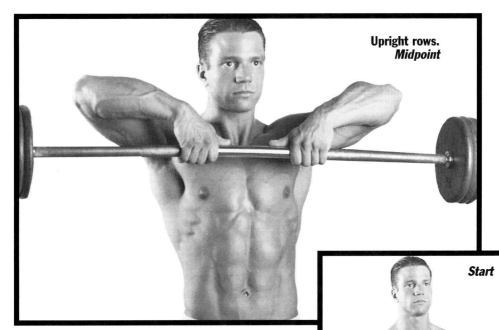

Upright rows.
Midpoint

Start

Generally, any hand spacing of 5 inches or less puts most of the stress on the traps. Widen the grip and the side deltoids come into play. In the routines presented above we are suggesting the exercise as a trap builder. But you can easily substitute upright rows for one of the delt exercises. Just remember to keep the grip wide when doing so.

If you have weak or injured wrists, you might want to think twice about performing this exercise. Upright rows place tremendous stress on the forearms and wrists. If you experience minor pain when doing the exercise, try wrapping the wrists with support bandages. This should enable you to complete your sets in comfort. Of course *you're* the only one who can determine if the pain is just a nuisance or representative of something more serious. If in doubt skip the exercise.

As with barbell curls, upright rows give you the option of adding a few cheat reps at the end of the set. Limit such cheat reps to 1 or 2. Don't make the mistake of cheating from rep one.

Muscles worked – With a narrow grip upright rows primarily work the traps, with some secondary deltoid stimulation. A wide grip (6 inches or more) will shift the strain to the side delts, with the traps now playing a secondary role. The forearms are worked no matter what grip you use.

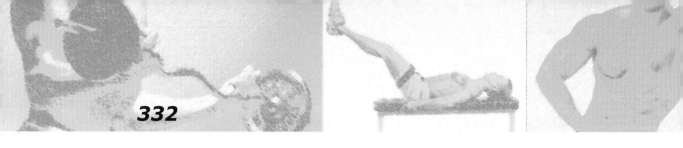

Lateral raises – You can perform this exercise seated or standing. Grab a pair of dumbells and, with the elbows slightly bent, raise them to the sides of the body. As you raise the bells, gradually rotate your wrists so that the little finger points up. Many bodybuilding authorities, including Robert Kennedy, liken the wrist action to pouring a jug of water.

Comments – You can do this exercise with the arms completely locked, but most bodybuilders find it more effective to bend the arms slightly and use more weight. Lateral raises can be done toward the front, side or rear (explained in detail later). Instead of using dumbells, a cable may be substituted. All versions may be performed with one or two arms at a time.

Muscles worked – You can do lateral raises to work any head of the deltoid muscle. Most intermediate bodybuilders use them for the side delts, as the front delts receive ample stimulation from various pressing movements. Side raises will give your delts that half-melon look. There's not much you can do to widen the clavicles, but you can increase your shoulder width by adding inches to the side delts.

Start

Bent-over laterals – This is the bent-over version of regular side raises. By bending over, the stress is shifted from the side to the rear delts. You can do the exercise free standing, seated, or with your head braced on a high bench. The latter is for those with lower back problems or individuals who have a tendency to swing the weight up.

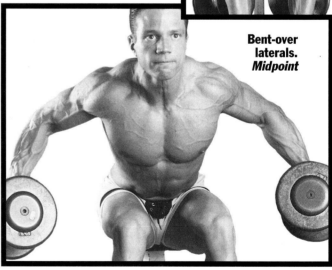

Bent-over laterals. Midpoint

Comments – Concentrate on lifting the dumbells with your rear delts and not your traps and lats.

Muscles worked – When performed properly, bent-over laterals primarily work the rear deltoids. There is, however, secondary triceps, trap and lat stimulation.

Front dumbell raises – Grab a set of dumbells and with the legs slightly bent, raise the dumbells forward and upward until your arms are parallel with the floor. Return to the starting position with the bells either by your sides (palms facing inward) or at the thighs (palms facing downward).

Comments – There are numerous variations of this exercise. You can raise both arms at the same time, or in an alternating fashion. As suggested above you can keep the palms facing in or down. Finally you may choose to grab one dumbell with both hands and raise it forward. Experiment and find what works best for you.

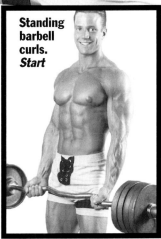

Biceps Exercises

Standing barbell curls – Perhaps the most used (and abused!) exercise performed in gyms. Grab the bar slightly wider than shoulder width and curl it up until the biceps are fully flexed. Try to keep your elbows close to your sides, and don't swing the weight up with your lower back. Lower the weight back to the starting position in good style. Don't simply let the thing drop! Not only would you lose half the movement, you'd also run the risk of tearing your biceps tendon.

Comments – Barbell curls are considered the ultimate biceps exercise. However, many people forget that the negative (lowering) section of the movement is just as important as the positive (hoisting) section. Try to lower the bar with about the same speed as you curl it up.

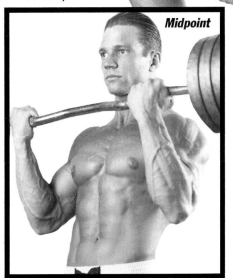

Midpoint

Standing barbell curls. Start

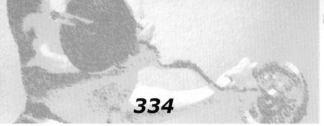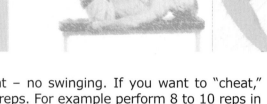

Keep your back straight – no swinging. If you want to "cheat," save it for the last couple of reps. For example perform 8 to 10 reps in good style and then cheat 1 or 2 more. Don't abuse a good thing, however. Forcing 1 or 2 cheat reps is fine, but cheating from the start is counterproductive.

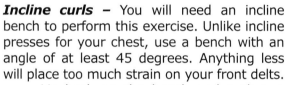
Start

Muscles worked – The barbell biceps curl works the entire biceps muscle. Also, because you have to forcibly grip the bar, this exercise will give you a great set of forearms. Finally, the front delts and lower back come into play for stabilizing purposes.

Incline curls – You will need an incline bench to perform this exercise. Unlike incline presses for your chest, use a bench with an angle of at least 45 degrees. Anything less will place too much strain on your front delts.

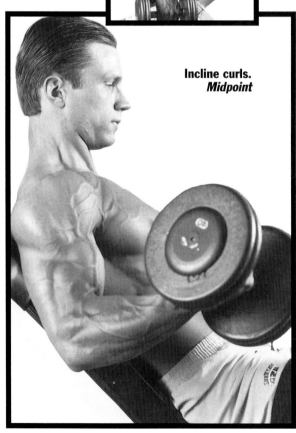
Incline curls.
Midpoint

Lie back on the bench and grab two dumbells. Curl the bells up until the biceps are fully flexed. All the tips suggested for standing dumbell curls apply here as well (rotate the hands from facing in, to a facing-up position, don't swing the weight up, etc.).

Comments – Once again you have the option of curling both dumbells simultaneously or curling alternately. When you lower the bells, be careful not to hit the side of the incline bench. In fact, this is another reason for starting with the dumbells in a forward-pointed position. If they were in the standard position, end to end, they would have less clearance from the bench.

The advantage of using the incline bench is that it limits the amount of cheating you can do. Let's face it, you can't swing very much if you have your back braced against a rigid board.

Muscles worked – Incline curls work the whole biceps region. The exercise does provide some forearm stimulation, but not to the same extent as the various barbell curls.

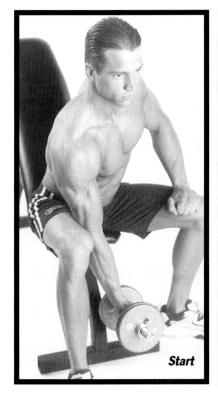

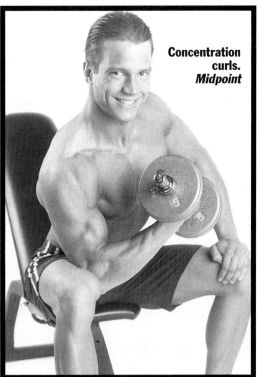

Concentration curls.
Midpoint

Start

Concentration curls – Sit down on the end of a bench and grab a dumbell. Rest the elbow of the working arm on your inner thigh. Curl the dumbell, flex, and lower it to a full stretch. Perform one set before switching arms.

Comments – Most people perform concentration curls in the seated position. A few (including the famous Arnold Schwarzenegger) like to do the movement standing, in a bent-over position. Instead of bracing the elbow against the thigh, it's held down and away from the body. Keep your shoulder on the exercising side lower than the one on the free side. Resist the urge to swing – use only biceps power. As with all dumbell curls, you may want to supinate the hands when performing the exercise.

Muscles worked – As with most dumbell exercises, concentration curls hit the entire biceps region. The forearms also come into play.

Standing dumbell curls – Instead of using a barbell, grab a pair of dumbells. Although it's possible to simultaneously raise both bells, most people do *alternate dumbell curls.* As the name implies, you curl the dumbells one at a time. Start with the dumbells by your sides with the ends pointing to the front and back (i.e. the dumbells are parallel to

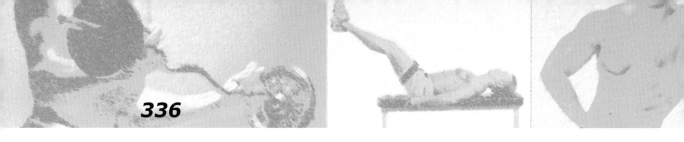

one another). As you curl, rotate your palms from the facing-in position to a facing-up position. This is called *supination.*

Many people are not aware that the biceps muscle has two main functions. Besides the more well-known curling movement, the biceps also rotate the forearms. You can see this motion if you hold your arm by your side and rotate the hand back and forth. Notice the biceps flexing as the hand approaches the palm-up position. By using dumbells, you can take advantage of this physiological trait. Now, we should add that you would have to use a very heavy dumbell (more than you could curl) to get the full effect of supination. Still every bit helps, so give it a try.

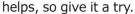

Comments – Once again, limit any swinging to the last rep or two. Anyway, cheating is probably not necessary at this stage of your development. Try to put total concentration into each and every rep.

Besides the psychological aspect of curling one dumbell at a time, there may be a physiological basis. Neurologists suggest that when two arms are used simultaneously, the brain has to split the nerve impulses. Whereas by alternating the dumbells, you get full nerve transmission to each arm. How much is fact and how much is theory? That's open to debate. And although you have no control over nerve impulses, you do have control over exercise performance. So choose the version that feels most productive.

Muscles worked – Dumbell curls are great for working the belly of the biceps. They also reduce the stress on the wrists and forearms. In fact many experts suggest starting your biceps workout with dumbells so as not to overstress the weaker areas.

Triceps Exercises

One-arm dumbell extensions **–** Grasp a dumbell and extend it above your head. Keeping the upper arm stationary, lower the dumbell behind the head. Try to perform the movement in a slow rhythmic manner.

Comments– It is possible to work up to 75-plus pound dumbells, but keep this in mind: The elbow joint and associated tissues (ligaments cartilage and tendons) were not designed to support huge poundages. Never bounce the dumbell at the bottom (arms in the bent position) of the exercise. Try to place the emphasis on style rather than weight.

Muscles worked – Although it works the whole triceps region, this exercise is great for the lower triceps.

Lying dumbell extensions – Sit on the end of a flat bench, and take hold of a dumbell in each hand. Lie down facing the ceiling and hold your arms straight upward. With the upper arms held still, bend at the elbows and lower the dumbells to the sides of your head to around ear level. Return to the starting point by extending the forearms back to the straight position, using the power of your triceps.

Comments – Lying dumbell extensions are great for those who are wary of using a barbell. (Let's face it, you have to stop the bar at the forehead. If you don't, you'll find out why the exercise is nicknamed "skullcrushers.") Dumbells also allow for an extra few degrees of movement. Finally some people find lying dumbell extensions much easier on the wrists and elbows.

Muscles worked – Lying dumbell extensions hit the entire triceps region – particularly the long rear head of the muscle.

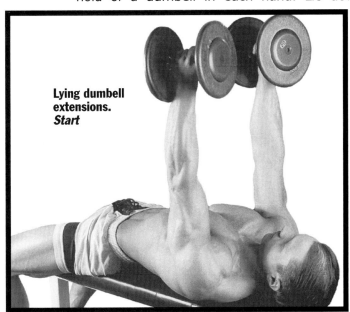

Lying dumbell extensions. *Start*

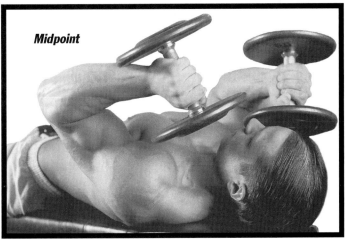

Midpoint

Triceps kickbacks – With your body braced on a bench, bend over and set your upper arm parallel with the floor. Grab a dumbell and extend the lower arm back until it's in the locked position (i.e. your whole arm is now parallel with the floor). Pause and squeeze at the top, and then lower back to the starting point.

Comments – Resist the urge to swing the dumbell up using body momentum. True, you can use more weight that way, but it won't give the same triceps development. Keep the upper arm locked against the side of the body. As with bent-over laterals, if you have trouble keeping stationary, or have a weak lower back, place your free hand on a bench or other such support.

Muscles worked – Triceps kickbacks are great for giving the triceps that horseshoe shape. They are especially useful for developing the long rear head of the triceps. Kickbacks are a favorite exercise during the precontest months.

Exercises for the Abdominals

Reverse crunches – Lie on your back and with the upper body held stationary draw the knees up toward the upper body. Return to the starting position with the legs stretched out.

Comments – To lessen the stress on your lower back, always keep a slight bend at the knees.

Muscles worked – Reverse crunches hit the entire abdominal region with special emphasis on the lower abdominals. The hip flexors also come into play.

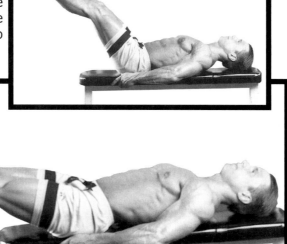

Midpoint

**Reverse crunches.
Start**

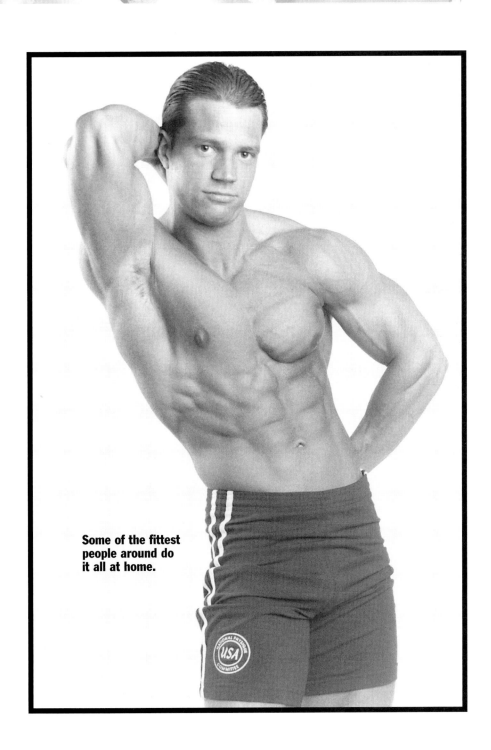

Some of the fittest people around do it all at home.

CHAPTER THIRTY

The Cardiovascular System

The cardiovascular system includes the heart and the blood vessels, and the respiratory system contains those organs which are responsible for carrying oxygen from the air to the bloodstream, and expelling the waste product of carbon dioxide. Blood is that sticky, red fluid that circulates throughout our bodies in veins and arteries. The heart pumps oxygen into the blood and collects carbon dioxide from it to be expelled through the lungs.

Cardiovascular Training

We usually think of respiration as the process of the lungs after air is breathed in through the mouth or nose. The lungs do play a very important role, but every living cell in the body is involved in this process. Respiration is the act of burning energy from oxygen. Breathing is an obvious part of respiration, but the respiratory passages are involved in the sense of smell as well, along with yawning, sneezing, coughing, hiccups, the power of speech, whereby the respiratory flow is "kidnapped" by the larynx (voice box), which uses the air flow to create a multiple range of sounds so that humans can communicate vocally. The tasks of the cardiovascular systems and the respiratory systems include organs which take up space in the face and neck, and most of the chest. These systems are basic to life and breathing, just as the beat of one's heart is a function which is automatically controlled by the brain.

Aerobic vs. Anaerobic Exercise

As you first start to exercise, no matter whether you are walking or running, your muscles immediately begin to use energy to allow them to work. For the first three minutes your muscles will burn glycogen, a special sugar which is stored in the muscles for a quick infusion of energy. Some glycogen is always stored within your muscle tissues. During this period fat is not burned. This process is called *anaerobic metabolism.* Often during the first few minutes of strenuous activity, especially during anaerobic metabolism, you may experience burning in muscles of your arms, legs or back. This is due to the creation of lactic acid, which occurs when glycogen is burned. This burning sensation will soon go away.

As you exercise more than three minutes you will eventually burn up all of the glycogen stored within the muscles and your muscles will move into *aerobic metabolism,* and lactic acid production is stopped. This occurs because the glycogen is now being burned in the presence of oxygen, which is brought to the muscles by way of the bloodstream. As long as you breathe correctly you will bring oxygen to the muscles and this process will continue.

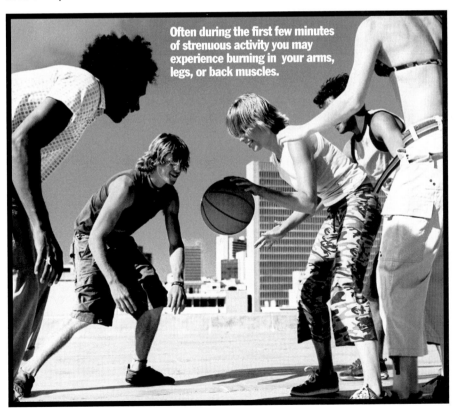

Often during the first few minutes of strenuous activity you may experience burning in your arms, legs, or back muscles.

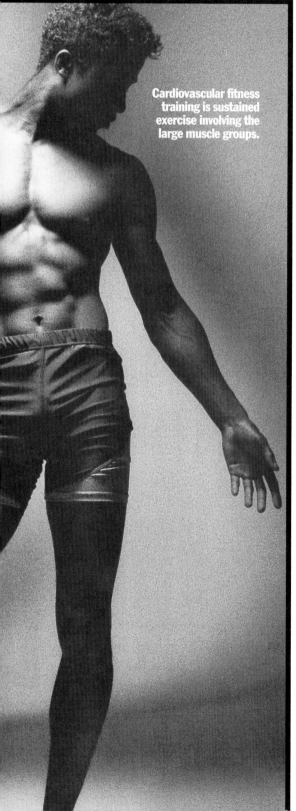

Cardiovascular fitness training is sustained exercise involving the large muscle groups.

Oxygen is essential to a muscle's ability to function correctly. With adequate oxygen the muscles can extract all the energy they need from blood sugar. During your workout session the liver and muscles will release their stored carbohydrate so that it can be used as energy by the muscles, hence allowing you to keep on exercising.

Once these stores of glycogen are used up – which usually occurs after about 20 minutes – the body will start burning its *fat stores* to produce blood sugar and ultimately glycogen. The longer you exercise the more fat burned. Fat, bodyfat and not dietary fat, can now be used virtually indefinitely to produce energy to support your exercise program.

While you are walking you do not directly burn fat, but once you stop walking the glycogen which has been burned up must be replaced. This can only be supplied by what you eat and by what the liver draws from the body's fat tissues. If you are on a limited caloric intake, then the food you ingest will be used basically for feeding your brain, and fat stores will have to be drawn on to replace the glycogen used up while exercising. Studies show that the fat-burning mode may last for anywhere from 6 to 24 hours after a regular exercise program – so even moderate exercise has long-term benefits for you.

Studies, however, also show us that the percentage of energy contributed from burning fat *decreases* as you increase the intensity of your exercise program. You do not have to exercise intensely or exert great effort – only mild to moderate exercise on a regular basis is needed.

Cardiovascular fitness training is sustained exercise involving the large muscle groups. This exercise should increase the heart rate to a designated range called the *target heart range* or exercise heart range.

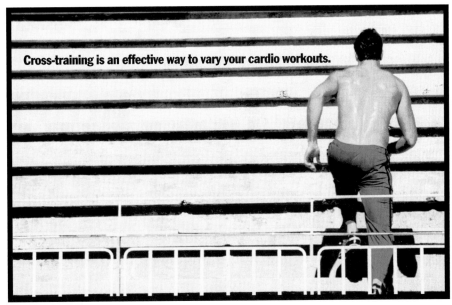

Cross-training is an effective way to vary your cardio workouts.

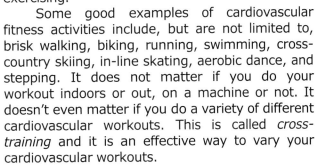

Sometimes you will see the terms "rate" and "range" used interchangeably, but "range" is generally a scope of numbers which encompass the more specific "rate," which is usually one number.

No matter which term is used, setting a range of goal numbers for the target heart rate is usually the best method of actually monitoring one's heart rate during activity. It is difficult to maintain and remain at one specific heart rate number. A range allows an individual to readily monitor his or her own target heart rate while exercising.

Some good examples of cardiovascular fitness activities include, but are not limited to, brisk walking, biking, running, swimming, cross-country skiing, in-line skating, aerobic dance, and stepping. It does not matter if you do your workout indoors or out, on a machine or not. It doesn't even matter if you do a variety of different cardiovascular workouts. This is called *cross-training* and it is an effective way to vary your cardiovascular workouts.

The bottom-line goal here is to raise your heart rate to your target range, keep it there for 30 minutes, and do so at least three times per week. If you are doing an activity like swimming or in-line skating, make sure your skill level is sufficient enough to allow you to do a proper cardiovascular workout. Start/stop activities, such as tennis, racquetball and basketball, are great supplemental workout fun, but do not provide enough sustained time in the target heart range to be used as your primary means of cardiovascular fitness.

In order to gain the benefits of cardiovascular training, one must do this sustained activity of the large muscle groups for a minimum of 20 to 30 minutes at least three times per week. Although some research has suggested shorter periods of 5 or 10 minutes can give the same benefits as longer sessions, we recommend 30 minutes of sustained cardio-vascular exercise three times per week as the best minimum for most people. This minimum is recommended only after safely building to this level. Of course, short periods of sustained exercise are better than remaining sedentary, but the "lack of time" reasoning that most people use for needing shorter workouts is lacking in substance. Certainly we can all find 30 minutes several times a week to invest in our health.

Oxygen is essential to a muscle's ability to function correctly.

Your target heart range is most accurately calculated in a laboratory setting but this is not feasible for the general public. Using a general formula, you can calculate your target heart range using your age, resting heart rate, and approximate fitness level. It is important to note that general guidelines based solely on a person's age and fitness level are guidelines only.

It is best to calculate your own target heart range using your individual resting heart rate since resting heart rates can vary significantly, even among people of the same age. Many factors such as hereditary tendencies, medical conditions, and even common medications can affect one's resting heart rate.

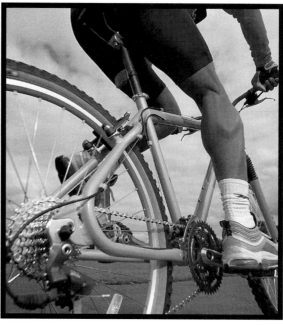

Calculating Your Target Heart Range

Exercise is most valuable from a cardiovascular point of view when the heart is not overtaxed but yet is challenged. The best way to get there is to bring the speed at which your heart beats (pulse taken in the lower extremities) into a range which is between 60 percent and 85 percent of your maximum heart rate. The maximum heart rate (measured in beats per minute) refers to that approximate level after which there is real or potential danger to the individual and where the heart is overtaxed. At this rate exercise is difficult and will cause fatigue within minutes or sooner. Below this and within the *target range* is where the heart is strengthened and made healthier. The target heart range is a calculated figure, which depends on age. The ability to reach and maintain a heart beat within the target range depends on the health of the heart, conditioning, frequency of exercise, and the length of time exercising.

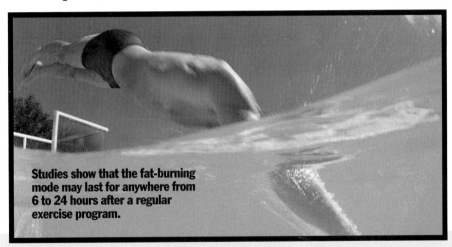

Studies show that the fat-burning mode may last for anywhere from 6 to 24 hours after a regular exercise program.

1. The first step is to subtract your age from 220 to get your maximum heart rate.

2. Multiply your maximum heart rate first by .60 (60 percent) and then by .85 (85 percent). This will give you your target heart range.

If you are 17 years of age, the calculations would look like this:

   220 - 17 = 203; then *203 x .60 = 122*; and *203 x .85 = 173*.

   Your target heart range would be *122 to 173* beats per minute.

Now you can calculate your own target heart range:

   220 - _____ = _____ x .60 = _____ x .85 = _____

   Your target heart range would be ____ *to* ____ beats per minute.

Exercise Machines You Can Take to Heart

We're the quirky civilization that rides elevators to the second floor and buys electronic stair-steppers to condition our thighs. We drive to nearby convenience stores and hurry back to our treadmills. Yes, we rely on machines to save us from working, then buy other machines to save our bodies from terminal flab. It's a roundabout way of staying in shape, and it's certainly not cheap. But if you want to get a good workout in front of the tube, an exercise machine may be the ticket.

There are plenty of marvels out there to work your pecs, quads, abs and glutes. All you need is several hundred to several thousand dollars. The ultimate focus is the most important muscle of all, *the heart.* Today's machines come with all sorts of snazzy panel displays that make heart-watching easier than ever. But one warning before you start: An estimated 50 percent of the machines people buy end up sitting idle in garages and spare bedrooms, abandoned after an initial burst of energy. (How many of you readers have such a machine in your attic or basement!)

So before you spring for one, get a doctor's okay and make sure you're ready to revamp your life to make room for this new routine. Next, see which equipment works best for you. After all, when you put down the money, you're committing yourself, in theory, to thousands of hours on this machine, perhaps tens of millions of steps, oar-strokes or revolutions. It had better be a motion your body likes. Most fitness machines replicate common real-world forms of exercise, from rowing to riding a bike to walking.

Treadmills

Treadmills are the most popular of all exercise machines, with 42 percent of the market. They sell well for a simple reason: *most humans know how to walk.* The nice thing about treadmills is that you can set the speed to your own pace. Instead of the machine telling you what you are going to do, you tell the machine what you are going to

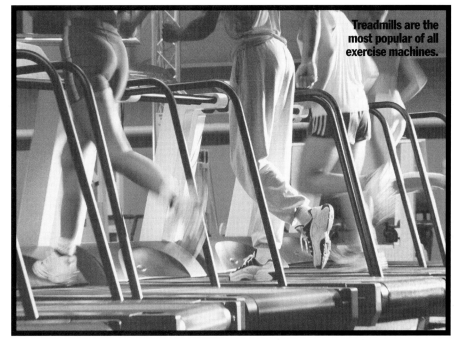

Treadmills are the most popular of all exercise machines.

do. As your fitness level improves it's just a matter of increasing the speed. Many treadmills also allow you to increase the angle from flat to an incline of 10 to 15 degrees. Now 15 degrees doesn't sound like much but try running uphill on such an incline. Not so easy any more is it?

If treadmills have a drawback it's that you have to support the entire body weight on the knees and ankles. For many people running or even walking is hard on the joints. Hopefully most readers don't fall into that category yet. Such problems tend to surface as we get older. But those of you who have knee or ankle problems from sports (or any reason for that matter) may want to consider another form of cardio machine.

Stationary Cycles

Although it's much more fun to ride outside in the fresh air, weather and time may force you to cycle indoors. No need to worry, though, as manufacturers have come up with an assortment of stationary cycles to make indoor bike riding fun.

Stationary bikes focus on the same muscles as treadmills but have several advantages. They occupy less space, and since the person is *sitting,* they place less stress on the ankles, knees and hips. They also average about half the price. The latest rage is the recumbent bike, where you sit in what looks like an office chair and pedal with your legs out front. In exercise clubs, you'll notice that the recumbents are

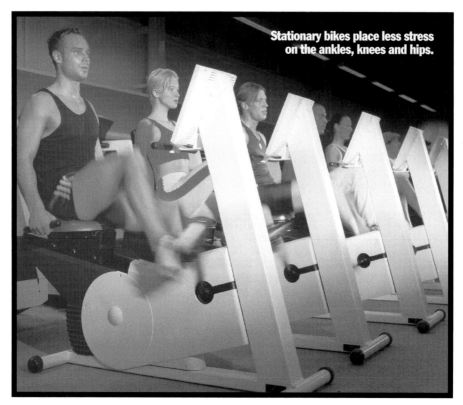

Stationary bikes place less stress on the ankles, knees and hips.

usually the ones you have to sign up for in advance. That's because they're easier on the back and the knees. Perhaps the ultimate form of indoor cycling is spinning. Read on.

Spinning

Spinning is a perfect example of a trendy new form of fitness that seems to have staying power. The name *"spinning"* is actually a trademark of the Schwinn Corporation, and refers to any group cycling class on stationary cycles. Just as most people refer to all forms of acetylsalicylic acid (ASA) as Aspirin (the trademark name held by the Bayer Corporation of Germany), so too are most group cycling classes called spinning classes.

What makes spinning so popular is that it offers numerous fitness-related benefits, as well as being gender neutral. Despite the advances made in the last couple of decades, weight training is still seen as masculine, and cardio as feminine. But spinning is for everyone, and most classes have an even mixture of men and women. In terms of conditioning, spinning is a great way to stimulate the cardiovascular system as well as strengthen and tone up the muscles, particularly the leg muscles.

A lesser-known reason for the popularity of spinning over other forms of fitness is that it is very motivational. A combination of small class size, a dynamic instructor, and suitable music all contribute to keep participants interested and determined to finish the class. In a large aerobics class it's easy to slack off and go through the motions, but in a spinning class there is no room for stragglers. Everyone is motivated to keep up.

A typical spinning class consists of one instructor and 10 participants. Instructors have different cycle arrangements but most use a semi circle pattern. As *Oxygen* consultant Lori Grannis put it, "It reminded me of the warm fuzzy feelings I experienced during storytime in first grade."

Other than the cycle, the only equipment recommended is a water bottle and maybe a towel. The cycle itself bears little resemblance to those $5000 cardio cycles that inhabit gyms these days. You won't find any bells or whistles either – in fact, no electronics of any kind. This is cycling at its purist. The cycle will have a lever located just beneath the handlebars that allows you to increase the tension on the pedals. Push the lever all the way down and it acts as a brake. Keep this in mind as the large front flywheel weighs 40 or 50 pounds and once it gets going you can't automatically stop it just by locking your legs. You either gradually slow down and stop or push the brake lever down.

If spinning cycles have one big disadvantage over regular cardio cycles it's lack of comfort. The seat on a typical cardio cycle is rather small and not blessed with the greatest amount of padding. After 10 or 15 minutes sitting on it your hindquarters are going to start to talk to you in unpleasant terms. Of course during a spinning class you'll be alternating sitting with standing and sprinting, so you won't be sitting on the seat for long.

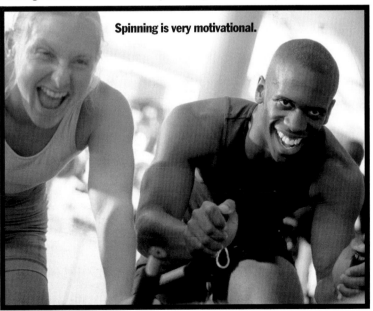

Spinning is very motivational.

The workout itself is like most forms of physical activity and can be divided into three phases, warmup, middle and cooldown. The warmup consists of various stretches that start while standing on the floor, and then progress to the cycle. Most instructors begin with a slow to moderate pace and then progress to the faster paced pedaling and sprinting, either seated or standing. During a typical class you'll alternate various speeds with different tensions on the wheels.

One thing we almost forgot to mention is the music. Besides the instructor yelling at you, and being surrounded by other "victims," spinning classes are conducted in the presence of music. Most gyms have the stereo system controls located next to the instructor's cycle so he or she can alternate various music tempos throughout the session. Typically slow music is used for the warmup and cooldown, and faster paced music for the heart of the class. Some instructors use rock music, while others go for upbeat dance music.

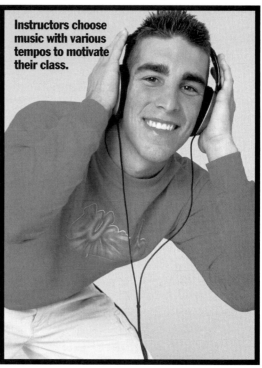

Instructors choose music with various tempos to motivate their class.

The average spinning class lasts 45 to 60 minutes, and is as good as it gets when it comes to cardiovascular conditioning. Where spinning has an advantage over many others forms of aerobics is in strengthening effects on the muscles. Most forms of cardio only use the weight of the body as resistance. For the first couple of weeks this may provide some strengthening benefits, but the leg muscles quickly adapt. But with spinning, the tension lever allows you to increase the resistance on demand. Many weight trainers report that their legs get as pumped from a spinning class as they do from a regular squat workout.

Most gyms don't charge extra for spinning. Others require you to pay a small fee. We suggest you check out different instructors. They should all have the same qualifications, but like anything else, personality often plays a role. One instructor may motivate you to the point you could go for two hours, while another may make you decide to give up after 15 minutes. Of course another gym member may find just the opposite. It may even come down to music selection. Finally, check with your gym to see if they offer teen spinning classes. If not you might want to round up eight or ten of your friends and approach the gym manager about offering such a class.

Rowers

Despite offering one of the quickest and most thorough cardiovascular workouts, rowers have fallen into disfavor as people worry about their lower backs. Rowers now account for less than 5 percent of the cardio equipment market. Still, they're among the best aerobic machines that also build full-body strength. With proper posture and technique, bending the legs with the sliding seat, the back shouldn't suffer. The standard for rowers is the Concept II Rowing Ergometer.

One of the nice things about rowers is their simplicity. There's no fancy programming to set up. No complicated technique to master. Simply sit down in the seat, grab the handlebar, and away you go!

A practical advantage to rowers is their ease of access. As we said earlier rowers are among the least popular forms of cardio equipment. That means you should have no problem accessing them when you go into the gym. Even at busy times there are usually a couple of rowers free to use.

Some good examples of cardiovascular fitness activities include, but are not limited to, brisk walking, biking, running, swimming, cross-country skiing, in-line skating, aerobic dance, and stepping.

Cross-Trainers

If treadmills and cycles were the most popular machines in the 1980s, cross-trainers are a product of the 1990s. For want of a better description, cross-trainers mimic cross-country skiing. You place your feet in a set of flat supports and grab

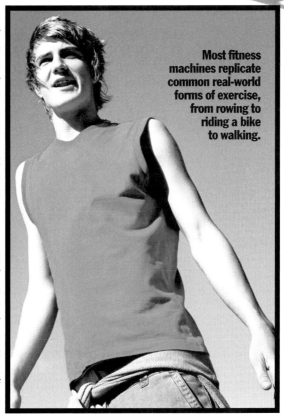

Most fitness machines replicate common real-world forms of exercise, from rowing to riding a bike to walking.

hold of a set of vertical poles or handles. On most cross-trainers the handles and foot supports are mechanically linked so coordination is not a problem. As the arms move back and forth the legs make an elliptical or circular pedaling-type motion. The advantage of this circular motion is that it places less stress on the knees and ankles than the older step machines. That's because your weight is being evenly distributed over the entire lower body rather than just pivoting on the knees and ankles.

Steppers

Although most machines in this category can be called steppers, the more popular name is StairMasters. That's because StairMaster became the leading manufacturer of such machines and most people nowadays refer to any stepping machine as a StairMaster.

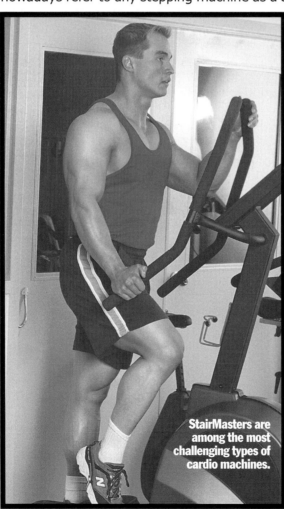

StairMasters are among the most challenging types of cardio machines.

StairMasters are among the most challenging types of cardio machines, and for anyone who doesn't have pre-existing knee or ankle problems, they are as good as it gets for indoor fitness. The problem with steppers is that the up and down stepping motion forces the knees and ankles to support virtually the entire bodyweight. If you are new to training, or have a pre-existing knee or ankle problem, we suggest you pass on the stepping machines until you strengthen up the area with other types of cardio exercise and strength training. In fact given the choices you have in cardio machines these days, you don't really ever have to use steppers.

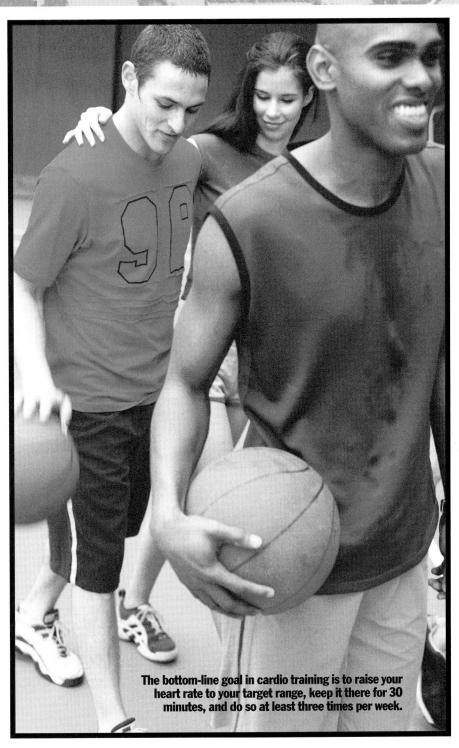

The bottom-line goal in cardio training is to raise your heart rate to your target range, keep it there for 30 minutes, and do so at least three times per week.

CHAPTER THIRTY-ONE

Weight training isn't a picnic or a walk in the park; it's sweaty, hard work that, if done correctly, has you treading the thin line between improvement and injury. If you train intensely – the only kind of training that stimulates success – you continually flirt with muscle damage. Injury is always just ahead for the careless weight trainer. Here are nine of the *most common causes of injury:*

1. Poor Exercise Technique

The most common weight training injuries are related to poor exercise technique. Incorrect technique can pull, rip or wrench a muscle, or tear delicate connective tissue quicker than you can strike a match. An out-of-control barbell or stray dumbell can cause serious damage in an instant.

Each human body has very specific biomechanical pathways. Arms and legs can only move in certain ways, particularly if you're stress-

Injuries

loading a limb with weight. Strive to become a technical perfectionist and respect the integrity of the exercise – no twisting, turning or contorting while pushing a weight. Either make the rep using perfect technique or miss the rep. Learn how to miss a rep safely; learn how to bail out.

2. Too Much Weight

Using too much weight in an exercise is a high-risk proposition loaded with injury potential. It's too heavy. If you can't control a weight as you lower it, it's too heavy. If you can't contain a

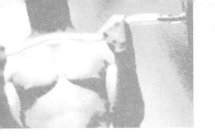

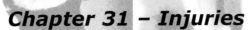

movement within its biomechanical boundaries, it's too heavy. And if you have to jerk or heave the weight in order to lift it, it's too heavy. An unchecked barbell or dumbell assumes a mind of its own; the weight obeys the laws of gravity and seeks the floor. Anything in its way (or attached to it) is in danger. Trust us, adding that extra 10 or 20 pounds to the bar just to impress the person next to you is just not worth it.

3. Poor Spotting

If you lift long enough, you'll eventually reach a point where you need to have a spotter for a number of exercises, including the squat and bench press. When you work as hard as you're supposed to, you occasionally miss a rep. Nothing is wrong with that – it's a sign that you're working to your limit, which is a good thing if you don't overdo it. Yet when you work this hard, you need competent spotters.

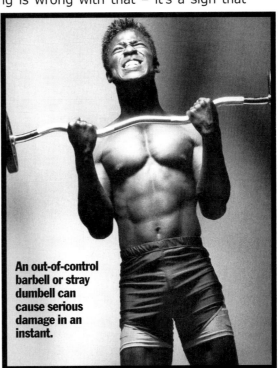

An out-of-control barbell or stray dumbell can cause serious damage in an instant.

A good spotter should conduct himself or herself at all times as though the lifter is on the verge of total failure. Your training partner can also lend a gentle touch that allows you to complete a rep you'd normally miss. A top spotter needs to be strong, sensitive and ever alert to the possibility of failure – not looking around or joking with friends. Don't ask a beginner to spot you either. Most people new to the gym are not familiar with proper spotting technique. Like most things there is a knack to it. Only ask someone you can trust. If there is any doubt, stop your set a couple of reps short of muscular failure, or use a machine or dumbells instead.

4. Incorrect Use of Advanced Techniques

Cheating and forced reps are advanced techniques that allow the lifter to train beyond normal. Taken past the point of failure, the muscle is literally *forced* to respond. When incorrectly performed, a cheating or forced rep can push or pull the lifter out of the groove. The weight collapses and a spotter must come to the rescue.

Cheating movements work. Yet cheating, by definition, is dangerous. Anytime you use momentum to artificially increase rep speed, thus allowing you to handle more poundage than when using strict techniques, you risk injury. To play it safe, use the bare minimum number of cheat reps to complete the set. On forced reps, make sure your training partner is on your wave length. Don't go crazy.

5. Overtraining

How does overtraining relate to injury? It negatively impacts the body's overall level of strength and conditioning. Overtraining saps energy, retarding progress. You can't grow when you're overtrained. It also interferes with the ability of both the muscles and the nervous system to recuperate – ATP (adenosine triphosphate, an energy compound in the cells) and glycogen stores are severely depleted when an agitated metabolic status is present. In such a depleted, weakened state, is it any wonder that injury is common, particularly if the athlete insists on handling big weights?

The solution is to cut back to three or four training sessions per week and keep session length to no more than an hour. If you are severely overtrained you might need to stop working out entirely for three or four weeks to let the body recharge.

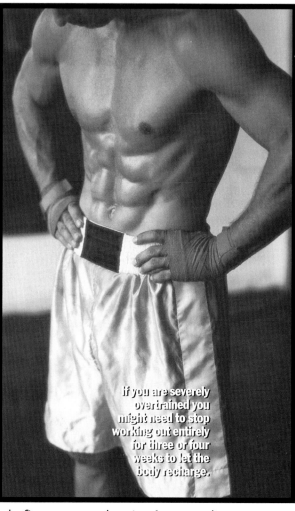

if you are severely overtrained you might need to stop working out entirely for three or four weeks to let the body recharge.

6. Not Enough Stretching

Stretching is different from warming up. Properly performed, a stretch helps relax and elongate a muscle after warmup and before and after your work sets. As a result of warming up and stretching, the muscle is warm, loose and neurologically alert – in its most pliable and injury-resistant state. In addition, stretching between sets actually helps build muscle by promoting circulation and increasing the elasticity of the fascia casing

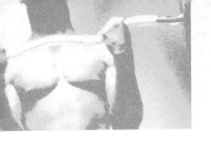
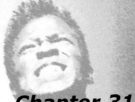

that surrounds the muscle. Finally, if you perform muscle-specific stretches at the end of your workout, you'll virtually eliminate next-day soreness.

7. Little or No Warmup

A warmup is usually a high-rep, low-intensity, quick-paced set used to increase blood flow to the muscle. This quick, light movement raises the temperature of the muscle while decreasing blood viscosity and promoting flexibility and mobility. How? Everyone knows that a warm muscle with blood coursing through it is more elastic and stretchable than a cold, stiff muscle. Recommended forms of warmup are riding a stationary bike, jogging, swimming, stair-climbing and some high-rep weight training.

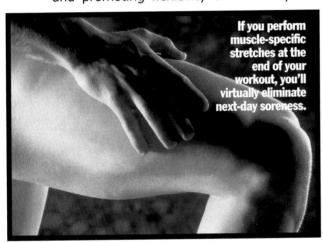

If you perform muscle-specific stretches at the end of your workout, you'll virtually eliminate next-day soreness.

Try a 5 to 10-minute formal warmup before stretching. If you choose high-rep weight training, perform 25 ultralight, quick reps in the following nonstop sequence: calf raise, squat, leg curl, crunch, pulldown, bench press and curl. Do one set each with no rest between sets. This can be accomplished in about 5 minutes and warms every major muscle in the body.

8. Poor Nutrition

Depending on who you consult, nutrition is anywhere from 50 to 90 percent of health and fitness. It makes no sense to be following a rigid training schedule and then derail everything with junk food – no matter how much cardio and strength training you perform.

9. Poor Concentration

If you're distracted, preoccupied or lackadaisical when you work out, you're inviting injury. Watch a champion bodybuilder train and one thing you'll notice is his or her intense level of concentration. This ability is developed over time. The athlete systematically develops a preset mental checklist that allows him or her to focus on the task at hand. More concentration equates to more poundage. More poundage equates to more growth. But watch out! More poundage can lead to injuries if you don't pay attention. *Train smart.*

CHAPTER THIRTY-TWO

Overtraining

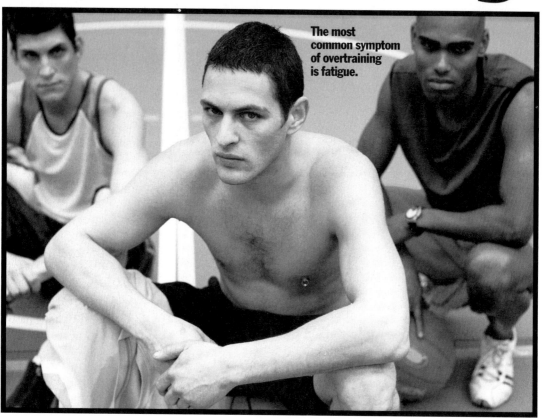

The most common symptom of overtraining is fatigue.

It is no secret among athletes that in order to improve performance you've got to work hard. However, hard training breaks you down and makes you weaker. *Rest improves your health.* Physiologic improvement in sports only occurs during the rest period following hard training. This adaptation is in response to maximal loading of the cardiovascular and muscular systems and is accomplished by improving efficiency of the heart, increasing capillaries in the muscles, and increasing glycogen stores and mitochondrial enzyme systems within the muscle cells. Basically, during recovery periods these systems build to greater levels to compensate for the stress that you have applied. The result is that you are now at a higher level of performance.

The Symptoms

If sufficient rest *is not* included in a training program, then regeneration cannot occur and the performance plateaus. If this imbalance between excess training and inadequate rest persists then performance will decline. Overtraining can best be defined as the state where the athlete has been repeatedly stressed by training to the point where rest is no longer adequate to allow for recovery. The "overtraining syndrome" is the name given to the collection of emotional, behavioral and physical symptoms due to overtraining that have persisted for weeks to months. Athletes and coaches also know it as a state of *burnout* or *staleness.* This is different from the day-to-day variation in performance and postexercise tiredness that is common among conditioned athletes. *Overtraining* is marked by *cumulative* exhaustion that persists even after recovery periods.

The most common symptom of overtraining is fatigue. This may limit workouts and may be present at rest. You may find yourself to be moody or easily irritated, have altered sleep patterns, become depressed, or lose the competitive desire and enthusiasm for the sport. You may also find you have a decreased appetite, and weight loss. Physical symptoms include persistent muscular soreness, increased frequency of viral illnesses, and increased incidence of injuries.

There have been several clinical studies done on athletes with the overtraining syndrome. Findings in these studies have shown decreased performance in exercise testing, decreased mood state, and, in some, increased cortisol levels – the body's "stress" hormone. A decrease in testosterone, altered immune status, and an increase in muscular breakdown products have also been identified.

Medically the syndrome of overtraining is classified as a neuroendocrine disorder. The normal fine balance in the interaction between the autonomic nervous system and the hormonal system is disturbed – and athletic "jet lag" results. The body now has a decreased ability to repair itself during rest. Heaping more workouts onto this unbalanced system only worsens the situation. Additional stress in the form of difficulties at school or work, or in your personal life also contributes to the problem.

The treatment for the overtraining syndrome is rest. The longer the overtraining has occurred, the more rest required. Therefore, early detection is very important. If the overtraining has only occurred for a short period of time (e.g., 3 to 4 weeks) then an interruption of training for 3 to 5 days is usually sufficient rest. After this, workouts can be resumed on an alternate day basis. The intensity of the training can be maintained but the *total volume* must be lower.

You *must* identify and correct the factors that led to your state of overtraining – that's very important. Otherwise, the overtraining syndrome is likely to *recur.* The alternate-day recovery period is continued for a few weeks and then an increase in volume is permitted. In more severe cases, the training program may have to be interrupted for many weeks, and recovery may take months. An alternate form of exercise can be substituted to help prevent the exercise withdrawal syndrome.

All of the medical studies and reports on overtraining have involved single-sport athletes. If you are involved in triathlon and other multi-sports the recovery

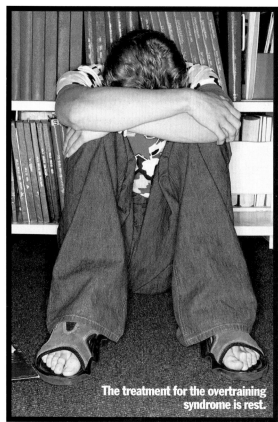

The treatment for the overtraining syndrome is rest.

process may be different depending on the circumstances. If you are sure the overtraining has occurred in only one discipline, then resting that discipline along with significant decreases in the other sports can bring about full recovery. Make sure you don't suddenly substitute more workouts in one sport in an attempt to compensate for rest in another – that's vitally important. Doing so will not heal the overtraining, but will drive you deeper into a hole. Overtraining affects both peripheral and central mechanisms in the body. Resting from overtraining on the bicycle by swimming more will help a pair of fatigued quadriceps, but to the heart, pituitary and adrenals, stress is stress.

As with almost everything else health-related, *prevention is the key.* Well-balanced gradual increases in training are recommended. A training schedule design called periodization varies the training load in cycles with built-in mandatory rest phases. During the high workload phase, you alternate between high-intensity interval work and low-intensity endurance work. This approach is used by a number of elite athletes in many sports.

Keep a training log – that's the best method to monitor progress. In addition to keeping track of distance and intensity, you can record your resting morning heart rate, weight, general health, how the workout felt, and levels of muscular soreness and fatigue. Significant progressive changes in any of these parameters may signal overtraining. Avoid monotonous training and maintain adequate nutrition – those are two more recommendations for prevention. Vigorous exercise during the incubation period of a viral illness may increase the duration and severity of that illness. If you feel you are developing a cold, try resting or reducing the training schedule for a few days.

Rest improves your health.

In conclusion, the prevailing wisdom is that it's better to be undertrained than overtrained. Rest is a vital part of your training. There is considerable evidence that reduced training (same intensity, lower volume) for up to 21 days will not decrease performance. A well-planned training program involves as much art as science and should allow for flexibility. Early warning signs of overtraining must be heeded and schedule adjustments made accordingly. Smart training is the path to faster times and good health.

Summary

Why does it happen?

Overtraining occurs when a person experiences stress and physical trauma from exercise before his or her body has had time to repair the damage caused by the last workout.

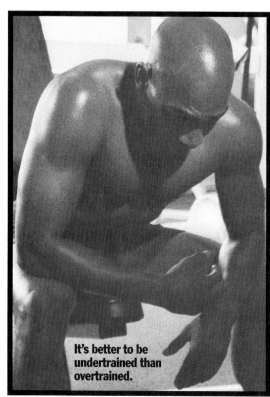

It's better to be undertrained than overtrained.

What happens?

The overtrained individual suffers from prolonged fatigue and underperformance. There is no easy test for overtraining, but the symptoms are:

Psychological:
- Fatigue
- Reduced concentration
- Apathy
- Insomnia
- Irritability
- Depression

Performance:
- Decreased performance
- Delayed recovery from training
- Intolerance to training

Physiological:
- Elevated morning resting pulse rate
- Increase in injuries
- Chronic muscle soreness
- Weight loss
- Frequent minor infections
- Appetite loss

Prevention and Treatment:
Less is More!

Recommended recovery program:
1. Five weeks of rest with low levels of exercise.
2. Correct nutrition.
3. Removing as much stress as possible.
4. Slow return to normal training levels.
5. Cross-training to avoid temptation of too much too soon.

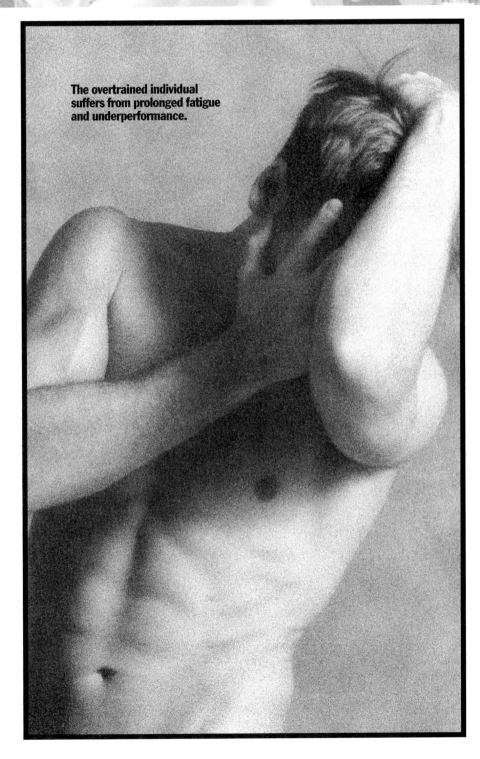

The overtrained individual suffers from prolonged fatigue and underperformance.

CHAPTER THIRTY-THREE

Getting In Shape Can Be Fun!

For those who dread going into the gym for another session of cardio or weight training, there are hundreds of outdoor sports to choose from to stimulate that system of yours. Some require expensive equipment and the right environmental conditions; other sports can be practiced for free at almost any time of the year. The following are some of the most popular sports and activities that you can try. Don't be afraid to experiment either. You may discover that a sport you initially thought was for sissies or jocks is in fact quite challenging ... and perhaps more important, *it's fun!*

Walking

Sometimes the best forms of exercise are the simplest and, perhaps more important, the cheapest. It often comes as a shock to most people that brisk walking offers almost the same degree of benefits as jogging or running without the same degree of stress on the joints. For example running places three to four times the weight of your body on each step, whereas walking produces one to one and a half times the weight of your body on each step.

For those who think walking offers little in the way of cardiovascular conditioning and calorie burning, take a look at these numbers. At a pace of 4 mph (15 minutes to do a mile), the average person burns 4 to 6 calories a minute. That works out to 240 to 360 calories per hour. At a slightly faster pace (5 mph, or 12 minutes to do a mile) the energy expenditure is 450 to 600 calories per hour. This means every six walking sessions burns off one pound (3600 calories).

The Way of the Walk

It may seem simple enough (after all, most of us have been doing it since we were one or two years old), but *walking* does have some do's and don'ts with regard to proper form – especially when you're going

Sometimes the best forms of exercise are the simplest.

at a faster than normal pace. Your posture should be erect with your abdominals tightened for good back support. Your feet should hit the ground squarely, heels first and toes lifted high. Also, to move faster don't increase your stride. Instead increase the number of steps per minute. To walk a mile in 12 minutes you will need to take approximately 160 steps. For a 15-minute mile you will need to make 135 steps a minute. Keep in mind speed burns calories.

As with sprinting, your arms should be bent at 90 degrees and your elbows tucked into your waist. A controlled arm swing does not allow your fingertips to cross the midline of your body or reach above your chest. You can close your fingers but don't clench them too tight.

As for the legs, try to step from the hips. And it's a good idea to do some light stretching *before and after* your walk to increase muscle flexibility and blood supply.

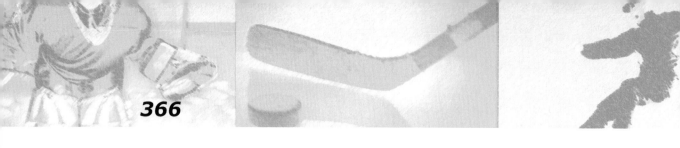

Get in the Habit

Psychologists tell us it takes about 3 weeks to form a habit, so don't let the first week throw you off. Make a commitment to walk three to five times a week for the next 3 weeks. Just three times per week is enough to maintain cardiovascular conditioning. For those relying on walking to improve their cardiovascular health, five or six times per week is recommended.

Get in the habit of walking. It's easy, it's fun, and it can be done just about anywhere, anytime. Try it and see!

Jumping Rope

Looking for a cheap and fun way to add variety to your conditioning? Try regressing a few years to your childhood. Remember how the girls couldn't wait for recess to get outside and jump rope with their friends? Well they were doing more than just having fun. They were engaging in one of the simplest yet most effective forms of physical activity, and it's not just for girls.

Jumping rope is practiced by everyone from playground kids to world-class boxers. If you want to see poetry in motion, take a look at some of Muhammad Ali's old tapes. The nice thing about skipping is that it costs only about $10. That investment, plus a good pair of shoes, is about all a person needs to start jumping rope. Fitness experts say that sessions of skipping can improve heart rate, breathing, endurance, upper and lower body strength, and coordination. That's something to keep in mind when someone starts bragging about the latest $5000 piece of equipment at his gym!

Learning the Basics

There are many different lengths of rope. To measure the right length for you, grab the handles, step on the middle of the rope with one foot, and bring both hands up to the chest. Your handles should reach just below chest high. Two of the most popular ropes are the colorful beaded ones and fast-speed leather ropes. Either one will do. When starting to jump, be sure to have enough room around you – and that includes ceiling space as well. Stay clear of hanging lights and fans!

Jumping Do's and Don'ts

• Wear aerobic or cross-training shoes at all times. Don't try to jump barefoot.

• Stay on the toes and balls of your feet when jumping. Your heels should barely touch, if at all. A wooden or matted floor is easier and preferred rather than carpet.

• Stand tall with abdominals tight, not hunched, with your knees slightly bent when landing. Use your calves as your shock-absorbers.

• Keep shoulders relaxed with elbows close to your sides.

• Always turn the rope from your wrists, without using your full arm.

• Don't try to jump too high. Keep the impact lower for your knees and ankles. Great jumpers need only about an inch of space off the ground.

• Don't look at your feet! Look straight ahead and concentrate on an even rhythm in your breathing.

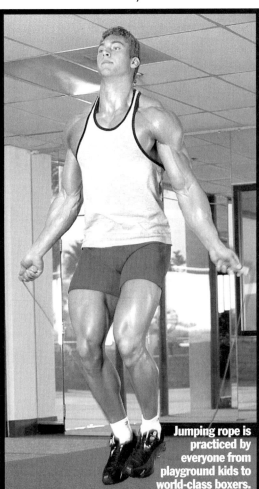

Jumping rope is practiced by everyone from playground kids to world-class boxers.

Practice Makes Progress!

If it's been a while since the last time you jumped rope, don't worry. You will be the one to see the most progress the quickest. There are two skills that just keep getting better and better when jumping rope: *cardiovascular endurance* and *coordination.* You may be starting at the very beginning with both or maybe you already feel inept at one. A great program to help you see your results in both is to keep a journal and mark your progress.

Endurance – Whether you are naturally trained for anaerobic or aerobic conditioning, jumping rope will help your heart pump more efficiently regardless. It doesn't matter how much time you have. Just start jumping. Put a clock in front of you with a second hand on it. Start with ten seconds at a time with a 10 second rest. Then move to 20 seconds with a 20-second rest ... and so on! You'll be jumping for minutes sooner than you think!

Coordination – Once you have mastered jumping for approximately 20 seconds at a time with a two-foot landing, it's time to move on to some more challenging moves. The reason is twofold: you want to keep challenging yourself physically with coordination tests and challenge yourself mentally due to the great boredom factor.

Try these variations:
• Two-foot landing with double hop between jumps
• Two-foot landing with single hop between jumps
• Single-foot landing: 8 each side, 4 each side,
  2 each side, single each side
• Jog knees up high
• Jog with hamstring curl
• Scissor legs on landing (front and back with switch)
• Jumping jack legs on landing (out and in)
• Jumping *backwards*
• Double jump (two spins of the rope with one hop)
• Crossovers (cross arms and jump and uncross over head)
• Swing rope side to side and jump in between
• Boxer's shuffle fast and slow

You may incorporate a skipping workout routine in with your weightlifting or other cardiovascular exercises. Jump to the beat of music and slowly speed it up. It's a great way to challenge yourself even more.

Skipping is simple, easy and fun. If you keep your jump rope by your bed and you are forced to trip over it or at least look at it every morning when you wake up, and every night before you retire, it may remind you to pick it up – even for as little as five minutes at a time.

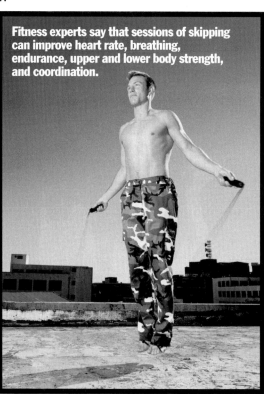

Fitness experts say that sessions of skipping can improve heart rate, breathing, endurance, upper and lower body strength, and coordination.

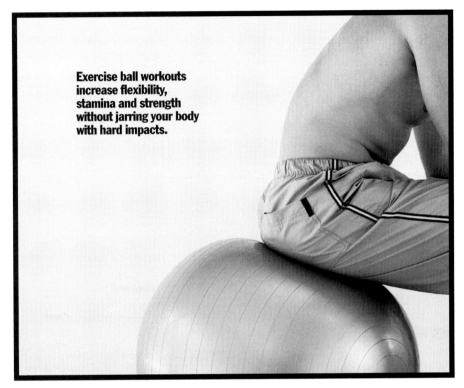

Exercise ball workouts increase flexibility, stamina and strength without jarring your body with hard impacts.

On the Ball with the Swiss

Every week a quick scan of the home shopping network reveals some new gizmo that supposedly is the greatest invention since sliced bread. You know the commercials, ... "just ten minutes three times a week for the midsection you've always dreamed about." Most of these crazy contraptions end up becoming nothing more than fancy clothes hangers. (One lady told the authors she put a blanket over hers and made it into an indoor doghouse!) Every now and then, however, one of these inventions actually stands the test of time. Case in point is the stability ball, or Swiss ball.

Swiss balls are large, inflated, rubber and vinyl balls used by physical therapists to enhance the neurodevelopment of their patients. More recently the Swiss ball has been introduced as a strength-training aid to athletes. Training in an unstable environment is said to strengthen stabilizer muscles, reduce chance of injury due to repetitive stress, and improve functioning of the nervous system, which leads to functional strength gains. The shape of the ball also facilitates multi-angle training and allows greater range of motion on some exercises; both potentially important factors in properly training certain muscle groups. Exercise ball workouts increase flexibility, stamina and strength without jarring your body with hard impacts.

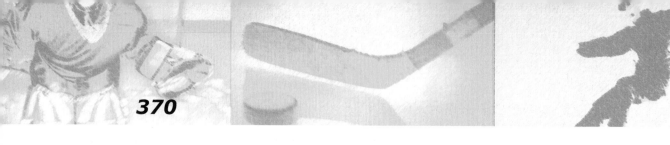

We recommend you use Swiss balls with an anti-burst system. Only these balls will guarantee the safety that is needed while exercising or sitting. These products have the highest quality and safety standards in the world. Due to new technology, these balls have extremely high weight limitations – most importantly they will not explode if punctured. When a sharp object penetrates the skin of the ball the air will escape *slowly* – which eliminates the risk of injuries.

Although you can use just about any size ball, the following chart makes recommendations based on height. Choose a ball that fits your body dimensions – that will make the exercises more effective.

How to determine the correct ball size:

BODY HEIGHT	SIZE	MAXIMUM INFLATION
up to 4'10" (up to 145 cm)	Small	18" (45 cm)
4'10" to 5'5" (145-165 cm)	Medium	22" (55 cm)
5'5" to 6'0" (165-185 cm)	Large	26" (65 cm)
6'0" to 6'5" (185-195 cm)	X-Large	30" (75 cm)
over 6'5" (over 195 cm)	XX-Large	33" (85 cm)

One of the biggest advantages of the Swiss ball over some of those other crazy TV contraptions is *cost*. An average Swiss ball costs $50 to $75. Compare that to "four easy payments of $99" for one of those useless home contraptions. There's also *versatility* to consider. For less than $100 you are getting a piece of equipment that can be used to train just about the entire body. Even the $3000 jobs in commercial gyms can't make that claim.

Another advantage to Swiss balls is their *convenience.* You can store them just about anywhere (although we'll admit storing the larger-sized balls will take some creative planning).

Finally, and laugh if you may, a Swiss ball makes a great conversation piece. Just think of all the creative and humorous comments your friends and relatives will make when they first lay eyes on your "big blue ball." Censors prevent us from repeating some of them here but we think you get the picture.

The Exercises

The following exercises for most of the major muscles in the body will get you started. As time goes on you can learn and add others. In fact there are videos available (they often come free with the ball) that will take you through dozens of exercises.

Wall squats – Stand with your back to a wall or vertical support. The ball should be pressed between your lower back and the wall. Walk your feet one or two steps out from your body and position them shoulder width apart. Slowly lower your body to a squat position as the ball rolls up your back. Pause when your thighs are parallel with the floor. Return to the starting position.

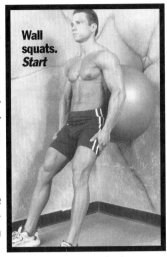

Wall squats. Start

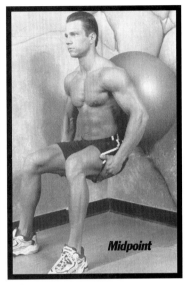

Midpoint

Muscle worked – quadriceps, hamstrings and glutes.

Hamstring curls – Lie on your back with your legs and feet on top of the ball. The closer the feet are together the harder the exercise will be. Lift your hips off the floor and roll the ball in toward your glutes. Roll the ball back to the starting position and lower your hips.
Muscles worked – hamstrings, glutes.

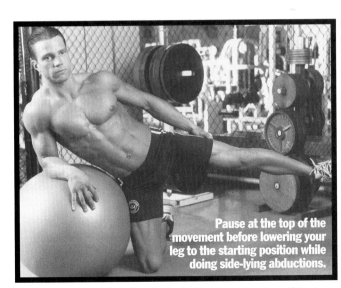

Pause at the top of the movement before lowering your leg to the starting position while doing side-lying abductions.

Side-lying abduction – Kneel on the floor or ground and place the ball at your side. Lean into the ball and extend your top leg to the side for balance. Keep your bottom leg bent for support. Firmly press your hip into the ball and maintain neutral posture. Try not to let your top hip roll forward or backward. Place your hand on the front of the ball for support. Slowly abduct the top leg until it is approximately parallel to the floor. Pause at the top of the movement before lowering your leg to the starting position.
Muscle worked – hip abductors.

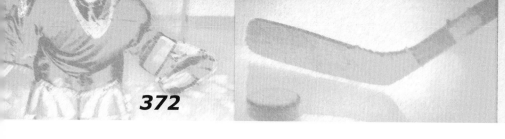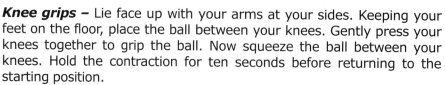

Knee grips – Lie face up with your arms at your sides. Keeping your feet on the floor, place the ball between your knees. Gently press your knees together to grip the ball. Now squeeze the ball between your knees. Hold the contraction for ten seconds before returning to the starting position.
Muscle worked – hip adductors.

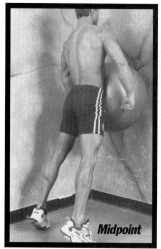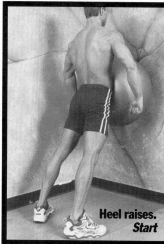

Midpoint

Heel raises.
Start

Heel raises – Stand with the ball pressed between your chest and a wall or vertical support. Walk your feet back one or two steps and lean into the ball. Place your hands by your sides. Keeping your weight balanced across the balls of your feet, lift your heels as high as possible. Lower to a starting position.
Muscles worked – gastrocnemius, soleus.

Abdominal curls – Sit on top of the ball. Keeping your feet about shoulder width apart, walk your feet away from the ball as it rolls up your back. Continue until your lower and middle back are fully supported by the ball. Place your fists at your temples (if your neck fatigues, place one or both hands behind your head for support). Slowly curl your trunk, lifting your shoulders and upper back off the ball. Return to the starting position.
Muscle worked – rectus abdominus, internal and external obliques.

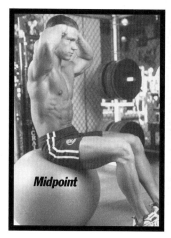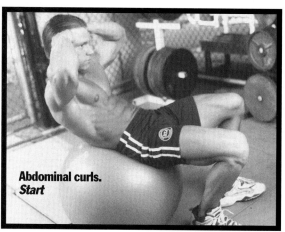

Midpoint

**Abdominal curls.
Start**

Trunk flexion – Kneel on the floor with the ball in front of your body. Place your hands on the ball and lower your body over the ball until your trunk is supported. Keeping your feet and knees on the floor, your head in line with your spine, and your hands to the sides of the ball, use the muscles in your lower back to lift your chest slightly off the ball. Return to the starting position.
Muscles worked – spinal erectors.

Pushups – Kneel with the ball in front of your thighs. Place your hands on each side of the ball and lower your torso until it's supported by the ball. Walk your hands forward on the floor as the ball rolls down your body. Stop when the ball is centered under your hips. Rest your toes on the floor, or to add intensity, lift your feet off the floor. Place your wrists under your shoulders. Maintain neutral posture and lower your chest to the floor. Pause at the bottom of the movement and return to the starting position.
Muscles worked – pectorals, anterior deltoid, triceps and serratus anterior.

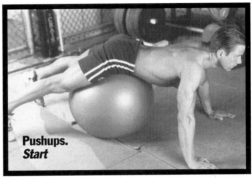

Pushups. Start

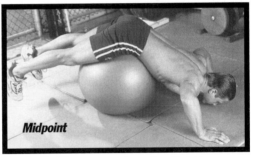

Midpoint

Seated triceps dips – Sit on top of the ball. Place your hands slightly behind and to the sides of your hips, fingers pointing down. Walk your feet two steps forward, allowing your hips to rest on the edge of the ball. Press your hands into the ball. At the same time, bend your elbows and lower your hips into the ball. Return to the starting position by extending the elbows.
Muscles worked – triceps, anterior deltoids, pectorals, lower trapezius.

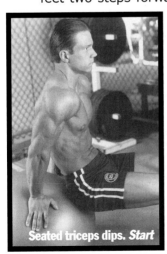

Seated triceps dips. Start

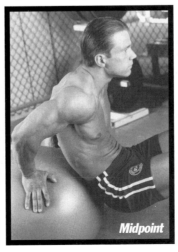

Midpoint

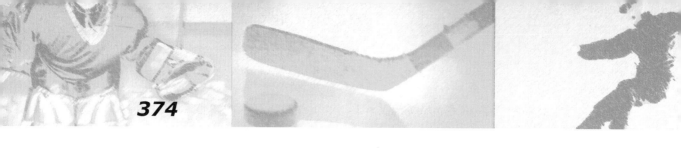

Snowboarding

It's been called *surfing on snow,* and it's one of the fastest rising of all winter sports. Instead of two long skis, you use a single wider *snowboard.* And like the California surfer, you don't get any help from ski poles for support. No, it's all balance. For those who think it's just a matter of standing on a board and "sliding" down the mountain, think again. It takes great skill, coordination and strength to remain upright on a snowboard. The downside is that you'll need to put in a fair amount of practice to get the hang of it. The upside, however, is that snowboarding strengthens and tones virtually the entire body. It also gives the cardiovascular system a great workout as well. Oh, and did we say – it's fun too! Here are a few tips to get you started in your snowboarding career.

What do I need to know before I start snowboarding?

Here are some tips from members of the US Snowboard Team, as well as from recreational snowboarders:

• *Get in shape first.* A regular general fitness program will make snowboarding easier and help protect you from injury.

• *Use the right equipment.* Buy or rent good snowboarding boots, an all-purpose snowboard, a helmet and wrist guards.

• *Pick the right time and place to learn.* Learn from a trained instructor in good weather (when there is good visibility and it's not too cold). Pick a skiing area that allows snowboarders. Use slopes that are not crowded and that have packed snow. Avoid icy slopes.

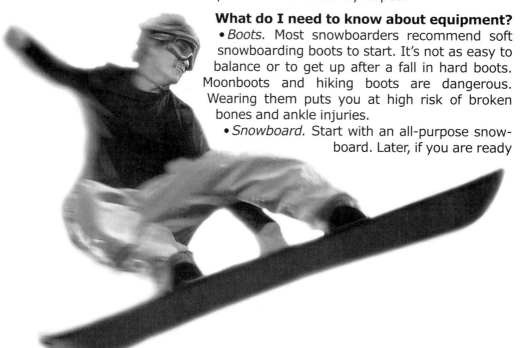

What do I need to know about equipment?

• *Boots.* Most snowboarders recommend soft snowboarding boots to start. It's not as easy to balance or to get up after a fall in hard boots. Moonboots and hiking boots are dangerous. Wearing them puts you at high risk of broken bones and ankle injuries.

• *Snowboard.* Start with an all-purpose snow-board. Later, if you are ready to race or do tricks, you can try a specialty board. Specialty boards are harder to turn and balance on.

• *Protective equipment.* Always wear wrist guards made for snowboarders or in-line skaters. Most racers and professional snowboarders wear helmets, wrist guards, arm guards and shin guards, as well as customized protective gear.

• *Ski poles.* You may want to use ski poles at first while you learn how to snowboard. Some teachers believe this is a good way for beginners to avoid wrist injuries. Learn how to use ski poles from a teacher who knows this technique, because snowboards are not actually designed to be used with ski poles.

How can I protect myself from injury?

Most falls in snowboarding are on the hands, buttocks and head, and only cause bruises and soreness. You can take a few precautions to reduce your chances of getting injured:

• *Protect your wrists.* Most snow-board injuries are to the wrists.

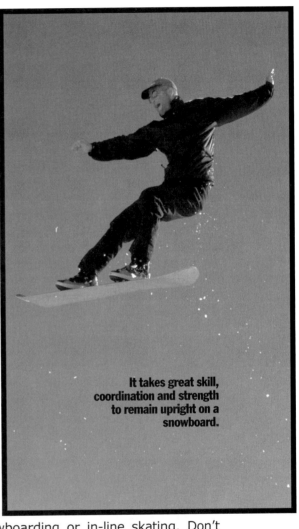

It takes great skill, coordination and strength to remain upright on a snowboard.

Wear wrist guards made for snowboarding or in-line skating. Don't break your fall with your open hands. Hold your hands in *closed fists* while you snowboard so you won't be tempted to break your fall with an open hand. Try to roll into a fall like a paratrooper would, spreading the force of the fall out over your body instead of taking all the force in one place.

• *Protect your head.* While you probably won't hit your head first, the back of your head may hit the ground at the end of a fall if you land on your buttocks. These head injuries usually aren't serious, but you can end up with quite a headache. Wear a helmet when learning, when racing, and when snowboarding on unmarked trails (collisions with trees cause some of the most serious injuries in this sport).

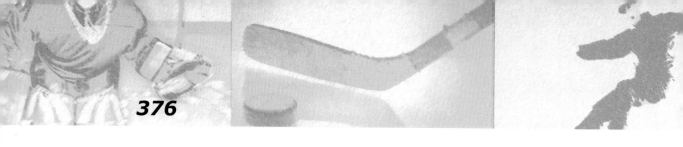

The Drills

The following drills are presented by Samantha Stenning, a highly sought after snowboarding instructor at Blackcomb Resort in Whistler, British Columbia, Canada.

Rocking but not rolling – According to Samantha, a balanced stance is the most important thing you need to learn in your snowboarding career, whether simple side-slipping or hanging big air. Your focus on day one is to learn how to balance your weight on a fast-moving object. Samantha suggests standing on the board on flat ground and rocking from toe to heel. The weight shift will illustrate how to keep your body centered on the board. Lean too far forward and you fall on your knees. Lean to far back and your butt kisses the ground. Try to keep your body aligned with the length of the board.

Heel-side stop – Once you've mastered the rocking technique it's time to hit the slopes. Stand with your torso facing downhill and the tip of the board at a slight downward angle. With even pressure kept on both feet, start moving down the hill with the slope on your heel edge. When you want to stop increase the pressure on your heel.

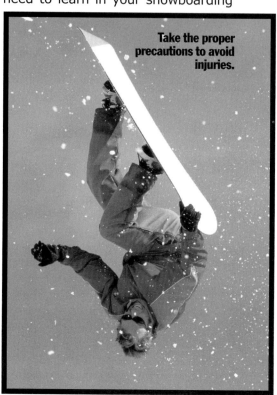

Take the proper precautions to avoid injuries.

Heel-side go – Samantha uses a car analogy to illustrate the physics of moving and stopping a snowboard. She compares the upper body to the car's steering wheel and the lower body to the gas pedal. By looking and pointing in a given direction you will automatically go in that direction. By the same argument the amount of pressure you apply to the corresponding foot will control your momentum. Try this drill. Position the board at a slight downward angle. Look toward your right and point your right hand in the same direction. Slowly apply pressure to you right heel and you will glide toward the right on your heel edge. To stop, apply pressure on both heels simultaneously. Repeat the drill with your left hand and head facing left. Put pressure on your left heel and ride to your left.

Toe-side stop – Start by standing on the board with your body facing up the mountain. Keeping even pressure on both feet, lift your heel edge and sideslip down the slope on your toes. It might be scary to slide backward down the mountain, but don't panic. Take your time and resist the temptation to bend forward at the waist. That would only send you to your knees. Apply pressure to both toes when you are ready to stop.

Toe-side go – Start with your torso facing up a gradual incline. Now turn your head to face the right and point your right hand toward the right end of the board. Slowly apply pressure to your right toe, and glide toward the right on your toe edge. Stop by increasing the pressure on both toes simultaneously. Repeat with your left hand and head pointing to the left end of the board. Apply pressure to your left toe and ride to your left on your left toe edge.

Turning – According to Samantha the key to an effective turn is to push on your front foot. This is what actually propels the turn. If you lean back on your heel, the nose of the board will come up and you will almost certainly lose control.

Before you can start practicing turning you need to determine your lead foot. For most people it's the one they would kick a soccer ball with. It's also the one that usually moves forward first to stop you from falling when pushed from behind.

With your dominant foot identified, it's time to start turning. Most beginners find it easier to turn from their toe side to their heels. Begin with a *toe-side go.* If you are regular-footed, point your arms toward the left, increasing pressure over your left toes as you glide in that direction. Now for the fun part. While still in motion, gradually decrease the pressure over your toes as you shift your hips. Simultaneously point your arms toward the right as you shift your weight to your heel edge. Let the board turn itself as you complete the transition. Once you've started, commit to the turn. If you don't follow through you may find yourself careening out of control down the mountain. The goal at this point is to ride across it.

Isolated turn, heel to toe – As with the toe-to-heel transition, a heel-to-toe turn calls for a gradual shift in weight from one edge to the other. Once again the adjustment should originate in your hips. Relax and keep your knees bent and your body aligned with the board. Don't flap your arms or double over.

> *Snowboarding strengthens and tones virtually the entire body.*

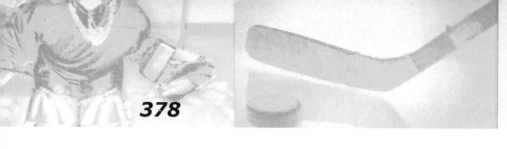

Linking your turns – Once you can perform each type of turn in isolation (and comfort!) it's no leap of faith to start linking them together. Well done and congratulations, you're a snowboarder! Samantha adds one final word of caution "Increased speed will come naturally with improvement. But there are tons of speed freaks out there whose style is as sloppy as they are fast. Take your time and you'll live to be a good rider."

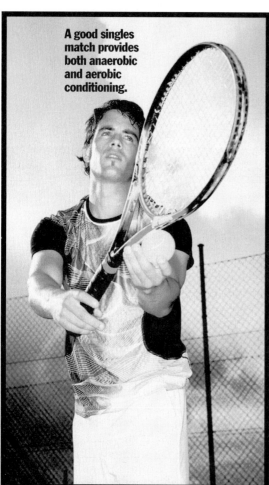

A good singles match provides both anaerobic and aerobic conditioning.

Tennis

Tennis is a superb sport. It requires excellent hand-eye coordination, good agility, and keen spatial awareness. In addition to the physical and mental challenge, a good singles match provides both anaerobic and aerobic conditioning. Although skill is essential for top-level tennis, technique development is easier if you are fit – which is also the critical factor for staying power during the second and third sets.

Fitness comes in many forms, and conditioning is specific to the training program. For example, joint flexibility is enhanced through stretching exercises, cardiovascular endurance is improved through aerobic activity, and muscular strength is increased through resistance training. Certainly, all of these fitness components may contribute to better tennis performance. If you were to focus on one area of physical conditioning for tennis, however, it should undoubtedly be strength exercise.

Basic Strength Exercises

Tennis play involves a lot of musculoskeletal activity, including all kinds of movements in the legs, midsection, upper body, and arms. You should therefore train all of the major muscle groups. This ensures overall strength and balanced muscle development to enhance performance power and reduce the risk of injuries. Here are a few suggestions:

Legs – Let's begin with the powerful leg muscles that generate the force for your ground strokes, as well as your movements across the court. Instead of training the quadriceps and hamstrings separately, replace the leg extension and leg curl with the leg press – it works both of these muscle groups and the gluteals simultaneously. The leg press permits heavier weight loads, and is the best exercise for developing functional leg strength. In addition to the quadriceps and hamstrings, the hip adductors and abductors play a major role in your weight shifts and lateral movements. These opposing muscle groups on the inner and outer thighs are best trained with the hip adductor and hip abductor machines, which should be added to your strength exercise program.

Due to the stop-and-go movements in tennis that require almost continuous force production and shock absorption in the lower leg muscles, it is prudent to perform some calf strengthening exercises. The calf machine or standing calf raises are highly effective for targeting the gastrocnemius and soleus muscles of the lower leg, and serve as an excellent supplement to the upper-leg exercises.

Midsection – The power generated by the large leg muscles is transferred to the upper body through the muscles of the midsection.

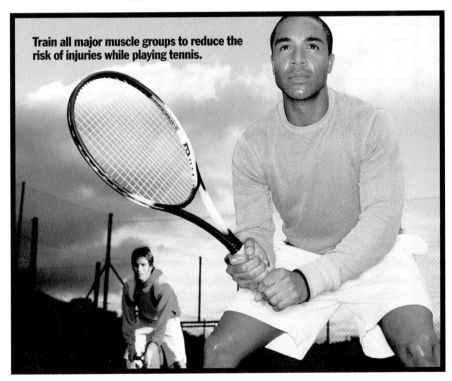

Train all major muscle groups to reduce the risk of injuries while playing tennis.

Swinging movements (ground strokes and serves) involve the internal and external oblique muscles on both sides of the midsection. These important muscles may be effectively strengthened on the dual-action rotary torso machine, which works the right internal and left external obliques on clockwise movements, and the left internal and right external obliques on counter-clockwise movements. Add the rotary torso exercise to the low back and abdominal machines for comprehensive midsection conditioning.

Upper body – The major upper body muscles involved in swinging a tennis racket are the pectoralis major, latissimus dorsi, and deltoids of the torso, and the biceps and triceps of the arms. While the basic strength-training program addresses these muscles individually, it may be advantageous to work some of the groups together. This is best accomplished by doing pushing and pulling exercises such as bench presses, seated rows, overhead presses and pulldowns.

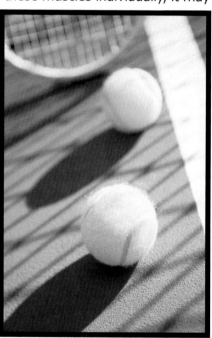

The bench press is a popular pushing exercise that strengthens the pectoralis major and triceps muscle at the same time. Conversely, the seated row is an effective pulling exercise that works the opposing latissimus dorsi and biceps muscles simultaneously. One of the best means for training the shoulder and triceps muscles together is the overhead press. The counterpart to this exercise is the pulldown that involves both the latissimus dorsi and the biceps muscles.

Replace the chest cross, pullover, lateral raise, biceps curl and triceps extension exercises with the bench press, seated row, overhead press and pulldown exercises. These provide a more comprehensive upper body workout that may have more practical benefit in terms of power production.

While both the basic and advanced strength-training programs should provide excellent tennis conditioning and reasonable injury protection, you should take one more step to address particularly vulnerable muscle groups that experience significant stress during tennis play.

Shoulder rotator muscles – The first of these smaller and frequently injured muscle groups is the rotator cuff complex that surrounds and stabilizes the shoulder joint. The shoulder rotator muscles lie beneath the large deltoid muscles, and enable us to turn our arms in various positions. Rotating the arm backward, called external rotation, uses the teres minor and infraspinatus muscles. Rotating the arm forward, called internal rotation, involves the subscapularis muscles. Keeping the arm within the shoulder joint structure is the primary function of the supraspinatus muscle. Together, the muscles of the rotator cuff surround the shoulder joint, providing both structural stability and the ability to produce forehand, backhand, and sewing movements.

Here's the good news: These four relatively small muscle groups respond very well to proper strength training. The bad news is, most people do not perform any specific exercises for their rotator cuff. This is unfortunate, because rotator cuff injuries occur frequently in tennis players and typically require a long recovery period.

Although the standard strength exercises offer some conditioning benefit, you should definitely do at least one workout per week for the shoulder rotator muscles. The best means for specifically training the rotator cuff muscles is the rotary shoulder machine, a dual-action exercise that provides full-range rotational resistance for both the external and internal shoulder rotator muscles.

If this machine is not available, you may also strengthen these important muscles with resistance bands. Simply attach the band to a door at waist level, stand with your left side toward the door, keep your left elbow against your left side, and pull the band across your midsection using your left hand. This works your left internal shoulder rotator muscles. Next, keep your right elbow against your right side and pull the band away from your midsection using your right hand. This works your right external shoulder rotator muscles. Repeat these two exercises standing with your right side toward the door and using the opposite hands.

Tennis requires excellent hand-eye coordination, good agility, and keen spatial awareness.

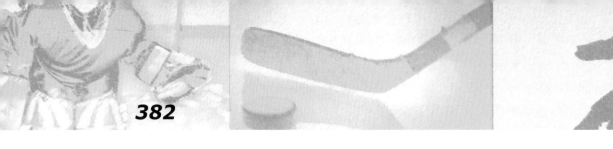

***Forearm Muscles* –** Due to the extensive wrist action required in tennis play, the forearm muscles can be easily overstressed, leading to injury at the elbow or wrist joints. The forearm machine provides five separate wrist movements to effectively condition all of the forearm muscles. Few exercises are better suited to tennis players, especially for increasing grip strength and reducing injury potential.

If you don't have access to this training device, an excellent alternative exercise is the wrist roller. Simply attach one end of a 2-foot rope to a 5-pound weight plate and tie the other end to a round wooden dowel. Holding the dowel in both hands, alternately turn your wrists clockwise to wind the rope around the dowel and lift the weight. This action addresses your forearm flexor muscles. When the weight touches the dowel, alternately turn your wrists counter-clockwise to unwind the rope and lower the weight. This action works your forearm extensor muscles.

Training your forearms will help increase your grip strength as well as reduce injury potential.

Program Design

If you play tennis three or four days per week, then it is probably best to do your strength training on two or three non-tennis days. That routine will permit plenty of recovery time after each activity. If you practice tennis every day, your strength training should probably be performed about four hours after your tennis training for best overall results. For example, if you play tennis every morning from 9 to 11, you may schedule your strength exercise around 3 p.m. Two or three equally spaced strength-training days per week are recommended for most practical purposes.

Remember that skill training is the most important factor in improving your tennis game. However, physical conditioning can certainly enhance your tennis playing efforts and outcomes. The cornerstone of physical conditioning is muscular strength, and a stronger tennis player will always be a better tennis player.

Baseball

Spring may herald the return of baseball/softball action for many little league, high school and recreational athletes. But the smart player begins his or her preparations for spring with an off-season workout program. All players can benefit from a training program that strengthens their throwing arm, increases their bat speed, and makes them faster base runners and fielders. More advanced athletes can ideally benefit from a "specificity" program tailored to their position.

An off-season strength and conditioning program can easily be set up for younger players utilizing dumbells. The basic exercises and suggested sets and reps outlined below are intended as general guidelines for the teenage athlete.

The primary "baseball muscles" **–** The force of the hips and legs, necessary in baseball for hitting and throwing, is transferred through the body to the arms and hands. If the torso is weak, energy transference is affected. A weight training regimen for younger athletes should include exercises that strengthen the torso, including the midsection, as well as the arms and legs.

Two exercises for the quadriceps are dumbell squats and lunges (with or without added weight). Dumbell squats reduce the chance of injury to the lower back and combined with lunges, strengthen hip and leg thrust. Bent-over one-arm dumbell rows and stiff-leg dumbell deadlifts strengthen the back, thereby helping energy transference. A side benefit from these exercises occurs for catchers, who need strong back muscles to hold their defensive position for long periods of time.

The chest area can be strengthened by performing dumbell presses on an incline bench. This exercise allows shoulder joints to rotate internally and greater freedom of movement as well. The shoulder muscles can be trained with the dumbell lateral raise movement. This exercise is very safe, while still effectively working all three areas of the shoulder muscles. Strong chest and shoulder areas provide the upper-body strength needed for speed, agility and hitting power.

Arm-training can be accomplished with two exercises. For the biceps we recommend incline dumbell curls, which allow a full range of motion without straining the wrists and elbows. The triceps can be worked with the dumbell kickback, another safe and effective

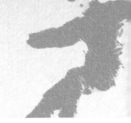
movement. The arms will also benefit from some of the specificity training we will outline later in the article.

The abdominals should not be neglected when training for baseball/softball. They are a key part of the energy transference from the lower body up through the torso, to the arms and hands. The abs can be trained with two exercises – crunches and reverse trunk twists. The crunch, done with the knees up, reduces the chance of straining the lower back, yet effectively strengthens the abdominal area.

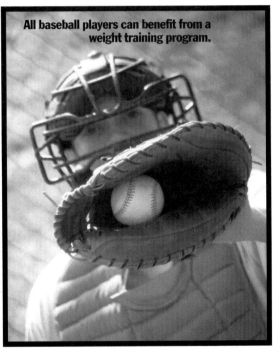

All baseball players can benefit from a weight training program.

The reverse trunk twist, although a little tougher to master, works not only the abdomen but the oblique areas of the midsection as well. These muscles are responsible for the rotation of the torso, which is used in the swinging of the bat and the overhand throwing motion. Initially this exercise should be performed with bent knees while lying on the back with the arms extended and thighs vertical. Slowly lower the knees, first to one side, then the other, while keeping the thighs perpendicular to the torso. The full general strength-training program for baseball/softball players is as follows:

Muscles and exercise:
Legs – dumbell squats and lunges
Back – one-arm dumbell rows, stiff-leg dumbell deadlifts
Chest – incline dumbell bench presses
Shoulders – dumbell lateral raises
Biceps – incline dumbell curls
Triceps – dumbell kickbacks
Abdominals – crunches (knees up), reverse trunk twists (knees up)

The general strengthening program for baseball/softball athletes can be supplemented by one or more specific programs. For a player trying to improve his or her batting speed and power, we'd suggest using one or more of the following exercises.

Practicing the swing of the bat is best simulated by the action of the cable pulley. With the cable angle set according to individual height, duplicate the swing of the bat. Simulate your actual swing as closely as possible using a sensible amount of weight. This movement has been shown to improve both bat speed for greater power and control for better accuracy.

For the wrist strength and grip needed to swing the bat effectively, there are several exercises. Wrist curls and its opposite movement, wrist extensions, both performed with dumbells, help develop forearm, wrist and hand strength. Squeezing hand rings, rubber balls or assorted grippers can also develop hand strength. A batting specificity program would look like this:

Sample Batting Specificity Program

Muscles and exercise:
Forearms – wrist curls (with dumbell), wrist extensions (with dumbell)
Hand/grip – squeeze hand rings/rubber ball, etc.
Torso/energy transference – simulated swing with cable pulley

A specificity program to improve the throwing motion can be useful to not only pitchers but all players. Studies have shown that both the velocity and accuracy of throws can be improved by such training. Exercises in this type of program include one or more of the following. Wrist curls and wrist extensions like those performed for the batting specific training, help forearm, wrist and hand strength.

We suggest seated dumbell pullovers (behind the neck) to strengthen the triceps. Extra effort should be taken to concentrate isolating the triceps, while performing this movement. Either an EZ-curl

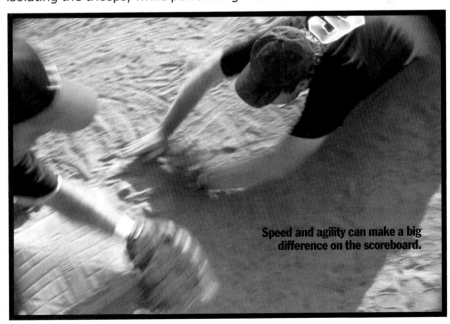

Speed and agility can make a big difference on the scoreboard.

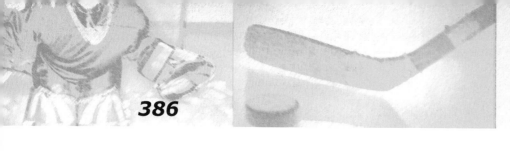

bar or a single dumbell may be used. Duplication of the actual throwing motion can be simulated with the cable pulley in much the same manner as the batting swing. Studies have shown that this simulation of the throwing motion also has an injury preventing effect. For softball pitchers, who deliver the ball underhanded, the throw should be simulated in that manner. A throwing specificity program would look like this:

Sample Throwing Specificity Program
Muscles and exercise:
Forearms – wrist curls (dumbell), wrist extensions (dumbell)
Triceps – overhead triceps extensions
Torso/arms – simulated throw with cable pulley
(overhand or underhand)

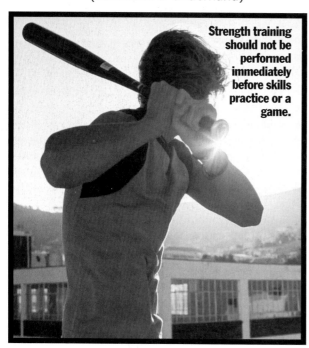

Strength training should not be performed immediately before skills practice or a game.

The sport-specificity workouts can be added to the general program and/or in place of the regular arm exercises. Frequency of course, depends on the time of the year and the direction of the coach/trainer. Usually twice weekly during the off-season and pre-season, reduced to once a week during the actual season is what we recommend.

Note: Strength training should not be performed immediately before skills practice or a game. Recent studies have cast doubt on the traditional on deck warmup activities of swinging several bats or a "bat donut." The studies have shown these motions to have a negative effect on the timing of the swing.

Hockey
Although it's a part of Canadian culture, and has been for most of the 20th century, hockey only took off in the US in the late 1980s. And even though others contributed, it was *Wayne Gretzky* who helped bring the NHL (National Hockey League) up to the level of other sports federations. Besides shattering most hockey records, Wayne was articulate and the perfect ambassador for the sport.

Hockey is one of the most demanding of all athletic pursuits, that's why professional hockey teams employ athletic trainers to get and keep their charges in shape. An injured or out of shape player doesn't serve the team that well. Here's a brief description of the three primary components of fitness, and the role they play for the hockey player.

Flexibility

Flexibility is important in any exercise program. It is especially important in ice hockey where the players use many different muscles to help them speed up, slow down, skate backwards, and change direction rapidly. A hockey player should get a good warmup before a game or practice. This warmup should include stretches that will loosen up the player's muscles. A well-planned stretching routine helps a player get his muscles ready for action – and it will decrease the risk of injury. Also, stretching increases the player's range of motion, which enables him to react to game situations quicker. In *Complete Conditioning for Ice Hockey*, Peter Twist recommends the following:

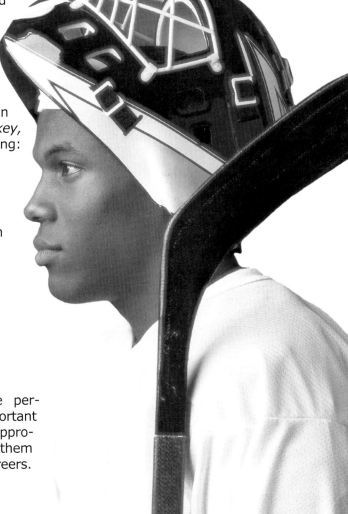

Flexibility exercises:
• T-stretch
• Wall stretch
• Arm across back stretch
• Triceps pulled across chest stretch
• Lateral seated trunk stretch
• Lying knee to chest stretch
• Lying gluteal stretch
• Seated hamstring stretch
• Groin stretch
• Snatch squats
• Kneeling lower-body stretch
• High leg swings
• Twists

All these stretches can be performed on and off the ice. It is important for hockey players to have an appropriate flexibility program to help them be successful and extend their careers.

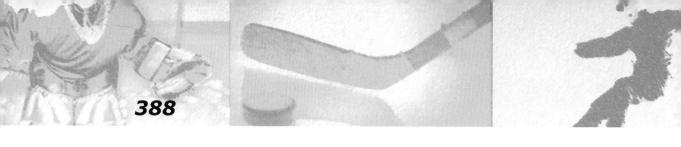

On-Ice and Off-Ice Weight-Training Exercises

Hockey players go through long and challenging seasons that require them to be in outstanding shape. The way the players accomplish their schedule of playing day in and day out is through strong on- and off-ice strengthening programs. On the ice the players must be able to give 100 percent on every shift. To achieve that goal, they must work hard not only on the ice, but also off the ice.

A good off-ice training program gives the players the base they need to go out and perform on the ice. The on-ice program helps sharpen their skills while making them stronger. Here are some basic exercises to improve your strength and power while playing this demanding sport.

Exercises to improve your strength and power:
- Power cleans
- Good mornings
- Crunches
- Lower-ab push-presses
- Lat pulldowns
- Seated rows
- Bench presses
- Dumbell flyes
- Push presses
- Upright rows
- Dips
- Standing barbell curls
- Squats
- Seated leg curls
- Lunges
- Lateral crossover box step-ups

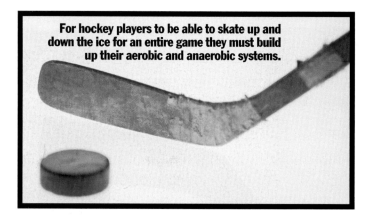

For hockey players to be able to skate up and down the ice for an entire game they must build up their aerobic and anaerobic systems.

Aerobic, Anaerobic and Cardiovascular Training

For hockey players to be able to skate up and down the ice for the duration of their shifts, the entire game and season, they must build up their aerobic and anaerobic systems. The *aerobic system* is used for long stretches on the ice while the *anaerobic system* is used for quick bursts of speed. Each is important for its own reasons.

Building an *aerobic* base gives an athlete greater energy to play longer and helps him recover quicker from lactic acid buildup. An *anaerobic* base gives the athlete the ability for quick energy surges. He is able to compete at a higher energy level. A well-conditioned anaerobic system helps delay the onset of lactic acid buildup.

The following exercises are suggested for aerobic conditioning:
• Stationary bicycling
• Bicycling
• Stair-climbing
• Running
• Aerobic skate
• Aerobic circle drill

The following exercises are for anaerobic training:
• Sprinting
• In-line skating
• Hill running/cycling
• Plyometrics
• On-ice ATP-PC sprint start relays
• Pair race drill
• Dot-to-dot drill
• Two-lap paced drill

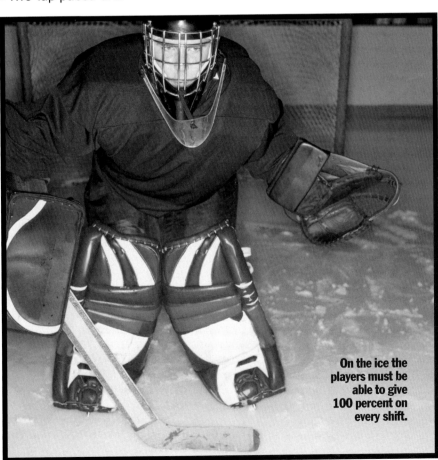

On the ice the players must be able to give 100 percent on every shift.

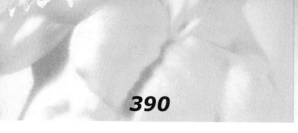

CHAPTER THIRTY-FOUR

Questions & Answers

Q. What can I do to excel in sports if I don't use steroids?

A. Focus on getting proper diet, rest, and good overall mental and physical health. These things are all factors in how your body is shaped and conditioned. Excelling in sports is achievable and done by millions of athletes without relying on steroids.

Q. How long do steroids stay in your system?

A. The length of time that steroids stay in the body varies from a couple of weeks to more than 18 months.

Q. Are steroids addictive?

A. Yes, they can be. Withdrawal symptoms include mood swings, suicidal thoughts and/or attempts, fatigue, restlessness, loss of appetite and sleeplessness.

Q. Is it possible to make a baby without having intercourse?

We were having dry sex and my boyfriend ejaculated into his boxers. He was also wearing shorts, but I had no underwear on.

A: Pregnancy is not likely to happen in this case. It seems as though clothing is a barrier. However, if the clothing were to be saturated and then pushed into the vaginal opening, then pregnancy could be possible.

Q. My friends don't like my new girlfriend.

She doesn't like me hanging around them and she's on my case over every little thing. Maybe it's not such a big deal. Is this a healthy relationship?

A. No, a healthy relationship is one part of a well-rounded life of friends, family, school, sports, hobbies, and a spiritual life. If she is trying to isolate you, it means she is trying to control you. Are you a man or a robot? Tell her how you feel and what you need. If she can't accept that you need time with others, then inform her you have no time for her.

Anyway, if she's on your case over every little thing, then she doesn't care for you. True affection means *acceptance*, especially when we make mistakes. Sounds like you can do a whole lot better!

Q. How do I get rid of bad breath?

I have always had bad breath. What causes this problem?

A. There are many conditions that can cause bad breath, besides the obvious one of forgetting to brush your teeth. The first is a sinus infection that causes infected drainage down the back of the throat. Second, a tooth abscess can cause you to have foul-smelling breath. Next, tonsillitis or a severely infected throat can make the breath smell bad. Finally, a foreign body in the nose, such as a piece of paper, toy, bead, raisin, etc. will cause an extremely foul smell that is hard to ignore.

The tomato has been proven to kill bacteria that cause bad breath.

Certain foods such as garlic are notorious for causing bad breath and body odor. Bad breath can also be caused by medications, dental problems and digestion. Speak to your doctor and your dentist. Breath fresheners are a billion dollar industry because it is such a common problem.

Want to know a quick breath freshener? Eat a nice fresh tomato! The enzymes in the tomato have been proven to kill bacteria that cause bad breath.

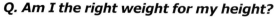

If there were a pill that could make you lose weight, *everyone* would be thin.

Q. Am I the right weight for my height?

A. Unfortunately, the height/weight charts are obsolete. We have found that there is no formula to determine your weight as compared to your age or height. Everyone develops at different rates, and with different stages of developmental growth, it is impossible and potentially damaging to force teens to conform to some average chart. No one is average – *everyone is unique!* So simply follow a healthy eating plan and active lifestyle, be happy and enjoy life. Keep active and feed yourself healthy food and you will never go wrong.

Q. How do I gain weight?

I'm a 16-year-old boy who is just starting to gain interest in weightlifting. I read on the Internet you should try to eat six small meals a day. I'm still in school so it would be hard to eat every three hours as the Web site recommends. Any suggestions?

A. Good question! The recommendation of six meals can be a little deceiving. "Meals" don't have to be a *big sit-down feast* – just something quick you can throw into your backpack to eat between classes or during a break. A sandwich, or cottage cheese with some fruit, or yogurt, or a protein bar – something that you can eat quickly to keep your body fueled with protein and carbs. The best choice is actually a protein bar you can eat anywhere, anytime.

Q. Are there any diet pills that work?

A. If there were a pill that could make you lose weight, *everyone* would be thin. So no, diet pills make some folks rich, but not thin. If you look at some ingredients in diet pills, you will find things like *caffeine,* which stimulates your metabolism, slightly. *Nothing* will work better than eating smaller meals, every 3 to 4 hours, and making better choices in *what you eat.* Exercise for 20 to 30 minutes every other day, and save your money, use it to buy healthy foods, like fruits and vegetables. Drink 8 glasses of water a day – that's better than any diet pill you can buy.

Q. At 14 am I old enough to work out? Will it stunt my growth?

A. We get this same question every day on e-mail. Read this and pass it along: Most teenagers are concerned about the fear of weight training and stunted growth. Steroids will definitely stunt your growth. No questions. However, weight training is very beneficial for teens to develop healthy and strong bodies. There are certain rules to follow while you are still growing and developing (under 18 years old).

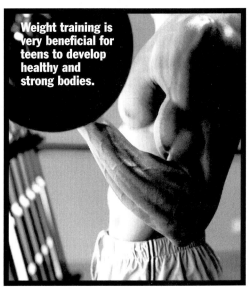

Weight training is very beneficial for teens to develop healthy and strong bodies.

Never lift heavy weights that overstress your joints. You will get wonderful results from using lighter weights and higher reps (15 to 20 reps per set). Keep in mind that pushups and pullups and situps are among the *best exercises* – and they can be done anywhere!

Q. I really like this girl but we're just friends.
Lately I am having really strong feelings toward her and I am afraid to tell her because it might ruin our friendship if she doesn't feel the same way. What should I do?
A. It is highly unlikely that you will ruin your friendship if you ask her out. Ask her if she would ever be interested in pursuing more with you? If she says no, then that's okay. At least you will know where you stand so you are no longer left wondering. If she says yes, then great!

Q. What can I do to gain some major weight and muscle?
I am almost 17 and I weigh 100 pounds at 5'3". I am clueless on what to do. Please help me.
A. In order to gain weight – muscular weight not fat – you must eat, eat, eat … low-fat low-sugar foods. But make sure you eat six small meals a day. Of those six, we would include two or three supplement shakes – it's an easy way to get calories. And you should be lifting weights three or four times a week.

Q. I'm thinking about getting a tattoo. Should I?
A. That depends on what, why and where. If it's a girlfriend's name, we suggest you don't. The tattoo is for life. And you're probably going to have more than one girlfriend before you settle down.

Why do you want a tattoo? Is it to make you look tougher? More mature? Does it hold some cultural or spiritual significance? There's a big difference between a religious symbol and a Tasmanian Devil cartoon character! The decision to get a tattoo should be taken very seriously.

Where do you want your tattoo? Facial and hand tattoos are a big mistake. They can be barriers to future job promotions. If you must get a tattoo, consider the upper arm, chest or back. And also keep this in mind: getting a tattoo hurts!

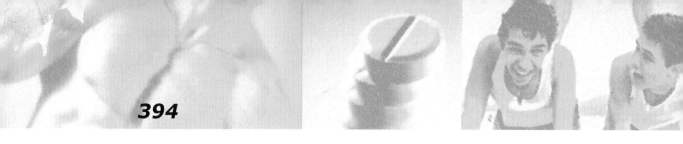

Q. I can't join a gym.

I don't have easy access to very much equipment for working my chest and I'm wondering how I could get in a good workout without going to the gym? I can't afford a membership. Any suggestions?

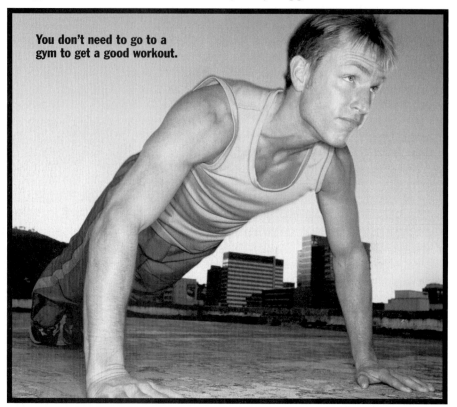

You don't need to go to a gym to get a good workout.

A. *Definitely* ... You don't need to go to the gym get a good workout. Some of the best exercises can be done at home with great results. Pushups work the upper body. Pullups work the back and arms. Situps for abs ... dips between two chairs can be done at home. If you can push or pull your bodyweight for 3 sets of 10 reps you are in great shape!

Q. How much exercise is too much?

And does regular exercise decrease or increase the number of hours you're supposed to sleep?

A. In general you should exercise no more than 3 to 5 days a week, with at least 48 to 72 hours for recovery before you work the same bodypart again. For example, if you work on your chest on Monday, then you should wait until Wednesday or Friday to do another chest workout. *Sleep is very important* – that is the only time your body can repair and build muscle. For best results, you must sleep about 8 hours per night.

Q. I am wondering if pornography is okay.
I try not to look at it but I seem to want to. Am I normal? I'm 14.
A. Are you "normal" – *yes!* Is what you're doing a good idea? Well, that's a different story. So you're at a point in your life when testosterone is just surging through your body. Like it or not, your mind is continually being bombarded with the urge to merge! Naturally, the opportunity to see some female flesh in the all-together is an attractive thought.

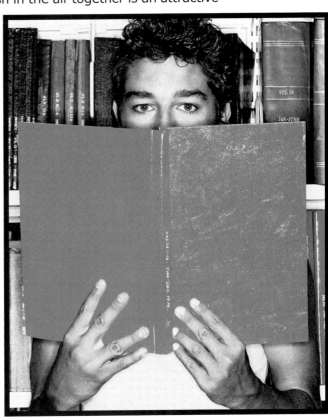

Pornography is a rather generic term. It runs the gambit from simple nudity to the most depraved behaviors imaginable. What is presented as "normal" in such media completely ignores the emotional aspects of relationships, and the values that maintain them. You must remember that pornography is classified as *adult* material which, in most cases, isn't appropriate for teenagers (or many adults for that matter). What may not have seemed inappropriate to you could be thought of by your parents as the greatest profanity they ever saw in their lives.

One compromise might be to order copies of *Victoria's Secret* catalogues or similar women's fashion magazines, filled with supermodels in revealing swimsuits. You won't offend your parents, or embarrass yourself.

Q. Is it good to exercise right before you go to sleep?
Or is there a certain length of time you should allow between exercising and going to bed? I am doing a project that involves nightly activities and their effect on sleep.
A. You should not exercise within 2 hours of bedtime. Your body needs this time to relax and for your heart rate to slow down, so you can fall asleep.

Q. Help! I'm a gambler.

I just got suspended (again) for gambling at school – which is just as well because I owe big money, and I'm scared some of the people I owe money to are going to beat me up the next time I show up at school! My parents have threatened to kick me out because I stole money from them to pay off debts. Why am I doing this?

A. Most people who wager don't have a problem. But a minority of the general population (an estimated 1 percent to 2 percent) become compulsive gamblers. People in this group lose control of their betting, often with serious and sometimes fatal consequences. What is compulsive gambling? The American Psychiatric Association (APA) classifies compulsive gambling as an impulse-control disorder. To meet the APA's diagnostic criteria for compulsive gambling, a person must show persistent gambling behavior as indicated by at least five of the following criteria:

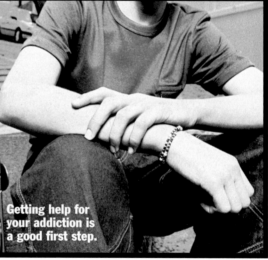

Getting help for your addiction is a good first step.

1. Preoccupation with gambling (for example being preoccupied with reliving past gambling experiences, handicapping or planning the next venture, or thinking of ways to get money with which to gamble).

2. Need to gamble with increasing amounts of money to achieve desired excitement.

3. Repeated unsuccessful efforts to cut back or stop gambling.

4. Restless or irritable when attempting to cut down or stop gambling.

5. Gambling is a way of escaping problems or of relieving a dysphoric mood (feelings of helplessness, guilt, anxiety, depression).

6. After losing money to gambling, the need to return another day to get even ("chasing" one's losses).

7. Lying to family members, therapist or others to conceal extent of involvement with gambling.

8. Committed illegal acts such as forgery, fraud, theft or embezzlement to finance gambling.

9. Jeopardized or lost a significant relationship, job or educational or career opportunity because of gambling.

10. Relying on others to provide money to relieve a desperate financial situation caused by gambling.

Here's the hardest part. You must tell your parents everything. Arrange a meeting with a guidance counselor, and speak to your doctor

Steroids will definitely stunt your growth.

about therapy. The sooner you seek treatment, the more likely you'll be successful in kicking this serious addiction. Depending on how much money you owe at school, consider getting transferred. A meeting with the guidance counselor, your principal, your parents and you can result in some positive actions to help you get things back together. They will all want to help you. (In addition, call Gamblers Anonymous. That organization has more than 1200 US locations and 20 international chapters.)

Q. I am training for volleyball season this summer. *I am wondering which aerobic activity would be best and for how long each day?*
A. Like many sports, volleyball requires strong legs to move quickly around the court. That means any activity that uses leg strength would benefit you. These include biking, rowing, hiking, running or speed-walking. Adding some weight training, such as squats, would definitely improve the power of your legs! Spend about 20 to 30 minutes every other day with aerobic activity.

Q. Tongue-piercing is so cool! *My friends say we should celebrate our high school graduation by getting our tongues pierced the day before the ceremonies! I think it will be so cool! Is it a good idea?*

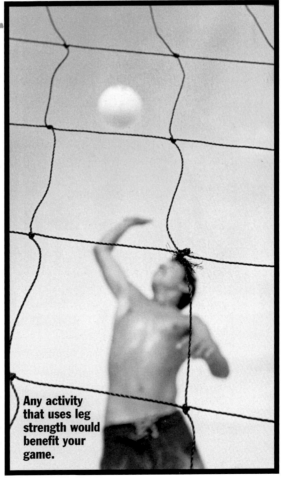

Any activity that uses leg strength would benefit your game.

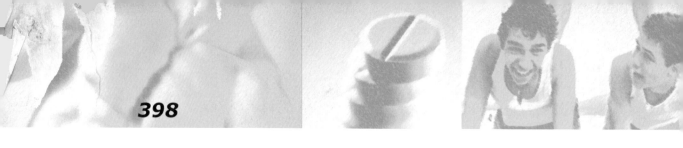

A. Depends on who's paying your dental bills. A new study shows extended wear of barbell-type tongue jewelry can cause receding gums and chipped teeth. The most common type of tongue jewelry is known as a *barbell.* It consists of a stem that goes through the tongue and is held in place with screw caps on both ends. Researchers say a short barbell is more likely to cause tooth-chipping because it's easier to position between the teeth. People with tongue jewelry tend to habitually play with it.

The study found receding gums (a problem that can lead to tooth loss) in 35 percent of those who had pierced tongues for four or more years and in 50 percent of those who had worn the long-stemmed barbells for two or more years. Researchers say that during tongue movement long-stemmed barbells are more likely to reach and damage the gums than short barbells.

So the answer is *no, tongue-piercing is not a good idea.* It looks stupid and will probably cause your teeth to fall out. And that is not cool!

Remember, if you find anything suspicious, report it to your doctor right away.

Q. I have one testicle that is bigger than the other.
Is this normal?
A. It may be normal for one testicle to be bigger than the other. However, it is important as a teenager to get this checked out by your doctor just to make sure everything is okay. Your doctor will do a testicular exam and instruct you on how to complete a monthly testicular self-exam, commonly referred to as TSE.

TSE is a simple examination that you can do on your testicles to help identify what is normal and not normal for your testicles, any changes in shape or size, pain or tenderness in the area, and any unusual lumps or bumps. Here's a brief description on how to do a TSE.

Perform your exam after a warm shower. This will help your testicles (scrotum area) to relax and drop down. Your testicles should be about the size of and shaped like an egg. It is normal for your left testicle to sometimes hang lower than the right one.

Examine each testicle using both hands. Your thumbs should be placed on the top side of your testicle and your index and middle finger should be place on the back side of testicle. Your testicles should feel smooth and rubbery. Gently roll each testicle between the thumbs and the fingers. You should not feel any lumps. Pay attention and look for any small, hard pea-shaped lumps.

Your testicles should not hurt or have any pain. You should not have a feeling of heaviness in your groin area. Visually inspect your genital area looking for any skin discoloration or bumps. Remember, if you find anything suspicious, report it to your doctor right away. Testicular cancer can be successfully treated, if it is caught in the early stages.

Q. I'm a jock and proud of it!

I play football, baseball and basketball. My dentist says I need braces. Can I still play sports, or do I have to hang out with the "Pocket-Protector" crowd?

A. Yes, you can still play football, baseball and basketball. Just make sure to wear a mouth guard, and try not to get hit in the face. We recommend that you avoid sports where you could get hit in the mouth. Fighting, boxing, wrestling, karate … they can be very painful when you have braces. By the way, do yourself a favor. Drop the superior "Jock" attitude and make friends with the "Pocket-Protector" crowd. Chances are you'll be working for them someday!

You can still play most sports if you wear braces, just make sure to wear a mouth guard.

Index

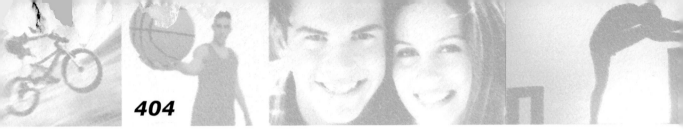

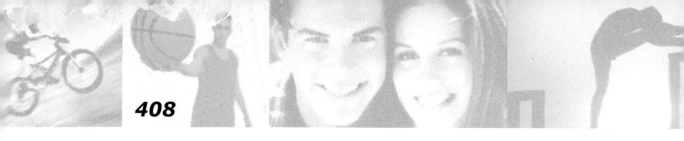

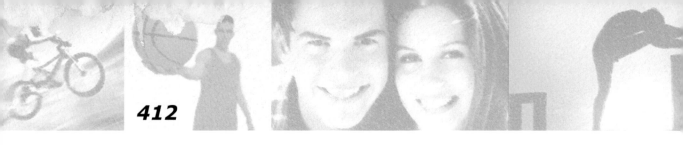

Contributing Photographers
Jim Amentler, Ralph DeHaan,
Irvin Gelb, Robert Kennedy